MW00397190

Therapeutic Neuroscience Education

Teaching Patients About Pain

A Guide for Clinicians

Adriaan Louw
PT, PhD (c), M.App.Sc (physio), CSMT

Emilio Puentedura
PT, DPT, PhD, OCS, GDMT, CSMT, FAAOMPT

Designed by OPTP.
optp.com
Copy edited by OPTP.
All images from ISPI, unless otherwise noted.

ISBN-978-0-9857186-4-0

Foreword

By Louis Gifford, FCSP
Chartered Physiotherapist

I'm honored to have been asked to write the foreword for this book. The authors were interested in my 'pain journey,' and both have kindly acknowledged the influence of my 'Mature Organism Model' on their clinical practice in the 1990's and their subsequent teaching. This book, *Therapeutic Neuroscience Education*, gives me a strong sense of personal satisfaction. Let me tell you why.

After completing my physiotherapy training, I always knew I wanted to specialize in the treatment of musculoskeletal pain. My father was a big influence – a physiotherapist, a natural communicator and a manual therapist who'd learned his trade from osteopaths and bone setters in the late 1940's and 50's. He was an impressive operator and my observations of him in work mode as a youngster left me in awe. I came to realize that he was way ahead of his time – not only for his exceptional hands and people skills but also for his diagnostic brilliance combined with his ability to instill physical confidence in his patients.

My father's influence led me to get immersed in manual therapy and within four years of qualifying as a Chartered Physiotherapist, Philippa Tindle and I moved to Adelaide, in Australia, to study and complete our Graduate Diploma in Manipulative Therapy. This was 1985. Being taught by Geoff Maitland was a dream come true and I learnt a great deal in the program and afterwards working in Geoff's practice for a couple of years. One of the greatest things I learnt from Geoff Maitland was his incredible ability to listen and communicate with his patients. However, manual therapy wasn't all I thought it was, and I felt a quietly growing skepticism and desire for rational explanations. I wasn't seeing the results I expected, especially with the large population of patients with chronic whiplash-associated disorders and repetitive strain injuries that frequented Geoff's practice. Due to the very nature of manual therapy, their problems were effectively reduced to some spinal joint 'comparable sign,' their range of movement to pain was observed, a very specific mobilization technique was performed and the range was reassessed. The range to pain invariably improved and the technique was repeated a few times during the session, and then the process was repeated. Patients were often seen three times a week, week in and week out and month in month out. I cannot ever recall exercise of any relevance being given to the patient. The treatment was entirely passive, and there was no patient responsibility in the whole process. The brunt of all therapist-patient interactions was in communicating the symptom behavior during the range of movement assessment. To me, the symptoms were very cleverly 'played with,' but the patient never moved on.

Remember, to provide a little fairness and balance, that we didn't know then what we know now. Reflecting, I now realize that I'd stumbled on a significant truth that would hugely influence my future. This was that chronic pain, or maybe even all pain, lacked an adequate explanation. The tissue- and biomechanical-centered explanations and the biomedical model that we were taught just didn't explain the broken lives and madly complicated body charts I continually witnessed!

Thanks to the course and Geoff, what I was learning and getting much better at was skilled physical examination of musculoskeletal tissues and the ability to think, reason and communicate at the level of knowledge we had back then.

In the early 1980's in the UK and while in the course in Adelaide in 1985, we were all learning the latest 'neural provocation' tests pioneered by the late Bob Elvey for the upper limb and the slump test pioneered by the late Geoff Maitland. What contemporary therapists now call an 'upper limb neurodynamic test' was called the 'Brachial Plexus Tension test of Elvey' and many of the students in the Adelaide manipulative therapy program studied normal responses of these tests for their research projects. I'm mentioning this because it was probably the start of a wider, bigger and better integration of science into manual therapy. David Butler, in particular, stands out and, as most now know, made a massive contribution by researching and integrating nerve biology, physiology, mechanics and many 'new' neural tests and treatment techniques in the later 1980's and early 1990's. David, along with Mark Jones, whose work on clinical reasoning is well known, were both classmates of mine on the 1985 course.

During the few years that followed the course, there was a heightened atmosphere of 'new direction' with the Adverse Mechanical Tension (AMT) analysis of chronic arm symptoms in patients with repetitive strain injuries and whiplash. David was responsible for a plethora of new AMT tests (since called neurodynamic tests) and later went on to publish his first book, 'Mobilisation of the Nervous system.' Here, at last, was a scientific and rationally based attempt to try and make better sense of those complex patients.

I have to say I enjoyed the fresh look at nerves as a 'moving' tissue, but in all honesty, I was never entirely convinced that adverse nerve mechanics and abnormal nerve movement was enough to account for the chronic pain symptom pictures I continued to puzzle over. My experience with these new techniques for repetitive strain injury and whiplash, while exciting to start with, still seemed to amount to 'playing with the symptom responses.' It was still passive manual therapy but applied to a 'new' tissue.

Philippa Tindle and I headed back to the UK in early 1988 where we both took over the family practice in Cornwall. I remained in contact with David, who by the early 1990's was travelling far and wide teaching AMT courses and bringing an exciting new era to physiotherapy. I occasionally assisted him on his courses when he was in Europe and the UK, and it was during one of these in Holland that I started reading a chapter by the late and famous pain scientist, Dr. Patrick Wall. The chapter title was 'Neuropathic pain and injured nerve: central mechanisms' (Wall 1991). It changed my professional life because it explained how the central nervous system could plastically change if it was given enough of an incoming 'afferent barrage' from an injured nerve or from inflamed and damaged tissues. These plastic changes could result in impulse barrages being self-generated from within the CNS, which then could result in massive spreads of inappropriate sensitivity and a massive enlargement of receptive fields.

This was a far better explanation for chronic whiplash and repetitive strain injury related pain! Pain and spread of pain not coming from the tissues but being generated in a maladaptive fashion from within the CNS! Wow! The pain meant nothing, it was useless, and this revelation meant that I suddenly lost my clinical fear of it. This was what I was going to tell my patients! No need to fear the pain. You're not broken; your pain processing system has gone mad!

These passive treatments that I'd rather denigrated as mere 'playing with pain,' I realized now were merely 'playing with processing'! I immersed myself in the literature, firstly of central mechanisms and then later, seeing the biological similarities, in the biology of memory. I actually met with Patrick Wall and we both agreed that the central pain mechanisms and the biology of memory were vastly similar, something he hadn't really thought about! I also enjoyed much discussion with the memory biologist Steven Rose, whose book 'The Making of Memory' was hugely influential. Memory involved synaptic plasticity in representational neural networks and increasing efficiency of those synapses – in effect, the formation of a memory was the formation of new neural circuit – and so was pain.

For me, chronic pain was like an 'annoying tune' playing in your head and this became very easy to explain to receptive patients. It also dawned on me that once something was committed to memory it was very hard to get rid of, and the same applied to ongoing chronic pain. Doing pain-focused passive manual therapy techniques to patients in 20-minute time slots was hardly enough to erase a pain memory! An exciting voyage of understanding and implementing had started. Those chronic pain presentations were beginning to make sense and a massive shift in my treatment and management strategies was clearly required.

Over the next 2-3 years, I obsessively reveled in the pain, memory, phantom-limb, placebo, and stress literature and started to integrate what I was learning into clinical practice. I started teaching the 'Clinical Biology of Aches and Pains' courses and so began my shift away from the purist manual therapy and passive dominated approach to pain problems. I sensed freedom and was excited by what I was discovering.

Clinically, one of the big things I started to do was spend plenty of time with the chronic pain patients, not only listening but also getting them to try and see their problem from a different perspective. Without really knowing it I was getting patients to shift their thinking about their problem from one of 'there's something seriously wrong with me... nobody's found the cause yet... when they do...they'll be able to fix what's wrong and I'll be better....' to one of 'there's a flaw in my processing system.... the tissues have healed.... they're safe to start loading...the pain has remained on when it shouldn't have.'

A few patients changed massively. They lost their concern and fear, and with guidance started to unlearn all the bad over-protective movement patterns and then got active and fitter. They got their lives back together. Some got fitter than they had ever been. I was starting to change a few lives, and my confidence was growing. Pain mechanisms made it all make sense, yet in a passive therapy dominated world I felt very alone. In my 'Aches and Pains' lectures, I introduced the pain science and meshed it with the ways I was explaining things to patients. I tried to get my audience of professionals to shift their thinking – which, for the most part, proved to be harder than shifting it with my patients!

The key was to demonstrate using real patients. Information doesn't change many people's hardened beliefs but witnessing change certainly can. I think it was around 1994 or 1995 when David Butler and I decided to start teaching a five-day course together using patients. The course was called 'The Dynamic Nervous System' and attracted a great many physiotherapists who were really expecting, at least in those early days, an 'Advanced' Butler AMT mobilization course with Louis Gifford assisting. Well, what they got from me was pain mechanisms, the integration of pain into clinical reasoning and me out in front with a live patient with chronic pain. I delved deeply into all the dimensions of their problem, examining them and then spending a great deal of time explaining their pain problem with the aim of shifting their thinking from 'my problem means I'm damaged in some way, I cannot move on...' to 'my body has healed but my pain processing system is at fault...'

I saw the patients over three days of the course and spent a great deal of time with them. Many of the patients made massive changes and, thankfully, helped many of the entrenched manual therapists to grasp what I was on about. I still hear from course participants that the course and the patients I grappled with were clinical life-changers.

Pleasingly, David saw what I was up to and came along. Those early courses in a way were a mismatch. I was emphasizing 'hands-off and start talking' – or at least 'top-down' (get the head right/accepting) before 'bottom-up' (doing any form of physical treatment). David was still emphasizing hands-on, teaching the tension tests and all the neural mobilizing sliders and tensioners that were all the rage then. Over the few years we taught the course, David also immersed himself in the pain literature and the course became more balanced with the passive mobilizing being placed much more comfortably and with less emphasis. Pain mechanisms were integrated into clinical reasoning. Time and again the course feedback indicated that it was the live patients and David's 'Pain, art and politics' lecture that left a deep impression, hugely challenged their beliefs and shifted them to see a much bigger picture.

By 1997 or 1998, we were taking the course all over Europe but also to South Africa and back to Adelaide! I can remember Lorimer Moseley in the Adelaide audience as well as a great many of the well-established manual therapy heavies there. As many of you will know, and will read about in this book, Lorimer went on to do a great deal of impressive research on pain education and also co-authored the 'Explain Pain' book with David. UK-based physiotherapist Mick Thacker added a massive amount of key declarative knowledge and was a great supporter of our exciting and revolutionary mission!

The integration of psychosocial factors into clinical practice forged ahead in the UK with the formation of the Physiotherapy Pain Association, the publication of its work in the Topical Issues in Pain series and later university-run courses headed by physiotherapists who were awarding Masters in Pain Science and Pain Management. The integration of Cognitive Behavioral Therapy (CBT) into mainstream physiotherapy has become significant.

In the last 15-18 years, there has been a pain revolution in physiotherapy, which I feel honored to have played a small part in. 'Therapeutic Neuroscience Education' is an excellent place to begin the journey of learning and change that started back in the early 1990's for physiotherapy and physical therapy. I hope this book sells worldwide and is soon considered as essential reading – not only for the naive and budding undergraduate but also for those who teach and educate and those whose role is to deal with the difficult and stubborn problem that is acute and chronic musculoskeletal pain.

For me this book represents something special. I worked very hard trying to understand pain in those early days. I worked hard trying to explain it to my colleagues and I worked very hard in explaining it to my patients. It is with a great sense of personal satisfaction that a very big part of my professional life – explaining and teaching about pain – has now gotten such excellent support from the research and clinical community. The authors have distilled and presented a great deal of this and their own research, and provided a first class guide to starting out on the 'explaining' voyage that is such an important part of good pain management.

I would like to finish with a simple appeal. When I first started teaching the Clinical Biology of Aches and Pains courses in 1993, I used to put a slide up with this on:

When I go to my Doctor, I have 4 questions that I'd like answered...
• 'Doc, what's wrong with me?'
• 'Doc, how long's it going to take to get better?'
• 'Doc, is there anything I can do to help myself?'
• 'Doc, is there anything that you can do to help me?'

If your treatment approach embraces these four questions and gives understandable answers that are based on rational medicine, science and biology, then you're doing a great service to the patient. Remember, every pain problem, acute or chronic, has a thinking, reasoning and emotional brain attached to it.

Enjoy and study this book; it will help you hugely.

Louis Gifford, FCSP
Chartered Physiotherapist
May 5th 2013

Reference

Wall, P. (1991). Neuropathic pain and injured nerve: Central mechanisms. *Br Med Bull, 47*(3): 631-643.

Preface

Our original goal for writing this text was to create a single, user-friendly resource for physical therapists and students learning to apply neuroscience education in the treatment of patients with chronic musculoskeletal pain complaints. We have taught seminars and presented at professional conferences on this topic for several years. Over the past few years, we have also begun a line of research into the use of therapeutic neuroscience education on patient outcomes. Our clinical and teaching experiences told us that this information needed to be shared not only within our particular profession but with all clinicians and personnel involved in patient care. Because of this, you will notice that we use the term 'therapist' throughout the text and not 'physical therapist.' Ultimately, we wanted to make pain neuroscience education accessible and relevant for therapists to be able to implement it in their clinical practice. Of course, once we began the process of writing this textbook, we realized it was easier said than done. We hope this final product achieves our original goal.

Therapeutic Neuroscience Education contains chapters that provide sufficient information about the neurobiology and neurophysiology of pain to allow all therapists engaged in patient care to understand and apply the concepts within the framework of movement-based therapy. The 'biopsychosocial approach' in the treatment of persistent musculoskeletal pain complaints has gained much deserved prominence in clinical practice, but we fear that most therapists may be wary of becoming de-facto psychologists in the process. This textbook emphasizes the value of *adding* neuroscience education to your regular clinical practice, not replacing it with an education-only approach.

In Chapter 1, we point out that clinicians are seeing more and more patients with chronic pain problems and how the current models of evaluation and treatment have been ineffective and insufficient. We stress the impact of cognitions on pain and, conversely, how persistent pain can adversely affect cognitions, beliefs, emotions and behaviors. Changing faulty patient cognitions regarding their pain is imperative for movement-based therapy to be effective, and we argue that therapists are capable and ideally situated to address faulty cognitions.

Chapter 2 provides all the details you need to know about therapeutic neuroscience education, including its development and the evidence for its effectiveness. We also report on our recent systematic review of therapeutic neuroscience education addressing pain, disability, anxiety, and stress in chronic musculoskeletal pain. It provided significant insight into the content, delivery methods, duration and frequency, and other aspects of its provision. In this chapter, we point out that our traditional biomedical education models have not been found to be helpful and may, in fact, make pain worse. We also note that the compelling evidence for a neuroscience approach gives us some direction and guidance regarding its clinical application.

In Chapter 3, we demonstrate how learning and understanding pain neuroscience and neurophysiology can be readily achieved through the analysis of the questions posed in the Neurophysiology of Pain Questionnaire (NPQ), developed by Lorimer Moseley. By systematically answering each of the original 19 questions, a clinician can easily develop a deeper and richer understanding of how pain works. We make the point that pain is not a simple matter of input. Pain is much more complex but our ever-increasing knowledge of how pain works can help us transfer a deeper understanding to our patients.

Is it easy to explain how pain works to a patient in pain? In Chapter 4, we argue that it can be made easier through the use of patient-friendly language and metaphors. In this chapter, we provide guidelines for the clinical application of therapeutic neuroscience education by covering all of the relevant topics from the viewpoint of the therapist and the patient, and detailing the kinds of images and clinical tools that may be helpful to ensure understanding of the concepts. This is our "how do you actually do it" chapter.

Chapter 5 covers important clinical application guidelines to ensure success with a therapeutic neuroscience education approach. We discuss the importance of time to ensure that the education can be provided but also the cost-effectiveness aspects of providing that time. We also cover billing issues, training clinical staff, development of tools and props to enhance the education and the various outcome measures available to measure progress with the approach. We emphasize the importance of combining therapeutic neuroscience education with other therapeutic modalities, especially exercise or movement-based therapies. We also briefly discuss the importance of 'deep learning' and some of the strategies currently available to promote it.

In Chapter 6, we present the bigger picture of pain and emphasize the various biological body systems that are engaged to protect during a pain experience. We feel this topic is extremely important for the patient with chronic pain to learn, as it can provide insight into why they might feel, act and behave in the manner that they do *because* of their persistent pain. It can be truly liberating for a patient in chronic pain to receive biological explanations for the various experiences associated with their persistent pain. The chapter provides guidelines for treating patients with chronic pain by addressing those biological body system changes and makes the point that understanding *why* a patient might have persistent pain can open so many avenues for treatment options. Therapists need not be stumped and left wondering what they can do when confronted with a patient with chronic musculoskeletal pain. Therapeutic neuroscience education opens many doors for treatment options and leaves therapists realizing they can offer so much more to their patients than just exercise and simple reassurance.

Chapter 7 allows us to provide a clinical example of how therapeutic neuroscience education can be applied to a patient with complex issues surrounding their chronic pain. We provide a case report to describe the process as well as report on the immediate and long-term results of therapeutic neuroscience education on a patient with a three-year history of chronic low back pain. This is just one of many case examples we could have provided. It is important to appreciate that successful outcomes can be expected with the appropriate application of therapeutic neuroscience education.

Finally, in Chapter 8, we provide a conclusion, summary and some thoughts on the future direction of therapeutic neuroscience education. We present a brief discussion on the benefit versus cost-effectiveness of group interventions as well as the need to take the message of how pain actually works to the general population. We conclude with a short preview of our research efforts on the use of preventive therapeutic neuroscience education.

Neither of us knew about how pain actually works until we attended a few seminars and presentations from leaders in research into this field. Until we had heard the messages from Louis Gifford, David Butler and Lorimer Moseley, our practice was stuck in the manual/mechanical therapy paradigm. We had our share of successful outcomes, but equally, we were left distressed by those more complex patients with pain that couldn't be explained by mechanical dysfunctions. Learning about the neuroscience and neurophysiology of pain was an eye-opening experience and required of us a significant paradigm shift. We found it truly liberating. Our hope is that, with this textbook, you will experience a similar sense of excitement and discover that there is so much we can offer to our more difficult patients – those with chronic pain.

Acknowledgements

Writing a book may appear to be solitary work. Nothing could be farther from the truth. It requires unlimited amounts of support and collaboration. This can be as intense and exhausting to those supportive, collaborative people as it is to the writers. We'd like to thank the following people and let them know, or at least be reminded of, how vital they have been in completing this project.

Thank you to the many influential supervisors, advisors, peers and authority figures within our profession. Not only have you provided wisdom, insight, vision and passion, but were kind enough to stop, listen, speak a kind word and spend time with us. This includes the late Geoff Maitland, the late Bob Elvey, Peter Rice, David Butler, Lorimer Moseley, Michael Shacklock, Louis Gifford, Ina Diener, Lance Twomey, Tim Flynn, Josh Cleland, Paul Mintken, Lynette Crous, Marietta Uys, Merrill Landers and many more.

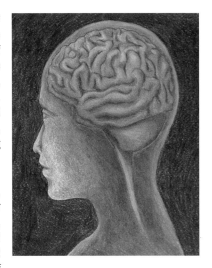

Illustration by Georgina Puentedura.

To every physical therapist, physician and patient who participated in our research, thank you for your willingness to be involved in these projects, your collegiality, your trust in us and your interest in being a part of the future of pain science.

To the International Spine and Pain Institute, thank you for your financial support of our research work.

To OPTP, thank you for your support in editing, designing, publishing and distributing this book. Also, thank you to Rod Bohner for your artwork.

To our parents and siblings, thank you for your steadfast support and encouragement and for providing us with our first examples of hard work and dedication.

To our children, Hailey and Samuel Louw; and Benjamin, Georgina and Alexander Puentedura, thank you for being patient with fathers who were too often tired and too often absent while in pursuit of projects like this book. You've never doubted how much we love each of you.

Lastly, but most importantly, we dedicate this book to our wives, Colleen Louw and Danielle Puentedura. Their continued support, enthusiasm and love made this book possible. Without it, there would be no book. Those countless days, being both a father and a mother to our children, you have grounded our families with your love and support.

Adriaan Louw
Emilio "Louie" Puentedura

Chapter 1

Cognitions and Pain

1.1: Chronic Pain and Therapy

Current research suggests that approximately 25% of the populations in developed countries experience chronic pain. Chronic pain can be defined as pain that persists beyond normal tissue healing time, which is generally thought to be between three and six months (Merskey & Bogduk, 1994; Wall & Melzack, 2005). In the United States (US), it is currently estimated that approximately 116 million Americans have persistent pain (IOM, 2011). A recent European study reported more than 1 in 3 people in Ireland (35%) live with persistent pain, suggesting a worldwide epidemic of pain (Raftery, Sarma, Murphy, De la Harpe, Normand, & McGuire, 2011). It is also important to recognize that chronic pain rates have been steadily increasing over time. Epidemiological data from the early 1990's shows 1 in 7 people were struggling with persistent pain, whereas the recent data indicates that it is now more like 1 in 4 (Merskey & Bogduk, 1994; Wall & Melzack, 2005).

This ever-increasing chronic pain epidemic comes at a cost. It is estimated that chronic pain costs the US economy about $635 billion a year (IOM, 2011). Apart from the financial burden of chronic pain, there is also a human, clinical cost. Treating people with chronic pain is difficult and poses significant challenges for clinicians, especially therapists. There is evidence that therapists struggle when treating patients with chronic pain (Latimer, Maher, & Refshauge, 2004; Nijs, Roussel, Paul van Wilgen, Koke, & Smeets, 2012; Timm, 1994). Although it is likely that many factors are involved, it is believed that a significant contribution to this clinical struggle is the lack of training and preparedness for treating chronic pain (Latimer, et al., 2004). Not only are therapists under-prepared to treat this challenging population, but the pain models they follow are outdated and treatment options that flow out of these models are often ineffective, leading to additional frustration. Therapy, especially orthopedic therapy, is traditionally rooted in a biomedical model that focuses on tissues and tissue injury (Henrotin, Cedraschi, Duplan, Bazin, & Duquesnoy, 2006; Houben, Ostelo, Vlaeyen, Wolters, Peters, & Stomp-van den Berg, 2005; Weiner, 2008). This traditional biomedical model of therapy suggests that every disease process (dysfunction) can be explained in terms of an underlying deviation from normal function, such as a pathogen or injury. The model implies that pathology and symptoms are correlated such that a greater expression of symptoms in patients would indicate greater underlying pathology (Figure 1.1 a). The model proposes that correction of the underlying pathology with treatment (for example, injection, surgery, manipulation or exercise) should result in elimination of the symptoms and subsequent restoration of normal function in the patient (Figure 1.1 b) (Haldeman, 1990). Clinical experience and pain science research tells us otherwise. Many patients will demonstrate physical and diagnostic signs that they have recovered from injury, yet they will continue to report symptoms/pain (Figure 1.1 c) (Haldeman, 1990; Iwamoto, Takeda, & Wakano, 2004).

Conversely, it has been well documented that many healthy asymptomatic people and patients often have significant tissue pathology (arthritis of the spine, bulging discs, bone spurs, etc.), yet experience little to no pain (Figure 1.1 d) (Alyas, Turner, & Connell, 2007; Haldeman, 1990; Waris, Eskelin, Hermunen, Kiviluoto, & Paajanen, 2007).

The time has come for therapists to take on the more comprehensive biopsychosocial model (Foster & Delitto, 2011; Linton & Shaw, 2011). The biopsychosocial model encompasses more than just the biological factors (anatomy, physiology and pathoanatomy) in human functioning by addressing the psychological (thoughts, emotions and behaviors) and social (work, culture and religion) factors, which are known to play a significant role in patients experiencing pain. A true biopsychosocial model includes a greater understanding of how the nervous system processes injury, disease, pain, threat and emotions (Louw & Butler, 2011).

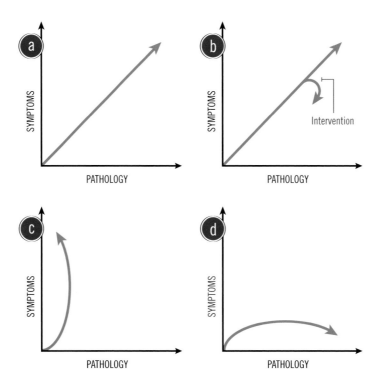

Figure 1.1: The failure of the biomedical model to predict pain (Haldeman, 1990).

1.2: Cognitions and Pain

There is significant debate about what constitutes a true biopsychosocial approach (Jull & Sterling, 2009; Weiner, 2008) and it could be argued that the list would vary, depending on each patient and his/her specific clinical presentation. At the heart of a true biopsychosocial approach is cognition. What a patient thinks, feels and believes about his or her condition will significantly impact their examination, treatment and prognosis (Vlaeyen, Kole-Snijders, Boeren, & van Eek, 1995). Many therapists attempting to practice a biopsychosocial approach may experience trepidation and concerns that they may be inappropriately entering the realm of psychotherapy. We should certainly acknowledge that serious debilitating psychological issues such as depression, abuse and various other psychological disorders, when noted in our examination, need referral to a professional for psychological counseling. However, therapists need to carefully re-think their role in helping these severely affected patients and not simply default to a 'for referral only' approach.

In its purist form, therapy can be seen as treating faulty human movement and function. Consider the following scenarios:

- A patient presents with pain and disability. After a skilled subjective and objective examination, the therapist determines a stiff joint or movement is associated with the pain and disability. Treatment incorporating manual therapy would be considered appropriate according to established clinical guidelines. It is hypothesized that manual therapy or passive joint movement may restore normal movement and this will then be associated with the observed clinical improvement.

- A patient presents with pain and disability. After a skilled subjective and objective examination, the therapist determines that altered muscle recruitment is associated with the pain and disability. In this case, a motor control strategy may be considered appropriate to alter motor control issues and, thereby, alleviate pain and disability.

- A patient presents with pain and disability. After a skilled subjective and objective examination, the therapist determines that there is a soft tissue problem, e.g., trigger point, which may be preventing optimal function and movement. Physical treatment of the trigger point via ischemic compression or mechanical disruption through the use of dry needling may be considered appropriate avenues to restore normal movement and function.

- A patient presents with pain and disability. After a skilled subjective and objective examination, the therapist determines that the main reason for their limited function and mobility is altered/inappropriate beliefs about their pain. Where are the clinical guidelines to cover such a clinical presentation and whose job is it to treat their altered beliefs?

It has been well established that cognitions such as fear, anxiety and pain catastrophization are strongly correlated to pain and disability (Meeus, Nijs, Van Oosterwijck, Van Alsenoy, & Truijen, 2010; G. L. Moseley, 2004; Vlaeyen, et al., 1995). This suggests that therapists working on restoring human movement should address these altered cognitions for patients to feel, move and function better. Furthermore, the notion that physical and psychological issues are separate and somewhat unrelated issues represents a classic flaw in medicine, based on the Cartesian model of pain that emphasizes the mind-body split (see later) (Goldberg, 2008). Therapists regularly engaged in clinical practice should readily agree that therapy can alter faulty cognitions. How can you treat any patient without providing education? Education is therapy. Such education may seem benign and informal, yet recent research has shown its powerful impact on patient pain and disability. A major theme of this textbook, which follows over 15 years of clinical research on therapeutic neuroscience education (TNE), is the concept of altering patients' beliefs to alter their pain experiences.

1.3: A Clinical Example

Here, we present a clinical example to illustrate the connection between cognitions and pain. This patient was sent to therapy to get help with her persistent pain (Louw, Puentedura, & Mintken, 2012):

'Suzy' is a doctor's wife with three years of spinal pain and recently diagnosed with fibromyalgia. She has seen numerous healthcare providers and her most recent treatment involves epidural steroid injections, radio-frequency denervation and stabilization exercises. She is now referred to physical therapy. She has good and bad days with her pain, but more bad days than good days. Her pain is in the low back and starting to spread down the legs (Figure 1.2). Her pain comes and goes and 'seems have a mind of its own.' Stress increases her pain considerably. She does not sleep well. She has had to stop cooking meals, as standing > 20 minutes increases the pain, which will then last 1-2 days. She is unable to sit > 60 minutes in a car during a road trip. She comes to physical therapy for help. Her Oswestry Disability Index and Fear Avoidance Beliefs Questionnaire scores are extremely high.

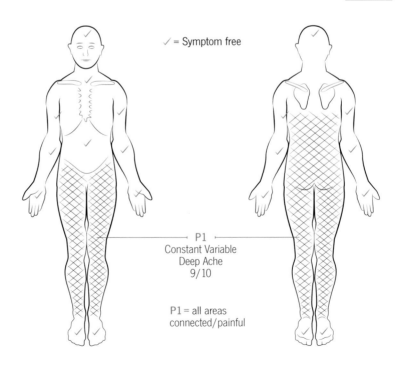

✓ = Symptom free

P1
Constant Variable
Deep Ache
9/10

P1 = all areas
connected/painful

Figure 1.2: Chronic Pain Body Chart (from the authors).

Additional:
- General health is good
- Works out: Pilates and Yoga
- No joint problems
- Family history of LBP
- Unable to work as a part-time office manager

Her physical tests reveal the following:
- Forward flexion: 10 degrees = pain (Figure 1.3)
- Extension: 10 degrees = pain
- SLR: sensitive at 45 degrees (L = R)
- Slump: leg pain with neck flexion
- *Palpation:*
  - ○ Tender L1 – L5
  - ○ Tender SIJ/PSIS palpation
  - ○ Tender – bilateral hips
- *Stabilization:* Unable to perform a coordinated deep corset contraction

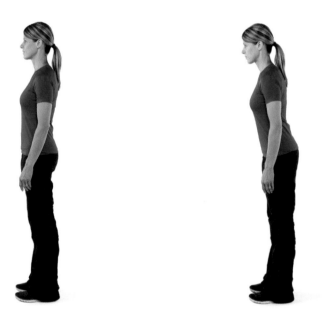

Figure 1.3: Chronic pain patient ('Suzy') at rest/neutral and maximum forward flexion (clinical images recreated).

In Figure 1.3, it is obvious that forward flexion is limited. The patient encountered increased pain and stopped further motion into forward flexion. When she was questioned about why she stopped, the patient answered *"I don't want the pain to get worse."* Further exploration of her thought processes and reasoning for stopping the movement elicited the following statement: *"If I bend more, the pain will increase; I have a bulging disc and it will get worse!"*

It should be clear from this case example that thoughts and beliefs can impact movement and function. The patient believes her bulging disc will get worse, bulge even more, and there is a real risk in bending more. This voluntary restriction is likely to impact physical treatments, which are the mainstay of therapy. How willing will this patient be to let a therapist apply passive (manual therapy) or active (exercise) movement to her spine to alleviate the pain, restricted ROM and disability?

Recent classification-based approaches to the treatment of LBP may be considered for this patient (Fritz, Cleland, & Childs, 2007). Is there a possibility that she may fit into a specific sub-group that might statistically predict her probability for success? A quick scan of clinical prediction rules for various LBP patients reveals that, in this case, it is unlikely she will benefit from spinal manipulation (Childs et al., 2004; Flynn et al., 2002), spinal stabilization (Hicks, Fritz, Delitto, & McGill, 2005), lumbar traction (Fritz et al., 2007), or directional preference (Hefford, 2008). Again, even if the patient met the requirements of a sub-group, the clinician would still need to convince her to participate in the proposed treatment. Furthermore, the clinician would likely be making the false assumption that there was a mechanical origin for the cause of the widespread pain. Pain is a lot more complex (Chapter 3).

Clearly, a deeper approach is needed. Evidence-based medicine has driven quantitative research to the forefront (Sackett, 1998). Quantitative research, with systematic reviews, randomized controlled trials (RCT) and meta-analyses, has led to experimentally designed, tested and "proven" treatment approaches for patients by delivering treatment protocols. Even though a particular treatment intervention may have high-level evidence to support it, and its use has been shown to statistically improve pain and function in appropriately selected patients, the clinician will still need to address the patient's fear. An often forgotten part of the evidence is that provided by qualitative research, especially when seeking what the patient wants. Qualitative studies and sound clinical reasoning, intuition and experience (see Gifford forward) show that patients want answers to the following (Verbeek, Sengers, Riemens, & Haafkens, 2004):

- What is wrong with me?
- How long will it take?
- What can I (the patient) do for it?
- What can you (the therapist) do for it?

These questions (and answers) are complicated. How would you answer these questions for this patient? How confident are you in your answers? To treat patients with chronic pain, we need to change cognitions. Two particular cognitions, fear and catastrophizing, have been linked to poor outcomes and need to be addressed by a therapist before engaging in a movement-based approach of therapeutic exercise, manual therapy, pacing and graded exposure.

1.4: Fear

Fear is defined as a distressing negative sensation induced by a perceived threat. Fear and its impact on pain have been discussed extensively, yet many therapists do not readily understand the debilitating effect of fear on movement and recovery (Cleland, Fritz, & Childs, 2008; George, Valencia, Zeppieri, & Robinson, 2009; Mintken, Cleland, Whitman, & George, 2010; Waddell, Newton, Henderson, Somerville, & Main, 1993). In a famous quote, it has been stated that

"the fear of pain is worse than pain itself"
(Arntz & Peters, 1995).

This statement is underscored by the fact that numerous studies evaluating LBP include the use of scales addressing fear, such as the Fear Avoidance Beliefs Questionnaire (FABQ) (Fritz & George, 2002; Fritz, George, & Delitto, 2001; George, Fritz, Bialosky, & Donald, 2003; George, Fritz, & McNeil, 2006). Fear within the general population is often associated with the belief that increased activity, movement or exercise will not only increase pain, but further damage tissues. Patients with LBP deal with the unknown, including diagnosis, how long the injury will take to heal, how long before they return to function, how the back pain may/may not influence income, etc. The clinical manifestation of these unknowns may present itself as increased fear.

It is clear that therapists need to not only take the patient's fear into consideration, but also find a way to quantify it. The most commonly used measure is the FABQ. (See Table 1.1). The FABQ is a 16-item questionnaire that was designed to quantify fear and avoidance beliefs in individuals with LBP. The FABQ has two subscales: 1) a four-item scale to measure fear avoidance beliefs about physical activity and 2) a seven-item scale to measure fear-avoidance beliefs about work. Each item is scored from 0 to 6 with possible scores ranging between 0 and 24 and 0 and 42 for the physical activity and work subscales, respectively, with higher scores representing an increase in fear-avoidance beliefs. The FABQ has demonstrated acceptable levels of reliability and validity in previous LBP studies (Cleland, et al., 2008; Grotle, Vollestad, & Brox, 2006a; Poiraudeau et al., 2006). Presence of avoidance behavior has been associated with increased risk of prolonged disability and work loss. It is proposed that a FABQ-PA >14 and FABQ-W >34 is associated with a higher likelihood of prolonged disability and not returning to work (Burton, Waddell, Tillotson, & Summerton, 1999; Fritz & George, 2002).

It is highly recommended therapists utilize outcomes measures such as the FABQ to objectively measure progress and perhaps flag patients who are more likely to need additional resources, i.e., multi-disciplinary treatment. Clinically skilled therapists may also wish to ask simple fear-related questions such as: *What are you afraid of? Are you afraid the pain will get worse?* and/or *Are you afraid therapy will increase your pain?* A skilled, thorough subjective examination should include listening for statements from patients regarding their fears (Maitland, 1986).

Table 1.1: The Fear Avoidance Beliefs Questionnaire (FABQ)

Name: _____   Date: _____/_____/_____
                                                      mm   dd   yy

Here are some of the things other patients have told us about their pain. For each statement, please circle the number from 0 to 6 to indicate how much physical activities such as bending, lifting, walking or driving affect or would affect your back pain.

		Completely Disagree			Unsure			Completely Agree
1.	My pain was caused by physical activity.	0	1	2	3	4	5	6
2.	Physical activity makes my pain worse.	0	1	2	3	4	5	6
3.	Physical activity might harm my back.	0	1	2	3	4	5	6
4.	I should not do physical activities which (might) make my pain worse.	0	1	2	3	4	5	6
5.	I cannot do physical activities which (might) make my pain worse.	0	1	2	3	4	5	6

FABQPA (2,3,4,5): _____ /24

The following statements are about how your normal work affects or would affect your back pain.

		Completely Disagree			Unsure			Completely Agree
6.	My pain was caused by my work or by an accident at work.	0	1	2	3	4	5	6
7.	My work aggravated my pain.	0	1	2	3	4	5	6
8.	I have a claim for compensation for my pain.	0	1	2	3	4	5	6
9.	My work is too heavy for me.	0	1	2	3	4	5	6
10.	My work makes or would make my pain worse.	0	1	2	3	4	5	6
11.	My work might harm my back.	0	1	2	3	4	5	6
12.	I should not do my regular work with my present pain.	0	1	2	3	4	5	6
13.	I cannot do my normal work with my present pain.	0	1	2	3	4	5	6
14.	I cannot do my normal work until my pain is treated.	0	1	2	3	4	5	6
15.	I do not think that I will be back to my normal work within 3 months.	0	1	2	3	4	5	6
16.	I do not think that I will ever be able to go back to that work.	0	1	2	3	4	5	6

FABQW (6,7,9,10,11,12,15): _____ /42

Vlaeyen and Linton (2000) introduced the fear-avoidance (FA) model to describe how pain disability, affective distress and physical disuse develop as a result of persistent avoidance behaviors motivated by fear. (See figure 1.4). It is interesting to note that after injury and the resultant pain experience, two very different pathways or choices lead to two very different outcomes.

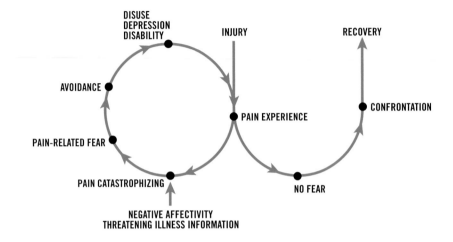

Figure 1.4: The fear-avoidance model. Image adapted from Vlaeyen & Linton (2000).

In figure 1.5, we extrapolate on the FA. Clinicians working with chronic pain patients will likely see several features that may appear to be quite familiar from the clinical point of view:

5a Could also be emotional overload—In the FA model, injury is set as an initiating event for the pain experience. Although injury may cause the start of the pain experience, many patients develop chronic pain in the absence of injury. Furthermore, injury and pain are not synonymous as we will discuss later in chapter 3. In the latest pain science terminology, pain is viewed as a defense, created by the brain when faced with danger (G. L. Moseley, 2003; G. Lorimer Moseley, 2007). Patients facing emotional issues related to work, family and life may have those stressful issues as the initiation of their pain experience and clinicians should be aware of this. The International Association on the Study of Pain (IASP) states pain can be from an emotional or physical issue and warrants inclusion in the FA model.

5b Choice made early—A human's experience and subsequent response to a threat, such as an injury or even emotional overload, can be very interesting. Some people may endure seemingly similar injuries, yet some develop no lasting pain experience, while others start a life of persistent pain. There are likely many factors impacting this "development" of pain (chapter 3) and these could include genetic coding, environmental issues, peer pressure, upbringing, knowledge, anxiety, and more. It is, therefore, clear that several factors will impact this development of a pain experience (F. Kovacs, Oliver-Frontera, Plana, Royuela, Muriel, & Gestoso, 2011; Staud, 2011; Wall & Melzack, 2005). More compelling is the fact that early intervention, especially education, may have a significant impact in the path chosen after injury (Buchbinder, Jolley, & Wyatt, 2001; Oliveira, Gevirtz, & Hubbard, 2006).

5c Knowledge—It is widely known that pain is more prevalent in patients with lower educational levels (Holm, Carroll, Cassidy, & Ahlbom, 2006; Schmidt et al., 2007). Conversely, it has been shown that healthcare providers who experience a similar injury to non-medically trained persons will report significantly less pain and disability (Virani, Ferrari, & Russell, 2001). Knowledge, in this case, may be seen as allaying any possible fears such that events may be confronted head-on with an expectation that recovery will follow.

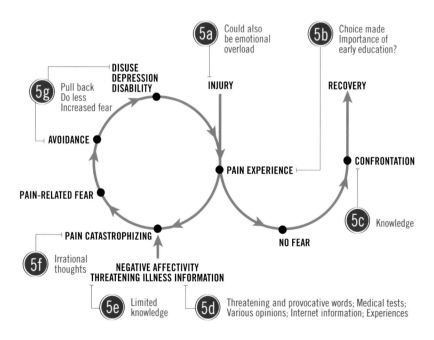

Figure 1.5: Clinical application of the fear-avoidance model.

5d Medical threats–Patients in pain invariably attend medical appointments, undergo tests and experience a variety of healthcare providers and their corresponding treatment interventions. During this medical journey, threatening and provocative terminology is likely to induce some level of fear and thereby increase the pain experience (Morr, Shanti, Carrer, Kubeck, & Gerling, 2010; Sloan & Walsh, 2010; Wilson, Williams, & Butler, 2009).

5e Limited knowledge–Pain and knowledge are intricately intertwined. Whereas having appropriate knowledge (5c) may allay fears and allow confrontation/dealing with the situation, limited or incorrect knowledge can have a powerful and negative effect on the pain experience.

5f Irrational thoughts–With limited or incorrect knowledge, poor decisions are likely to be made. This limited or incorrect information may lead to an inability to foresee anything other than the worst possible outcome. Pain catastrophizing is such an example.

5g Pull back–With persistent pain and limited help, patients in persistent pain may start a social withdrawal process. The social withdrawal is likely due to pain, lack of energy, limited mobility, family issues, lack of goals and more. This withdrawal process can further reinforce the notion of how badly they are affected and can propel the pain experience into a downward spiral.

1.5: Catastrophizing

Catastrophizing is defined as the inability to foresee anything other than the worst possible outcome, however unlikely, or experiencing a situation as unbearable or impossible when it is just uncomfortable. Catastrophizing due to pain is often associated with chronic pain (Garcia-Campayo et al., 2009; F. M. Kovacs, Seco, Royuela, Pena, & Muriel, 2011).

The most commonly used measuring tool for measuring catastrophization is the Pain Catastrophizing Scale (PCS) (Table 1.2). The PCS is a self-report questionnaire that assesses inappropriate coping strategies and catastrophic thinking about pain and injury. The PCS has been used in previous TNE studies (G. L. Moseley, 2004; G. L. Moseley, Nicholas, & Hodges, 2004) for chronic LBP and has been shown to have strong construct validity, reliability and stability (Sullivan, Bishop, & Pivik, 1995). As with fear, clinicians should train themselves to listen for catastrophizing phrases, which may include: *"That's it…life is over, might as well bury me now…"*; *"Now that I have a bulging disc, I will never walk again"*; *"Because of my arthritis, I will be in a wheelchair soon"* or *"I've got arthritis. I will never run again."*

Table 1.2: Pain Catastrophizing Scale

Name: _____ Date: _____ / _____ / _____
                                                    mm   dd   yy

Age: _____ Gender: ☐ Male   ☐ Female

Everyone experiences painful situations at some point in their lives. Such experiences may include headaches, tooth pain, joint or muscle pain. People are often exposed to situations that may cause pain such as illness, injury, dental procedures or surgery.

Instructions: *We are interested in the types of thoughts and feelings that you have when you are in pain. Listed below are thirteen statements describing different thoughts and feelings that may be associated with pain. Using the following scale, please indicate the degree to which you have these thoughts and feelings when you are experiencing pain.*

Rating	0	1	2	3	4
Meaning	Not at all	To a slight degree	To a moderate degree	To a great degree	All the time

Number	Statement	Rating
1.	I worry all the time about whether the pain will end.	
2.	I feel I can't go on.	
3.	It's terrible and I think it's never going to get any better.	
4.	It's awful and I feel that it overwhelms me.	
5.	I feel I can't stand it anymore.	
6.	I become afraid that the pain will get worse.	
7.	I keep thinking of other painful events.	
8.	I anxiously want the pain to go away.	
9.	I can't seem to keep it out of my mind.	
10.	I keep thinking about how much it hurts.	
11.	I keep thinking about how badly I want the pain to stop.	
12.	There's nothing I can do to reduce the intensity of the pain.	
13.	I wonder whether something serious may happen.	

1.6: Beliefs

Apart from fear and pain catastrophizing, various other maladaptive beliefs may be in need of change to allow for normal movement, exercise and function, let alone participation in rehabilitation (Mutsaers, Peters, Pool-Goudzwaard, Koes, & Verhagen, 2012; Sloan & Walsh, 2010). Impaired beliefs include the following:

- *Belief that pain is always bad*
- *Belief that all pain must be gone before engaging in normal activity, movement and therapy*
- *Belief that passive treatment is the answer*
- *Belief that pain will increase with any/all activity*
- *Belief that work is potentially harmful*

Along with altered cognitions such as fear, beliefs and pain catastrophizing, several other impaired psychosocial issues have been found to correlate to pain, development of chronicity, healthcare expense and compliance with treatment (Grotle, Vollestad, & Brox, 2006b; N. Kendall & Watson, 2000; Watson & Kendall, 2000). These factors are often referred to as "Yellow Flags" (N. Kendall & Watson, 2000).

1.7: Yellow Flags

Although yellow flags have evolved considerably, it is worth spending some time outlining them. Yellow flags are psychosocial factors that have been shown to correlate to the development of chronic pain (Figure 1.6). LBP is the most widely reported musculoskeletal disorder in western civilization and estimated to be second only to the common cold in reasons for seeking medical care (Cherkin, 1998; Deyo, Mirza, & Martin, 2006; Lurie, Birkmeyer, & Weinstein, 2003; Waddell, 1991). Epidemiological data indicates approximately 80% of people will develop LBP in life (Cherkin, 1998; Deyo, et al., 2006; Lurie, et al., 2003; Waddell, 1991) and that, at any given point, 40% of people at a large gathering will have some form of LBP (Cherkin, 1998; Deyo, et al., 2006; Lurie, et al., 2003; Waddell, 1991).

Additionally, the recurrence rate of LBP shows that 70% of people who have suffered an episode of LBP are still not satisfied with their condition one year later (Croft, Macfarlane, Papageorgiou, Thomas, & Silman, 1998). The most alarming epidemiological data, however, lead to the research and development of the yellow flags. It was alarming to discover that 6% of LBP sufferers consume greater than 50% of the cost associated with LBP (Linton, Hellsing, & Hallden, 1998; Linton & Nordin, 2006). With the huge financial impact of such a sub-group, scientists set out the determine if there were psychosocial issues that may have been predictive of persistent LBP and if subsequent tailored treatment may lessen the burden of LBP (N. A. S. Kendall, Linton, & Main, 1997). The subsequent use of the FABQ and PCS is an extension of the original 'yellow flags' research.

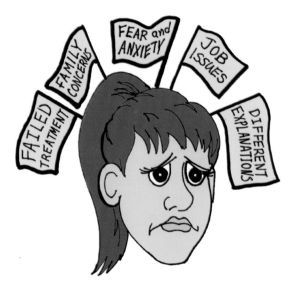

Figure 1.6: Psychosocial yellow flags. Image from Louw, 2013.

Apart from the previously discussed issues of fear, pain catastrophizing and beliefs; yellow flags like various emotions, behaviors, family and work issues, as well as medical examinations and treatment issues were also identified in regards to pain and recovery (N. Kendall & Watson, 2000; N. A. S. Kendall, et al., 1997). These factors are listed in Table 1.3.

Table 1.3: Additional psychosocial yellow flags

Behaviors
- Extended rest
- Withdrawal from social life, daily life and people
- Compliance issues with therapy
- Report of extremely high intensity of pain, e.g., 15 on a 0-10 Visual Analog Scale
- Excessive reliance on use of aids or appliances
- Problems sleeping
- High intake of alcohol and medication
- Smoking

Work
- History of manual work
- Job dissatisfaction
- Problems with peers and supervisors
- Low educational background
- Low socioeconomic status
- High physical demand
- Working shifts – especially at night
- Negative experience of workplace management of pain or injury

Compensation issues
- Lack of financial incentive to return to work
- History of claims due to other injuries or pain problems

Emotions
- Fear of increased pain with activity, work or therapy
- Depression
- Irritability
- Anxiety

Diagnosis and treatment
- Health professional sanctioning disability
- Conflicting diagnoses
- Diagnostic language leading to catastrophization and fear
- Number of healthcare providers visited
- Expectation of a 'techno-fix'
- Lack of satisfaction with treatment

Family
- Overprotective spouse
- Punitive responses from spouse

As stated before, yellow flags have evolved. Some factors, e.g., fear and catastrophizing, have been studied in greater depth. Additional flags have also been identified (Figure 1.7).

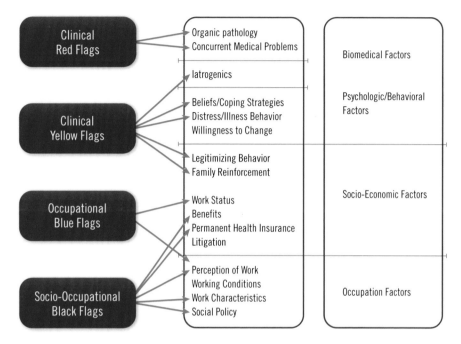

Figure 1.7: Additional flags identified as representing barriers to recovery (from Mark Jones).

- **Red Flags:** There are many different "flags" therapists need to consider. Probably the most well-known flags are 'red flags' (Boissonnault, 1994; Goodman & Boissonnault, 1998), keeping to the fundamental first rule of medicine: Do No Harm.

- **Blue Flags:** These are specific occupational issues and involve perceived features of work that are often associated with higher rates of symptoms, ill-health and work loss. High physical or emotional (stress) demands of the job, low ability to control the work environment, problems with management, poor social support from colleagues, perceived time pressure, and lack of job satisfaction are examples of blue flags.

- **Black Flags:** These are considered socio-occupational issues, such as national healthcare policy, rates of pay, negotiated entitlements, employer policy, sickness policy, restricted duties policy, management style, organization size and structure, trade union support, content-specific aspects of work, ergonomics, hours and shift work.

It should be noted that there is considerable overlap between the yellow, blue and black flags.

1.8: Returning to the Patient

Considering the discussion thus far, let's revisit our case example. It could easily be argued that this patient may have various cognitive issues that are limiting her ability and willingness to flex forward. They are also likely to limit her ability/willingness to fully participate in therapy. These issues include fear, pain catastrophizing, different explanations for her pain, failed treatments, social withdrawal and, perhaps, the effect of provocative language used to describe why she has her pain.

Clinicians should not label her as a "difficult" patient or a "malingerer." Because of the issues she has faced, this patient believes there is serious danger in flexing forward. It might even be more correct to suggest that her brain believes it is dangerous. This belief is based on all the available information the brain has regarding the "bulging disc." In this case, the brain uses pain to protect. Other systems are used to protect as well, e.g., muscle guarding, possibly some adrenaline, faster and shallower breathing and even a linguistic response of "ooooooooh" as she flexes forward.

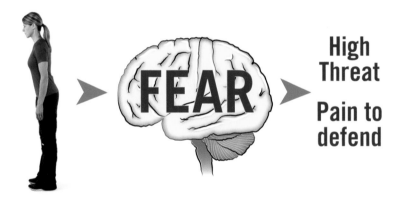

This psychosocial interpretation of her forward flexion is in line with the current neuroscience definition of pain:

Pain is a multiple system output activated
by the brain based on perceived threat.
(G. L. Moseley, 2003)

1.9: Key Points from Chapter 1

- Clinicians have seen and will continue to see many patients with chronic pain
- Current models of evaluation and treatment are insufficient
- Cognitions impact pain
- Persistent pain affects cognitions, beliefs, emotions and behaviors
- Changing cognitions must occur to allow movement-based approaches to be effective
- Therapy should address faulty cognitions

Chapter 1 References

Alyas, F., Turner, M., & Connell, D. (2007). MRI findings in the lumbar spines of asymptomatic, adolescent, elite tennis players. *Br J Sports Med, 41*(11), 836-841; discussion 841.

Arntz, A., & Peters, M. (1995). Chronic low back pain and inaccurate predictions of pain: is being too tough a risk factor for the development and maintenance of chronic pain? *Behaviour Research and Therapy, 33*(1), 49-53.

Boissonnault, W. G. (1994). *Examination in Physical Therapy Practice*. New York: Churchill Livingstone.

Buchbinder, R., Jolley, D., & Wyatt, M. (2001). 2001 Volvo Award Winner in Clinical Studies: Effects of a media campaign on back pain beliefs and its potential influence on management of low back pain in general practice. *Spine (Phila Pa 1976), 26*(23), 2535-2542.

Burton, A. K., Waddell, G., Tillotson, K. M., & Summerton, N. (1999). Information and advice to patients with back pain can have a positive effect. A randomized controlled trial of a novel educational booklet in primary care. [Clinical Trial Randomized Controlled Trial]. *Spine, 24*(23), 2484-2491.

Cherkin, D. C. (1998). Primary care research on low back pain. The state of the science. *Spine, 23*(18), 1997-2002.

Childs, J. D., Fritz, J. M., Flynn, T. W., Irrgang, J. J., Johnson, K. K., Majkowski, G. R., & Delitto, A. (2004). A clinical prediction rule to identify patients with low back pain most likely to benefit from spinal manipulation: a validation study. *Annals of Internal Medicine, 141*(12), 920-928.

Cleland, J. A., Fritz, J. M., & Childs, J. D. (2008). Psychometric properties of the Fear-Avoidance Beliefs Questionnaire and Tampa Scale of Kinesiophobia in patients with neck pain. *Am J Phys Med Rehabil, 87*(2), 109-117.

Croft, P. R., Macfarlane, G. J., Papageorgiou, A. C., Thomas, E., & Silman, A. J. (1998). Outcome of low back pain in general practice: a prospective study. *Bmj, 316*(7141), 1356-1359.

Deyo, R. A., Mirza, S. K., & Martin, B. I. (2006). Back pain prevalence and visit rates: estimates from U.S. national surveys, 2002. *Spine, 31*(23), 2724-2727.

Flynn, T., Fritz, J., Whitman, J., Wainner, R., Magel, J., Rendeiro, D., . . . Allison, S. (2002). A clinical prediction rule for classifying patients with low back pain who demonstrate short-term improvement with spinal manipulation. *Spine, 27*(24), 2835-2843.

Foster, N. E., & Delitto, A. (2011). Embedding Psychosocial Perspectives Within Clinical Management of Low Back Pain: Integration of Psychosocially Informed Management Principles Into Physical Therapist Practice — Challenges and Opportunities. *Phys Ther.*

Fritz, J. M., Cleland, J. A., & Childs, J. D. (2007). Subgrouping patients with low back pain: evolution of a classification approach to physical therapy. *J Orthop Sports Phys Ther, 37*(6), 290-302.

Fritz, J. M., & George, S. Z. (2002). Identifying psychosocial variables in patients with acute work-related low back pain: the importance of fear-avoidance beliefs. *Phys Ther, 82*(10), 973-983.

Fritz, J. M., George, S. Z., & Delitto, A. (2001). The role of fear-avoidance beliefs in acute low back pain: relationships with current and future disability and work status. *Pain, 94*(1), 7-15.

Fritz, J. M., Lindsay, W., Matheson, J. W., Brennan, G. P., Hunter, S. J., Moffit, S. D., . . . Rodriquez, B. (2007). Is there a subgroup of patients with low back pain likely to benefit from mechanical traction? Results of a randomized clinical trial and subgrouping analysis. *Spine, 32*(26), E793-800.

Garcia-Campayo, J., Serrano-Blanco, A., Rodero, B., Magallon, R., Alda, M., Andres, E., . . . del Hoyo, Y. L. (2009). Effectiveness of the psychological and pharmacological treatment of catastrophization in patients with fibromyalgia: a randomized controlled trial. *Trials, 10*, 24.

George, S. Z., Fritz, J. M., Bialosky, J. E., & Donald, D. A. (2003). The effect of a fear-avoidance-based physical therapy intervention for patients with acute low back pain: results of a randomized clinical trial. *Spine (Phila Pa 1976), 28*(23), 2551-2560.

George, S. Z., Fritz, J. M., & McNeil, D. W. (2006). Fear-avoidance beliefs as measured by the fear-avoidance beliefs questionnaire: change in fear-avoidance beliefs questionnaire is predictive of change in self-report of disability and pain intensity for patients with acute low back pain. *Clin J Pain, 22*(2), 197-203.

George, S. Z., Valencia, C., Zeppieri, G., Jr., & Robinson, M. E. (2009). Development of a Self-Report Measure of Fearful Activities for Patients With Low Back Pain: The Fear of Daily Activities Questionnaire. *Phys Ther.*

Goldberg, J. S. (2008). Revisiting the Cartesian model of pain. *Med Hypotheses, 70*(5), 1029-1033.

Goodman, C. C., & Boissonnault, W. G. (1998). *Pathology. Implications for the Physical Therapist.* Philadelphia: Saunders.

Grotle, M., Vollestad, N. K., & Brox, J. I. (2006a). Clinical course and impact of fear-avoidance beliefs in low back pain: prospective cohort study of acute and chronic low back pain: II. *Spine, 31*(9), 1038-1046.

Grotle, M., Vollestad, N. K., & Brox, J. I. (2006b). Screening for yellow flags in first-time acute low back pain: reliability and validity of a Norwegian version of the Acute Low Back Pain Screening Questionnaire. [Comparative Study]. *The Clinical Journal of Pain, 22*(5), 458-467.

Haldeman, S. (1990). North American Spine Society: failure of the pathology model to predict back pain. *Spine (Phila Pa 1976), 15*(7), 718-724.

Hefford, C. (2008). McKenzie classification of mechanical spinal pain: profile of syndromes and directions of preference. *Man Ther, 13*(1), 75-81.

Henrotin, Y. E., Cedraschi, C., Duplan, B., Bazin, T., & Duquesnoy, B. (2006). Information and low back pain management: a systematic review. *Spine, 31*(11), E326-334.

Hicks, G. E., Fritz, J. M., Delitto, A., & McGill, S. M. (2005). Preliminary development of a clinical prediction rule for determining which patients with low back pain will respond to a stabilization exercise program. *Arch Phys Med Rehabil, 86*(9), 1753-1762.

Holm, L. W., Carroll, L. J., Cassidy, J. D., & Ahlbom, A. (2006). Factors influencing neck pain intensity in whiplash-associated disorders. *Spine, 31*(4), E98-104.

Houben, R. M., Ostelo, R. W., Vlaeyen, J. W., Wolters, P. M., Peters, M., & Stomp-van den Berg, S. G. (2005). Health care providers' orientations towards common low back pain predict perceived harmfulness of physical activities and recommendations regarding return to normal activity. *Eur J Pain, 9*(2), 173-183.

IOM, I. o. M. (2011). Relieving Pain in America: A Blueprint for Transforming Prevention, Care, Education and Research, The National Academies Press. (Vol. 2012). Washington DC: The National Academies Press.

Iwamoto, J., Takeda, T., & Wakano, K. (2004). Returning athletes with severe low back pain and spondylolysis to original sporting activities with conservative treatment. *Scand J Med Sci Sports, 14*(6), 346-351.

Jull, G., & Sterling, M. (2009). Bring back the biopsychosocial model for neck pain disorders. *Man Ther, 14*(2), 117-118.

Kendall, N., & Watson, P. (2000). Identifying psychosocial yellow flags and modifying management. In L. S. Gifford (Ed.), *Topical Issues in Pain 2.* Falmouth: CNS Press.

Kendall, N. A. S., Linton, S. J., & Main, C. J. (1997). *Guide to assessing psychosocial yellow flags in acute low back pain: risk factors for long term disability and work loss.* Wellington: Accident Rehabilitation & Compensation Insurance Corporation of New Zealand and the National Health Committee.

Kovacs, F., Oliver-Frontera, M., Plana, M. N., Royuela, A., Muriel, A., & Gestoso, M. (2011). Improving schoolchildren's knowledge of methods for the prevention and management of low back pain: a cluster randomized controlled trial. [Randomized Controlled Trial Research Support, Non-U.S. Gov't]. *Spine, 36*(8), E505-512.

Kovacs, F. M., Seco, J., Royuela, A., Pena, A., & Muriel, A. (2011). The correlation between pain, catastrophizing, and disability in subacute and chronic low back pain: a study in the routine clinical practice of the Spanish National Health Service. [Multicenter Study Research Support, Non-U.S. Gov't]. *Spine, 36*(4), 339-345.

Latimer, J., Maher, C., & Refshauge, K. (2004). The attitudes and beliefs of physiotherapy students to chronic back pain. *Clin J Pain, 20*(1), 45-50.

Linton, S. J., Hellsing, A. L., & Hallden, K. (1998). A population-based study of spinal pain among 35-45-year-old individuals. Prevalence, sick leave, and health care use. *Spine (Phila Pa 1976), 23*(13), 1457-1463.

Linton, S. J., & Nordin, E. (2006). A 5-year follow-up evaluation of the health and economic consequences of an early cognitive behavioral intervention for back pain: a randomized, controlled trial. *Spine, 31*(8), 853-858.

Linton, S. J., & Shaw, W. S. (2011). Impact of Psychological Factors in the Experience of Pain. *Phys Ther.*

Louw, A., & Butler, D. S. (2011). Chronic Pain. In B. S.B. & R. Manske (Eds.), *Clinical Orthopaedic Rehabilitation* (3rd Edition ed.). Philadelphia, PA: Elsevier.

Louw, A., Puentedura, E. L., & Mintken, P. (2012). Use of an abbreviated neuroscience education approach in the treatment of chronic low back pain: a case report. [Case Reports]. *Physiother Theory Pract, 28*(1), 50-62.

Lurie, J. D., Birkmeyer, N. J., & Weinstein, J. N. (2003). Rates of advanced spinal imaging and spine surgery. *Spine, 28*(6), 616-620.

Maitland, G. D. (1986). *Vertebral Manipulation* (6th ed.). London: Butterworths.

Meeus, M., Nijs, J., Van Oosterwijck, J., Van Alsenoy, V., & Truijen, S. (2010). Pain Physiology Education Improves Pain Beliefs in Patients With Chronic Fatigue Syndrome Compared With Pacing and Self-Management Education: A Double-Blind Randomized Controlled Trial. *Arch Phys Med Rehabil, 91*(8), 1153-1159.

Merskey, H., & Bogduk, N. (1994). *Classification of Chronic Pain* (2nd ed.). Seattle: IASP Press.

Mintken, P. E., Cleland, J. A., Whitman, J. M., & George, S. Z. (2010). Psychometric properties of the Fear-Avoidance Beliefs Questionnaire and Tampa Scale of Kinesiophobia in patients with shoulder pain. [Clinical Trial Research Support, Non-U.S. Gov't]. *Archives of Physical Medicine and Rehabilitation, 91*(7), 1128-1136.

Morr, S., Shanti, N., Carrer, A., Kubeck, J., & Gerling, M. C. (2010). Quality of information concerning cervical disc herniation on the Internet. *Spine J, 10*(4), 350-354.

Moseley, G. L. (2003). A pain neuromatrix approach to patients with chronic pain. *Man Ther, 8*(3), 130-140.

Moseley, G. L. (2004). Evidence for a direct relationship between cognitive and physical change during an education intervention in people with chronic low back pain. *Eur J Pain, 8*(1), 39-45.

Moseley, G. L. (2007). Reconceptualising pain according to modern pain science. *Physical Therapy Reviews, 12*(3), 169-178.

Moseley, G. L., Nicholas, M. K., & Hodges, P. W. (2004). A randomized controlled trial of intensive neurophysiology education in chronic low back pain. *Clin J Pain, 20*(5), 324-330.

Mutsaers, J. H., Peters, R., Pool-Goudzwaard, A. L., Koes, B. W., & Verhagen, A. P. (2012). Psychometric properties of the Pain Attitudes and Beliefs Scale for Physiotherapists: A systematic review. *Man Ther.*

Nijs, J., Roussel, N., Paul van Wilgen, C., Koke, A., & Smeets, R. (2012). Thinking beyond muscles and joints: Therapists' and patients' attitudes and beliefs regarding chronic musculoskeletal pain are key to applying effective treatment. *Man Ther.*

Oliveira, A., Gevirtz, R., & Hubbard, D. (2006). A psycho-educational video used in the emergency department provides effective treatment for whiplash injuries. *Spine, 31*(15), 1652-1657.

Poiraudeau, S., Rannou, F., Baron, G., Le Henanff, A., Coudeyre, E., Rozenberg, S., . . . Ravaud, P. (2006). Fear-avoidance beliefs about back pain in patients with subacute low back pain. *Pain, 124*(3), 305-311.

Raftery, M. N., Sarma, K., Murphy, A. W., De la Harpe, D., Normand, C., & McGuire, B. E. (2011). Chronic pain in the Republic of Ireland--community prevalence, psychosocial profile and predictors of pain-related disability: results from the Prevalence, Impact and Cost of Chronic Pain (PRIME) study, part 1. [Research Support, Non-U.S. Gov't]. *Pain, 152*(5), 1096-1103.

Sackett, D. L. (1998). Evidence-based medicine. *Spine, 23*(10), 1085-1086.

Schmidt, C. O., Raspe, H., Pfingsten, M., Hasenbring, M., Basler, H. D., Eich, W., & Kohlmann, T. (2007). Back pain in the German adult population: prevalence, severity, and sociodemographic correlates in a multiregional survey. *Spine (Phila Pa 1976), 32*(18), 2005-2011.

Sloan, T. J., & Walsh, D. A. (2010). Explanatory and diagnostic labels and perceived prognosis in chronic low back pain. *Spine, 35*(21), E1120-1125.

Staud, R. (2011). Evidence for shared pain mechanisms in osteoarthritis, low back pain, and fibromyalgia. [Review]. *Curr Rheumatol Rep, 13*(6), 513-520.

Sullivan, M. J. L., Bishop, S. R., & Pivik, J. (1995). The Pain Catastrophizing Scale: Development and validation. *Psychological Assessment, 7*(4), 524-532.

Timm, K. E. (1994). A randomized-control study of active and passive treatments for chronic low back pain following L5 laminectomy. *J Orthop Sports Phys Ther, 20*(6), 276-286.

Verbeek, J., Sengers, M. J., Riemens, L., & Haafkens, J. (2004). Patient expectations of treatment for back pain: a systematic review of qualitative and quantitative studies. *Spine, 29*(20), 2309-2318.

Virani, S. N., Ferrari, R., & Russell, A. S. (2001). Physician resistance to the late whiplash syndrome. *J Rheumatol, 28*(9), 2096-2099.

Vlaeyen, J. W., Kole-Snijders, A. M., Boeren, R. G., & van Eek, H. (1995). Fear of movement/(re)injury in chronic low back pain and its relation to behavioral performance. *Pain, 62*(3), 363-372.

Vlaeyen, J. W., & Linton, S. J. (2000). Fear-avoidance and its consequences in chronic musculoskeletal pain: a state of the art. *Pain, 85*(3), 317-332.

Waddell, G. (1991). Low back disability: A syndrome of western civilisation. *Neurosurgical Clinics of North America, 2*, 719-738.

Waddell, G., Newton, M., Henderson, I., Somerville, D., & Main, C. J. (1993). A Fear-Avoidance Beliefs Questionnaire (FABQ) and the role of fear-avoidance beliefs in chronic low back pain and disability. *Pain, 52*(2), 157-168.

Wall, P. D., & Melzack, R. (2005). *Textbook of Pain* (5th edn ed.). London: Elsevier.

Waris, E., Eskelin, M., Hermunen, H., Kiviluoto, O., & Paajanen, H. (2007). Disc degeneration in low back pain: a 17-year follow-up study using magnetic resonance imaging. *Spine, 32*(6), 681-684.

Watson, P., & Kendall, N. (2000). Assessing psychosocial yellow flags. In L. S. Gifford (Ed.), *Topical Issues in Pain 2*. Falmouth: CNS Press.

Weiner, B. K. (2008). Spine update: the biopsychosocial model and spine care. *Spine, 33*(2), 219-223.

Wilson, D., Williams, M., & Butler, D. (2009). Language and the pain experience. [Review]. *Physiother Res Int, 14*(1), 56-65.

Chapter 2

Patient Education

2.1: Education

Education is therapy. Knowledge is therapy. Chapter 1 clearly indicates patients need education. The question now arises as to what education is needed; this includes content and educational delivery methods. Patient education is defined as any set of planned educational activities designed to improve a patient's health behaviors, health status or both. Such activities are aimed at facilitating the patient's knowledge base (Lorig, 2001; Oshodi, 2007). Patient education has always had a strong history in nursing and in therapy; it has always been seen as a non-specific intervention. In Table 2.1, we highlight some common styles of education, including their reported benefits and pitfalls. The list is by no means an authoritative review of patient education, but likely an introductory listing for most therapists.

Most therapists reviewing Table 2.1 will likely identify styles of education they commonly utilize in clinical practice. Do they work? The systematic reviews on the efficacy of education show it to provide only little benefit:

- May have benefit for acute and sub-acute LBP, but not chronic (Engers, Jellema et al., 2008).
- Helps with anxiety prior to surgery (Galaal, Deane et al., 2007).
- No evidence for any neck pain disorders (Gross, Aker et al., 2000).
- No evidence for neck pain with or without radiculopathy (Haines, Gross et al., 2008).
- No evidence for preoperative education for knee or hip replacement (McDonald, Hetrick et al., 2004).
- Helpful in kids with asthma (Wolf, Guevara et al., 2003).

The list continues. In general, there is a lack of convincing evidence for the usefulness of education in acute/sub-acute conditions. For chronic pain, the evidence seems even less. The real question therapists (and all healthcare providers) should ask is: why does it not work? Review Table 2.1 again, and then view Figures 2.1 and 2.2. These images, taken from the Internet, display two common injuries: whiplash and an ankle sprain. Would viewing these images help a patient recover faster or even help ease pain, fear or anxiety? Although the answer might seem to be quite simple, it is instead rather complex. It is also, likely, one of the biggest reasons why therapists struggle to effectively treat patients with chronic pain.

Table 2.1: Summary of common patient education styles

Education Style	Positives	Negatives
1. **Verbal one-on-one education** (Moseley, 2005; Louw, Puentedura et al., 2012)	• Personal • Patient and condition specific • Ability to answer questions	• Expense • Time consuming • Limited recall
2. **Video/DVD** (Brison, Hartling et al., 2005; Oliveira, Gevirtz et al., 2006)	• Cheap and easy to produce • Mass education • Standard message	• Impersonal • Limited for Q & A • Variability in conditions
3. **Booklets/pamphlets** (Burton, Waddell et al., 1999; McGregor, Burton et al., 2007)	• Cheap and easy to produce • Mass education • Standard message	• Boring; low compliance • Limited Q & A • Standard message
4. **TV advertising** (Buchbinder, Jolley et al., 2001; Buchbinder and Jolley, 2005)	• Mass communication • May change behaviors • Visual and auditory	• Expensive • Short times • Generalization
5. **E-mail** (Lorig, Laurent et al., 2002; Louw, 2012 – Submitted for publication)	• Quick, fast • Keeping up with technology • Personal	• Can be time consuming • Technological limitations • Invasion of personal space
6. **Internet/Web** (Saryeddine, Levy et al., 2008; Morr, Shanti et al., 2010)	• Easy, free • Visually appealing • Interactive	• Technological limits • Poor quality information • Competing for attention
7. **Joint models** (Louw, et al., 2012 – accepted for publication)	• Visual • Realistic • Accompanies verbal	• Can induce fear • Biomedical information
8. **Back School** (Brox, Storheim et al., 2008)	• Standardized training	• Little evidence for efficacy (Maier-Riehle and Harter 2001; Brox, Storheim et al., 2008)

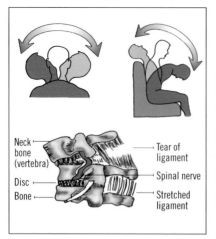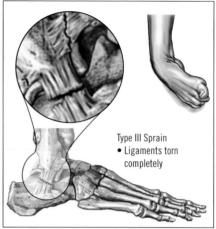

Figures 2.1 and 2.2: Common provocative injury pictures from the Internet.

Therapy is deeply rooted in a biomedical model focusing on tissues and tissue injury (Houben, Ostelo et al., 2005; Henrotin, Cedraschi et al., 2006; Weiner, 2008). The biomedical model seeks to find the anatomy or biomechanics at fault. If the faulty biomechanics or pathoanatomy can be corrected, it is then expected that the pain and disability will be recovered (Houben, Ostelo et al. 2005; Henrotin, Cedraschi et al., 2006; Weiner, 2008). Not only have these models shown limited efficacy in decreasing pain and disability, they may have increased fear in patients, which in turn may increase their pain (Greene, Appel et al., 2005; Morr, Shanti et al., 2010).

To add to this dilemma, patients have been indoctrinated in this biomedical model, as well. In a classic experiment, patients who underwent lumbar discectomy and shown their "damaged disc" material that was removed in the surgery recovered significantly better than those who were not shown their excised disc material (Tait, Levy et al., 2009).

- Leg pain (91.5 vs. 80.4%; p<0.05)
- Back pain (86.1 vs. 75.0%; p<0.05)
- Limb weakness (90.5 vs. 56.3%; p<0.02)
- Paresthesias (88 vs. 61.9%; p<0.05)
- Reduced analgesic use (92.1 vs. 69.4%; p<0.02)

The educational strategies employed in Table 2.1 are likely limited due to the content of their message. These educational sessions use only biomedical information (anatomy, biomechanics and physiology) to educate patients about their pain. Instead, this newly acquired biomedical education may reinforce the anatomical source of pain and even induce fear. The dichotomy that arose was as follows:

*Patients in pain want to know more
about pain, not anatomy.*

Patients in pain want to know more about pain (Louw, Louw et al., 2009). Healthcare providers underestimate patients' ability to understand pain (Moseley, 2003).

2.2: Neuroscience Education

A new model to educate patients as a means to modulate pain and disability was needed. Early work conducted by Gifford (1998) indicated the need for a much broader view of pain. In a series of articles on pain mechanisms (see Chapter 3), therapists were made more aware of a bigger and more biological view of pain and pain processing (Gifford and Butler, 1997; Gifford, 1998; Gifford, 2001). Anecdotal clinical evidence implied a possible use for these scientific, biological explanations for pain experiences to patients. These scientific, biological explanations for pain were referred to as neuroscience education.

The first published study involving neuroscience education was conducted by Dr. Lorimer Moseley (2002). By concealed randomization, 57 patients with chronic LBP were allocated to either a four-week combined physiotherapy and education program or management as directed by their general practitioners (usual care). The dependent variables of interest were pain and disability. Assessors were blind to group allocation. Outcome data from 49 subjects (86%) showed a significant treatment effect. The four-week combined physiotherapy and education program reduced pain and disability by a mean of 1.5/10 points on a numerical rating scale and 3.9 points on the 18-point Roland Morris Disability Questionnaire respectively. The number needed to treat in order to gain a clinically meaningful change was 3 for pain and 2 for disability. A treatment effect was maintained at one-year follow-up. The findings support the efficacy of combined physiotherapy and education program in producing symptomatic and functional change in moderately disabled patients with chronic low back pain. What exactly did they do for education?

"Each subject participated in a one-hour education session, once per week for four weeks. The education session was in a one-to-one seminar format, conducted by an independent therapist, and focused on the neurophysiology of pain with no particular reference to the lumbar spine."

In its purest form, the neuroscience education session educated patients about pain but at the same time de-focused anatomical issues. Since 2002, there have been a dozen randomized controlled trials (RCT), case studies and case series published on the use of therapeutic neuroscience education for chronic LBP, chronic whiplash, chronic fatigue syndrome, post-lumbar surgery and, more recently, pre-lumbar surgery (Figure 2.3).

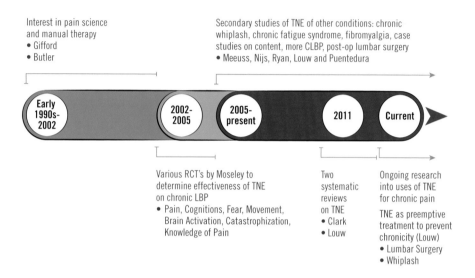

Interest in pain science and manual therapy
• Gifford
• Butler

Secondary studies of TNE of other conditions: chronic whiplash, chronic fatigue syndrome, fibromyalgia, case studies on content, more CLBP, post-op lumbar surgery
• Meeuss, Nijs, Ryan, Louw and Puentedura

Early 1990s-2002

2002-2005

2005-present

2011

Current

Various RCT's by Moseley to determine effectiveness of TNE on chronic LBP
• Pain, Cognitions, Fear, Movement, Brain Activation, Catastrophization, Knowledge of Pain

Two systematic reviews on TNE
• Clark
• Louw

Ongoing research into uses of TNE for chronic pain

TNE as preemptive treatment to prevent chronicity (Louw)
• Lumbar Surgery
• Whiplash

Figure 2.3: Proposed timeline of therapeutic neuroscience education (TNE).

2.3: Evidence for Therapeutic Neuroscience Education

With all the attention surrounding therapeutic neuroscience education (TNE), the question was posed: Does it work? To answer the question, a systematic review of RCT's was warranted. In 2011, a systematic review of TNE was conducted for musculoskeletal pain (Louw, Diener et al., 2011). The objective was to evaluate the evidence for the effectiveness of TNE for pain, disability, anxiety, and stress in chronic musculoskeletal (MSK) pain. The systematic review ultimately comprised six high-quality RCTs, one pseudo-RCT, and one comparative study involving 401 subjects (Table 2.2).

Table 2.2: RCT's of TNE studies included in the systematic review

Year	Author	Journal	Title
2002	Moseley, G.L	Australian Journal of Physiotherapy	Combined physiotherapy and education is efficacious for chronic low back pain.
2003	Moseley, G.L.	The Journal of Pain	Unraveling the barriers to reconceptualization of the problem in chronic pain: the actual and perceived ability of patients and health professionals to understand the neurophysiology.
2003	Moseley, G.L.	Journal of Manual and Manipulative Therapy	Joining forces – combining cognition-targeted motor control training with group or individual pain physiology education: a successful treatment for chronic low back pain.
2004	Moseley, G.L.	European Journal of Pain	Evidence for a direct relationship between cognitive and physical change during an education intervention in people with chronic low back pain.
2004	Moseley, Hodges and Nicholas	Clinical Journal of Pain	A randomized, controlled trial of intensive neurophysiology education in chronic low back pain.
2010	Meeus, Nijs, et al.	Archives of Physical Medicine and Rehabilitation	Pain Physiology Education Improves Pain Beliefs in Patients With Chronic Fatigue Syndrome Compared With Pacing and Self-Management Education: A Double-Blind Randomized Controlled Trial.
2010	Ryan, Gray et al.	Manual Therapy	Pain biology education and exercise classes compared to pain biology education alone for individuals with chronic low back pain: a pilot randomized controlled trial.
2011	Van Oostervijk, Nijs, et al.	Journal of Rehabilitation Research and Development	Pain neurophysiology education improves cognitions, pain thresholds, and movement performance in people with chronic whiplash: A pilot study.

2.4: Therapeutic Neuroscience Education Addressing Pain

Six of the eight studies in the review examined the effectiveness of TNE addressing issues associated with pain (Moseley, 2002; Moseley, 2003; Moseley, 2003; Meeus, Nijs et al., 2010; Ryan, Gray et al., 2010; Van Oosterwijck, Nijs et al., 2011). Methodological quality of the six studies addressing pain ranged from 11 (good) (Moseley, 2002) to 15 (excellent) (Ryan, et al., 2010; Meeus, et al., 2010), with a mean score of 13/16.

- A neuroscience education session for patients with chronic LBP by itself produces a more favorable immediate effect on decreasing pain ratings (out of 100) (39.3 ± 26.2 to 8.4 ± 7.5) than a program combining neuroscience education and an exercise program (28.1 ± 20.4 to 23.9 ± 23.3) ($p < 0.025$), but loses its superior efficacy at three-month follow-up (Ryan, Gray et al. 2010).

- Neuroscience education for patients with chronic LBP decreased pain in both short term (one month) and long term (one year) ($p < 0.01$) compared to patients receiving ongoing medical care without physiotherapy (Moseley, 2002). Mean improvement of the neuroscience education session was 1.5 points on the numeric rating scale (NRS).

- Neuroscience education sessions for chronic LBP patients delivered as single one-on-one sessions or as group sessions decreased pain significantly ($p < 0.05$), yet individual one-on-one education sessions were associated with a more favorable outcome compared to the group educational sessions ($p = 0.004$) (Moseley, 2003). Average reduction in pain was 3.1 (1.8-4.2) for the individual education group versus 2.7 (1.6-3.9) for the group education session.

- Following a neuroscience education session, patients with chronic whiplash associated disorders (WAD) had a significant reduction in pain (VAS) during a neck extension test without fixation ($p = 0.04$) and with fixation ($p = 0.04$) (Van Oosterwijck, Nijs et al., 2011). Perceived pain on the VAS was decreased 43.5% for the test without fixation and 59.2% with fixation.

- In patients with chronic fatigue syndrome (CFS), a 30-minute neurophysiology education session is able to increase knowledge of pain, compared to a program focused on pacing and self-management ($p < 0.001$) (Meeus, Nijs et al., 2010).

- A single neuroscience educational session will increase the knowledge of pain in patients with chronic LBP (Moseley, 2003).

- Neuroscience education did not improve pressure pain thresholds (PPT) in patients with CFS (Meeus, Nijs et al., 2010), while PPT was significantly increased (decreased sensitivity of the nervous system) in patients with chronic WAD (trapezius $p = 0.03$ and calf $p = 0.04$) (Van Oosterwijck, Nijs et al., 2011).

- Of all the self-report WAD symptoms on the WAD symptoms list (photophobia, neck mobility and sweating), neuroscience education showed a significant effect only on decreasing photophobia ($p = 0.04$) (Van Oosterwijck, Nijs et al., 2011).

2.5: Therapeutic Neuroscience Education Addressing Function and Disability

Five of the eight studies in the review examined the effectiveness of TNE addressing issues associated with function and disability (Moseley, 2002; Moseley, 2003; Moseley, Nicholas et al., 2004; Ryan, Gray et al., 2010; Van Oosterwijck, Nijs et al., 2011). Methodological quality of the five studies addressing pain ranged from 11 (good) (Moseley, 2002) to 15 (excellent) (Ryan, et al., 2010), with a mean score of 12.6/16.

- Neuroscience education sessions for patients with chronic LBP delivered as single one-on-one sessions or as group sessions decrease disability (Roland Morris Disability Questionnaire – RMDQ) significantly (p < 0.05; average 5.5 points), yet individual one-on-one education sessions were associated with a more favorable outcome, compared to the group educational sessions (p = 0.004) (Moseley, 2003). The change in RMDQ in this study was clinically meaningful and comparable to studies showing manipulation (3 RMDQ points) (Cherkin, Deyo et al., 1998) and exercise's (2.9 RMDQ points) (Klaber Moffett, Torgeson et al., 1999) effect on changing disability.

- Neuroscience education session for patients with chronic LBP alters disability as measured by RMDQ (p = 0.02), but due to effect size (< 2 points on the RMDQ), was clinically insignificant.

- Neuroscience education for patients with chronic LBP decreased perceived disability in both short term (one month) and long term (one year) (p < 0.01), compared to patients receiving ongoing medical care without physiotherapy (Moseley, 2002). The mean improvement on the RMDQ was 3.9 points for the experimental group, which is clinically significant (Moseley, 2002).

- Neuroscience education reduced perceived disability in patients with chronic LBP, but failed to reach significance (p = 0.127). The immediate effect leveled off at three-month follow-up.

- In measuring perceived disability following whiplash, Van Oosterwijck, Nijs et al. (2011) showed that neuroscience education was able to decrease perceived disability (p = 0.046) from 28.26% to 22.72%, which is comparable to disability decrease by Moseley (2002).

2.6: Therapeutic Neuroscience Education Outcomes Related to Psycho-Social Issues

2.6a: Tampa Scale of Kinesiophobia (TSK)

- Three of the eight studies used the TSK as the outcome measure to assess fear of (re)injury due to movement (Meeus, Nijs et al., 2010; Ryan, Gray et al., 2010; Van Oosterwijck, Nijs et al., 2011).

- A single neuroscience education session for patients with chronic WAD decreased fear of (re)injury ($p = 0.03$) (Van Oosterwijck, Nijs et al., 2011).

- A neuroscience education program alone compared to a neuroscience education and exercise program failed to show any significant difference in pain-related fear, as measured by the TSK ($p > 0.05$) (Ryan, Gray et al., 2010).

- In a study on patients with CFS, a neuroscience education session failed to show a significant difference in fear of (re)injury compared to a pacing and self-management program ($p > 0.05$) (Meeus, Nijs et al., 2010).

2.6b: Pain Catastrophizing Scale (PCS)

- Four of the eight studies used the PCS as an outcome measure to assess pain catastrophizing (Moseley, 2004; Moseley, Nicholas et al., 2004; Meeus, Nijs et al., 2010; Van Oosterwijck, Nijs et al., 2011).

- The study by Meeus, Nijs et al. (2010) evaluating the effect of neuroscience education compared to pacing and self-management for patients with CFS showed that neuroscience education changes one of the PCS factors (ruminating) by a statistically significant difference, compared to the control group ($p < 0.05$).

- A single neuroscience education session for patients with chronic WAD showed no effect on pain catastrophizing ($p > 0.05$) (Van Oosterwijck, Nijs et al., 2011).

- A RCT of patients with chronic LBP comparing neuroscience education to a back education program showed a statistical significant effect in decreasing pain catastrophizing ($P < 0.001$) (Moseley, Hodges et al., 2004).

- Neuroscience education has shown to decrease pain catastrophizing ($p < 0.001$), which was correlated to increased SLR and trunk forward bending (Moseley, 2004).

2.6c: Pain Coping Inventory (PCI)

- Two of the eight studies used the PCI as an outcome measure to assess cognitive and behavioral pain-coping strategies (Meeus, Nijs et al., 2010; Van Oosterwijck, Nijs et al., 2011).

- In a study evaluating the effect of neuroscience education on patients with chronic WAD, neuroscience education changed passive coping strategies (p = 0.03), but not any of the other PCI categories of retreating and worrying.

- The study by Meeus, Nijs et al. (2010) evaluating the effect of neuroscience education compared to pacing and self-management for patients with CFS, neuroscience education failed to produce a significant change in PCI (p > 0.05) (Meeus, Nijs et al., 2010).

2.6d: Pain Attitudes (SOPA(R))

- Two of the eight studies used the SOPA(R) as an outcome measure of attitudes and beliefs regarding pain (Moseley, 2004; Moseley, Hodges et al., 2004).

- In a RCT comparing neuroscience education to back education, the neuroscience education session provided a significant change in patient attitudes and beliefs regarding pain, compared to a back education group (p < 0.001). Patients who received neuroscience education were less likely to seek care from others when they experienced pain, more likely to believe that they could control their pain, more likely to believe pain is affected by emotional distress and less likely to believe pain is due to tissue injury (Moseley, Hodges et al., 2004).

- The study by Moseley (2004) showed that a neuroscience education session altered two SOPA(R) factors significantly (p < 0.05) – harm and disability, which in turn was associated with increased physical performance (Moseley, 2004).

2.6e: Pain Self Efficacy Questionnaire (PSEQ)

- Only one of the eight studies used the PSEQ as an outcome measure to determine an individual's beliefs regarding their ability to carry out activities and function despite their pain (Ryan, Gray et al., 2010).

- In a study comparing neuroscience education to neuroscience education plus exercise, no statistical significant changes were found between the groups (p > 0.05) (Ryan, Gray et al., 2010).

2.7: Therapeutic Neuroscience Education Addressing Physical Movement

Four of the eight studies in this review examined the effectiveness of neuroscience education addressing issues associated with physical movement (Moseley, 2004; Moseley, Hodges et al., 2004; Ryan, Gray et al., 2010; Van Oosterwijck, Nijs et al., 2011). Methodological quality of the four studies addressing physical movement ranged from 12 (good) (Moseley, 2004) to 15 (excellent) (Ryan, et al., 2010), with a mean score of 13.5/16.

- **Neurodynamic tests** – Neuroscience education compared to back education causes an immediate increase in SLR ROM ($p < 0.01$) (Moseley, 2004; Moseley, Hodges et al., 2004), taking into consideration measurement error (Coppieters, Alshami et al., 2006) and decreased pain perception during a BPPT (Brachial Plexus Provocation Test) in patients with chronic WAD (Van Oosterwijck, Nijs et al., 2011).

- **Spine movements** – Neuroscience education compared to back education causes an immediate increase in trunk forward flexion in patients with chronic LBP ($p < 0.01$) (Moseley, 2004; Moseley, Hodges et al., 2004), and decreased pain perception during neck extension movements in patients with chronic WAD (Van Oosterwijck, Nijs et al., 2011).

- **Motor control** – Neuroscience education compared to back education resulted in no statistical difference between the groups ($p > 0.05$) (Moseley, Hodges et al., 2004).

- **Physical performance** – Neuroscience education compared to a neuroscience education plus exercise program did not show a statistically significant difference ($p > 0.05$) (Ryan, Gray et al., 2010).

CONCLUSION

For chronic MSK pain disorders,
there is compelling evidence that
an educational strategy addressing
the neurophysiology and neurobiology
of pain can have a positive effect
on pain, disability, catastrophizing,
and physical performance.

The systematic review showed that educating people in pain about their pain may be a more advantageous approach than traditional biomedical education. TNE has also been used in case studies showing similar effect in reducing pain and disability (Puentedura, Brooksby et al., 2009; Louw, Puentedura et al., 2011) as well as reduction in widespread brain activation (Moseley, 2005).

Apart from the positive effect of TNE on pain, function, disability, catastrophizing and physical performance, the study by Moseley (2003) also began a process of measuring participants' knowledge of pain. Originally designed for medical students, Moseley adapted a Pain Neurophysiology Questionnaire (Table 2.3) to determine a healthcare provider's knowledge of pain in general, and after a three-hour TNE session. The same was done for the general population. Overall, healthcare providers tend to underestimate the general population's ability to comprehend TNE. The Pain Neurophysiology Questionnaire has since been used to measure a patient's knowledge of pain (Moseley, 2003) and could potentially be correlated to their level of pain. Additionally, in two studies, the Pain Neurophysiology Questionnaire was used as the basis of the neuroscience education. By going through each of the questions and then discussing answers, patients were provided neuroscience education (Meeus, Nijs et al., 2010; Van Oosterwijck, Nijs et al., 2011).

Table 2.3: Pain Neurophysiology Questionnaire (Moseley, 2003)

Questions	True	False	Unsure
1. Receptors on nerves work by opening ion channels (gates) in the wall of the nerve.			
2. When part of your body is injured, special pain receptors convey the pain message to your brain.			
3. Pain only occurs when you are injured.			
4. The timing and intensity of pain matches the timing and number of signals in nociceptors (danger receptors).			
5. Nerves have to connect a body part to your brain in order for that body part to be in pain.			
6. In chronic pain, the central nervous system becomes more sensitive to nociception (danger messages).			
7. The body tells the brain when it is in pain.			
8. The brain sends messages down your spinal cord that can increase the nociception (danger message) going up your spinal cord.			
9. The brain decides when you will experience pain.			
10. Nerves adapt by increasing their resting level of excitement.			

Questions	True	False	Unsure
11. Chronic pain means that an injury hasn't healed properly.			
12. Nerves can adapt by making more ion channels (gates).			
13. Worse injuries always result in worse pain.			
14. Nerves adapt by making ion channels (gates) stay open longer.			
15. Second-order nociceptor (messenger nerve) post-synaptic membrane potential is dependent on descending modulation.			
16. When you are injured, the environment that you are in will not have an effect on the amount of pain you experience.			
17. It is possible to have pain and not know about it.			
18. When you are injured, chemicals in your tissue can make nerves more sensitive.			
19. In chronic pain, chemicals associated with stress can directly activate nociception pathways (danger messenger nerves).			

2.8: Content of Therapeutic Neuroscience Education

The systematic review by Louw, Diener et al. (2011) also included a comprehensive description of the content and materials used in neuroscience education. This level of detail was sorely needed. What exactly does TNE consist of? What material needs to be discussed with the patient? In summary, TNE session contents included the following:

- Neurophysiology of pain (Moseley, 2002; Moseley, 2003; Moseley, 2003; Moseley, 2004; Moseley, Hodges et al., 2004; Meeus, Nijs et al., 2010; Ryan, Gray et al., 2010; Van Oosterwijck, Nijs et al., 2011).

- No reference to anatomical or pathoanatomical models (Moseley, 2002; Moseley, Hodges et al., 2004).

- No discussion of emotional or behavioral aspects of pain (Moseley, Hodges et al., 2004).

- Nociception and nociceptive pathways (Moseley, 2004; Moseley, Hodges et al., 2004; Van Oosterwijck, Nijs et al., 2011).

- Neurons (Moseley, 2004; Van Oosterwijck, Nijs et al., 2011).

- Synapses (Moseley, 2004; Moseley, Hodges et al., 2004; Van Oosterwijck, Nijs et al., 2011).

- Action potential (Moseley, 2004; Van Oosterwijck, Nijs et al., 2011).

- Spinal inhibition and facilitation (Moseley, 2004; Moseley, Hodges et al., 2004; Van Oosterwijck, Nijs et al., 2011).

- Peripheral sensitization (Moseley, 2004; Moseley, Hodges et al., 2004; Van Oosterwijck, Nijs et al., 2011).

- Central sensitization (Moseley, 2004; Moseley, Hodges et al., 2004; Van Oosterwijck, Nijs et al., 2011).

- Plasticity of the nervous system (Moseley, Hodges et al., 2004; Van Oosterwijck, Nijs et al., 2011).

2.9: Delivery Methods of Therapeutic Neuroscience Education

Neuroscience education is relatively new and described as an educational intervention which aims to reduce pain and disability by explaining the biology of the pain experience to a patient (Moseley, 2005; Ryan, Gray et al., 2010).

In our review, it is noteworthy that the authors differed in the terminology they used to describe the intervention of explaining the biological processes behind a patient's pain state. Terms used were as follows:

- *Neurophysiology of pain education*
- *Pain physiology education*
- *Pain biology education*
- *Pain neurophysiology education*

Considering that the aim of providing neuroscience education is to gain the observed therapeutic effects, we have proposed that therapists utilize the term 'Therapeutic Neuroscience Education' (TNE). The neuroscience education provided in the studies included in our systematic review was done almost exclusively by physical therapists. Only one study failed to clearly identify the qualifications or professional designation of the educator (Meeus, Nijs et al., 2010).

2.10: Patient Characteristics

In our review, TNE was administered to 401 patients, of which 63% were women (n = 252). The average age of the patients ranged from 24 ± 10 years (Moseley, Hodges et al., 2004) to 45.5 ± 9.5 years (Ryan, Gray et al., 2010), giving a mean age (calculated as the mean of the mean reported ages) of the patients receiving TNE as 38.2 years. TNE was provided to patients with LBP, chronic fatigue syndrome (CFS), widespread pain and chronic whiplash-associated disorders (WAD). The LBP studies primarily focused on chronic LBP with average duration of symptoms ranging from 13.7 ± 10.2 months (Ryan, Gray et al., 2010) to 48 ± 18 months (Moseley, 2003), giving an average duration (calculated as a mean of the mean scores) of 31.2 months.

2.11: Duration and Frequency of Therapeutic Neuroscience Education

The duration and frequency of the TNE sessions were quite varied. Educational sessions lasted as long as four hours (Moseley, 2003), while more recent studies reported sessions lasting 30 minutes (Meeus, Nijs et al., 2010; Van Oosterwijck, Nijs et al., 2011). Educational sessions were also varied between single educational sessions (Moseley, 2003; Moseley, 2003; Moseley, 2004; Moseley, Hodges et al., 2004; Meeus, Nijs et al., 2010; Ryan, Gray et al., 2010) and multiple sessions (Moseley, 2002; Moseley, 2003; Van Oosterwijck, Nijs et al., 2011). The most common frequency between multiple educational sessions was one week (Moseley, 2002; Moseley, 2003; Van Oosterwijck, Nijs et al., 2011). Because studies varied between single and multiple educational interventions, total education time was also determined. On the high end, one study spent eight hours on TNE (Moseley, 2002) while the two studies with the least amount of total time only spent 30 - 60 minutes on TNE (Meeus, Nijs et al., 2010; Van Oosterwijck, Nijs et al., 2011). The remainder of the studies averaged between two and a half and four hours total education time.

2.12: Educational Format

The format in which the TNE was delivered was primarily by means of one-on-one verbal communication (Moseley, 2002; Moseley, 2003; Moseley, 2004; Moseley, Hodges et al., 2004; Meeus, Nijs et al., 2010; Van Oosterwijck, Nijs et al., 2011). Only two studies utilized group sessions (Moseley, 2003; Moseley, 2003). It's important to note one-on-one educational sessions tended to result in superior outcomes compared to the group sessions.

2.13: Educational Tools

TNE sessions are accompanied by prepared pictures (Moseley, 2004; Moseley, Hodges et al., 2004; Meeus, Nijs et al., 2010; Ryan, Gray et al., 2010; Van Oosterwijck, Nijs et al., 2011), examples (Moseley, Hodges et al., 2004; Meeus, Nijs et al., 2010; Van Oosterwijck, Nijs et al., 2011), metaphors (Van Oosterwijck, Nijs et al., 2011), hand drawings (Moseley, 2003; Moseley, 2004; Ryan, Gray et al., 2010), workbooks with reading/question-answer assignments (Moseley, 2002; Moseley, Hodges et al., 2004), and the Neurophysiology Pain Questionnaire (Van Oosterwijck, Nijs et al., 2011).

2.14: Adjunct Treatment to the Therapeutic Neuroscience Education

Several different research designs were included in the systematic review. In all the studies, patients received various forms of other therapeutic interventions at various stages of the studies for various reasons. TNE was therefore preceded, combined with, or followed by various therapeutic activities. The therapeutic activities that accompanied TNE included the following:

- Manual therapy, including spinal mobilization and manipulation (Moseley, 2002).
- Soft tissue treatment/massage (Moseley, 2002).
- Neural tissue mobilization (Moseley, 2002).
- Spinal stabilization exercises (Moseley, 2002; Moseley, 2003; Ryan, Gray et al., 2010).
- Home exercises (Moseley, 2002).
- Circuit training (Ryan, Gray et al., 2010).
- Aerobic exercise (Ryan, Gray et al., 2010).
- None (TNE only) (Moseley, 2003; Moseley, 2004; Moseley, Hodges et al., 2004; Meeus, Nijs et al., 2010; Van Oosterwijck, Nijs et al., 2011).

Considering the evidence for TNE and following the extensive review of content and delivery methods, TNE can be best applied as follows:

> *Therapists should educate patients in a one-on-one session using various examples, metaphors and drawings explaining the neurobiology and neurophysiology of their pain experience while simultaneously defocusing anatomical tissues. Additionally, patients should attend such a one-on-one session, be provided with homework to reflect on their learning experience, and return to therapy to answer questions and progress. This educational approach should include physical movement, especially aerobic exercise (Louw, Diener et al., 2011; Nijs, Paul van Wilgen et al., 2011).*

Best summary for TNE–Current best-evidence research indicates that when a therapist explains to a patient the neurobiology and neurophysiology (neuroscience) of their pain experience and the patient truly understands it, they have less pain, less disability, move better, perform better with rehabilitation, have better cognitions regarding their pain and experience decreased sensitization of their nervous system.

2.15: Managing Pain

Based on the current evidence for TNE, we believe we *treat* chronic pain, not merely *manage* chronic pain. Manage infers a maintenance of the status quo or, at least, making sure it does not get any worse. If a patient starts with an average pain rating of 8 out of 10 on a visual analog scale (VAS) and six months later it is 5 and one year later at 3, is it purely *managing* pain? We believe not. Review some of the data from the RCT's regarding pain ratings at least six to twelve months after TNE (Figure 2.4):

- One year later, pain improved by almost 3 points on a 10 point scale (Moseley, 2002).

- Average reduction in pain was 3.1 (1.8-4.2) for the individual education group versus 2.7 (1.6-3.9) in the group education session at one year (Moseley, 2003).

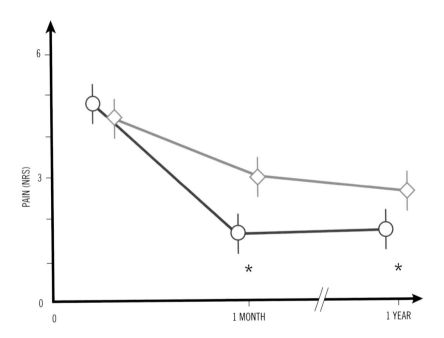

Figure 2.4: Pain rating changes in one year after TNE. The TNE plus physical therapy group (circles) demonstrated statistically significant differences in pain ratings compared to a control group (diamonds). Asterisks denote statistical significance (p<0.025). Graph adapted from Moseley (2002).

2.16: Key Points from Chapter 2

- Biomedical education models are not helpful in altering pain
- Biomedical education may actually make pain worse
- Compelling evidence for the neuroscience education approach
- Some direction and guidance for clinical application

Chapter 2 References

Brison, R. J., L. Hartling, S. Dostaler, A. Leger, B. H. Rowe, I. Stiell and W. Pickett (2005). A randomized controlled trial of an educational intervention to prevent the chronic pain of whiplash associated disorders following rear-end motor vehicle collisions. *Spine, 30*(16): 1799-1807.

Brox, J. I., K. Storheim, M. Grotle, T. H. Tveito, A. Indahl and H. R. Eriksen (2008). Systematic review of back schools, brief education, and fear-avoidance training for chronic low back pain. *Spine J, 8*(6): 948-958.

Buchbinder, R. and D. Jolley (2005). Effects of a media campaign on back beliefs is sustained 3 years after its cessation. *Spine, 30*(11): 1323-1330.

Buchbinder, R., D. Jolley and M. Wyatt (2001). 2001 Volvo Award Winner in Clinical Studies: Effects of a media campaign on back pain beliefs and its potential influence on management of low back pain in general practice. *Spine* (Phila Pa 1976), 26(23): 2535-2542.

Burton, A. K., G. Waddell, K. M. Tillotson and N. Summerton (1999). Information and advice to patients with back pain can have a positive effect. A randomized controlled trial of a novel educational booklet in primary care. *Spine, 24*(23): 2484-2491.

Cherkin, D. C., R. A. Deyo, M. Battie, J. Street and W. Barlow (1998). A comparison of physical therapy, chiropractic manipulation, and provision of an educational booklet for the treatment of patients with low back pain. *N Engl J Med, 339*(15): 1021-1029.

Coppieters, M. W., A. M. Alshami, A. S. Babri, T. Souvlis, V. Kippers and P. W. Hodges (2006). Strain and excursion of the sciatic, tibial, and plantar nerves during a modified straight leg raising test. *J Orthop Res, 24*(9): 1883-1889.

Engers, A., P. Jellema, M. Wensing, D. A. van der Windt, R. Grol and M. W. van Tulder (2008). Individual patient education for low back pain. *Cochrane Database Syst Rev*(1): CD004057.

Galaal, K. A., K. Deane, S. Sangal and A. D. Lopes (2007). Interventions for reducing anxiety in women undergoing colposcopy. *Cochrane Database Syst Rev*(3): CD006013.

Gifford, L. (1998). Pain, the Tissues and the Nervous System: A conceptual model. *Physiotherapy, 84*(1): 27-36.

Gifford, L. (2001). Acute low cervical nerve root conditions: symptom presentations and pathobiological reasoning. *Man Ther, 6*(2): 106-115.

Gifford, L. S. and D. S. Butler (1997). The integration of pain sciences into clinical practice. *Journal of Hand Therapy: Official Journal of the American Society of Hand Therapists, 10*(2): 86-95.

Greene, D. L., A. J. Appel, S. E. Reinert and M. A. Palumbo (2005). Lumbar disc herniation: evaluation of information on the internet. *Spine (Phila Pa 1976), 30*(7): 826-829.

Gross, A. R., P. D. Aker, C. H. Goldsmith and P. Peloso (2000). Patient education for mechanical neck disorders. *Cochrane Database Syst Rev*(2): CD000962.

Haines, T., A. Gross, C. H. Goldsmith and L. Perry (2008). Patient education for neck pain with or without radiculopathy. *Cochrane Database Syst Rev*(4): CD005106.

Henrotin, Y. E., C. Cedraschi, B. Duplan, T. Bazin and B. Duquesnoy (2006). Information and low back pain management: a systematic review. *Spine, 31*(11): E326-334.

Houben, R. M., R. W. Ostelo, J. W. Vlaeyen, P. M. Wolters, M. Peters and S. G. Stomp-van den Berg (2005). Health care providers' orientations towards common low back pain predict perceived harmfulness of physical activities and recommendations regarding return to normal activity. *Eur J Pain, 9*(2): 173-183.

Klaber Moffett, J. A., D. Torgeson, S. Bell-Syer, D. L. Jackson and H. Llewellyn-Phillips (1999). Randomised controlled trial of exercise for low back pain: clinical outcomes, costs and preferences. *BMJ, 319*: 279-283.

Lorig, K. (2001). *Patient Education: A Practical Approach*. California, Sage Publications, Inc.

Lorig, K. R., D. D. Laurent, R. A. Deyo, M. E. Marnell, M. A. Minor and P. L. Ritter (2002). Can a Back Pain E-mail Discussion Group improve health status and lower health care costs?: A randomized study. *Arch Intern Med, 162*(7): 792-796.

Louw, A., I. Diener, D. S. Butler and E. J. Puentedura (2011). The effect of neuroscience education on pain, disability, anxiety, and stress in chronic musculoskeletal pain. *Archives of Physical Medicine and Rehabilitation, 92(12): 2041-2056.*

Louw, A., Q. Louw and L. C. C. Crous (2009). Preoperative Education for Lumbar Surgery for Radiculopathy. *South African Journal of Physiotherapy, 65*(2): 3-8.

Louw, A., E. L. Puentedura and P. Mintken (2011). Use of an abbreviated neuroscience education approach in the treatment of chronic low back pain: A case report. *Physiotherapy Theory and Practice.*

Louw, A., E. L. Puentedura and P. Mintken (2012). Use of an abbreviated neuroscience education approach in the treatment of chronic low back pain: a case report. *Physiotherapy Theory and Practice, 28*(1): 50-62.

Maier-Riehle, B. and M. Harter (2001). The effects of back schools--a meta-analysis. *Int J Rehabil Res, 24*(3): 199-206.

McDonald, S., S. Hetrick and S. Green (2004). Pre-operative education for hip or knee replacement. *Cochrane Database Syst Rev*(1): CD003526.

McGregor, A. H., A. K. Burton, P. Sell and G. Waddell (2007). The development of an evidence-based patient booklet for patients undergoing lumbar discectomy and un-instrumented decompression. *Eur Spine J, 16*(3): 339-346.

Meeus, M., J. Nijs, J. Van Oosterwijck, V. Van Alsenoy and S. Truijen (2010). Pain Physiology Education Improves Pain Beliefs in Patients With Chronic Fatigue Syndrome Compared With Pacing and Self-Management Education: A Double-Blind Randomized Controlled Trial. *Arch Phys Med Rehabil, 91*(8): 1153-1159.

Morr, S., N. Shanti, A. Carrer, J. Kubeck and M. C. Gerling (2010). Quality of information concerning cervical disc herniation on the Internet. *Spine J, 10*(4): 350-354.

Moseley, G. L. (2003). Joining forces - combining cognition-targeted motor control training with group or individual pain physiology education: a successful treatment for chronic low back pain. *J Man Manip Therap, 11*(2): 88-94.

Moseley, G. L. (2003). Unravelling the barriers to reconceptualisation of the problem in chronic pain: the actual and perceived ability of patients and health professionals to understand the neurophysiology. *J Pain, 4*(4): 184-189.

Moseley, G. L. (2004). Evidence for a direct relationship between cognitive and physical change during an education intervention in people with chronic low back pain. *Eur J Pain, 8*(1): 39-45.

Moseley, G. L. (2005). Widespread brain activity during an abdominal task markedly reduced after pain physiology education: fMRI evaluation of a single patient with chronic low back pain. *Aust J Physiother, 51*(1): 49-52.

Moseley, G. L., M. K. Nicholas and P. W. Hodges (2004). A randomized controlled trial of intensive neurophysiology education in chronic low back pain. *Clin J Pain, 20*(5): 324-330.

Moseley, L. (2002). Combined physiotherapy and education is efficacious for chronic low back pain. *Aust J Physiother, 48*(4): 297-302.

Nijs, J., C. Paul van Wilgen, J. Van Oosterwijck, M. van Ittersum and M. Meeus (2011). How to explain central sensitization to patients with 'unexplained' chronic musculoskeletal pain: practice guidelines. *Man Ther, 16*(5): 413-418.

Oliveira, A., R. Gevirtz and D. Hubbard (2006). A psycho-educational video used in the emergency department provides effective treatment for whiplash injuries. *Spine, 31*(15): 1652-1657.

Oshodi, T. O. (2007). The impact of preoperative education on postoperative pain. Part 1. *Br J Nurs, 16*(12): 706-710.

Puentedura, E. J., C. L. Brooksby, H. W. Wallmann and M. R. Landers (2009). Rehabilitation following lumbosacral percutaneous nucleoplasty: a case report. *J Orthop Sports Phys Ther, 40*(4): 214-224.

Ryan, C. G., H. G. Gray, M. Newton and M. H. Granat (2010). Pain biology education and exercise classes compared to pain biology education alone for individuals with chronic low back pain: a pilot randomised controlled trial. *Man Ther, 15*(4): 382-387.

Saryeddine, T., C. Levy, A. Davis, J. Flannery, S. Jaglal, L. Hurley, R. McGlasson and N. Mahomed (2008). Patient education as a strategy for provider education and engagement: a case study using myJointReplacement.ca. *Healthc Q, 11*(1): 84-90.

Tait, M. J., J. Levy, M. Nowell, C. Pocock, V. Petrik, B. A. Bell and M. C. Papadopoulos (2009). Improved outcome after lumbar microdiscectomy in patients shown their excised disc fragments: a prospective, double blind, randomised, controlled trial. *J Neurol Neurosurg Psychiatry, 80*(9): 1044-1046.

Van Oosterwijck, J., J. Nijs, M. Meeus, S. Truijen, J. Craps, N. Van den Keybus and L. Paul (2011). Pain neurophysiology education improves cognitions, pain thresholds, and movement performance in people with chronic whiplash: A pilot study. *J Rehabil Res Dev, 48*(1): EPub ahead of print

Weiner, B. K. (2008). Spine update: the biopsychosocial model and spine care. *Spine, 33*(2): 219-223.

Wolf, F. M., J. P. Guevara, C. M. Grum, N. M. Clark and C. J. Cates (2003). Educational interventions for asthma in children. *Cochrane Database Syst Rev*(1): CD000326.

_____ Notes

Chapter 3

The Neuroscience of Pain

3.1: Educating the Patient

In Chapter 2, we presented the current evidence for TNE. That evidence indicates therapists need to be able to adequately explain various aspects of the neuroscience of pain to their patients (Moseley, Hodges et al., 2004; Louw, Diener et al., 2011). In order to explain the complex neurobiology and neurophysiology that underpins a patient's pain experience, a therapist "needs to be smarter than their patient." The information used in educating the patient is supported by years of knowledge of anatomy, biomechanics, tissue healing, neurobiology, neurophysiology, kinesiology, ethics, etc., as well as clinical experience by the therapist.

3.2: Traditional and Old Pain Models

Our knowledge of pain and pain processing has evolved considerably (Melzack, 1999), and it really is foolish for any therapist to believe that what we currently know about pain is not that much different from what was known in the past. The interesting thing is that many of the current treatment approaches aimed at treating pain are still based on old, outdated models (Moseley, 2007; Louw and Butler, 2011), including the Cartesian model of pain (Goldberg, 2008), the pain gate (Melzack, 1999), and the belief in a hardwired brain (Doidge, 2007). As well as appreciating that there are far more complex pain models, therapists should also revisit basic biology, i.e., A and C-fibers, to develop an understanding of pain. As a simple example, therapists are well versed in the notion of "pain fibers." A patient sprains his or her ankle, the "pain fibers" send "pain messages" to the brain, pain is perceived by the brain and the patient tends to the injured and painful ankle. How does this explain pain in the absence of injury? How does this explain pain in the absence of the body part, e.g., amputated leg? How does this explain ankle sprains with no pain, e.g., an athlete performing despite pain? It doesn't, and this is why we need to explore and update our models of pain.

3.3: Cartesian Model of Pain
(René Descartes 1596 – 1650)

The Cartesian model of pain (1664) is likely to blame for many of the misconceptions about pain, yet it continues to be a driving force in the delivery of Medicine today (Wade, 2006; Goldberg, 2008). The Cartesian model very simplistically proposed that if you placed your foot into or too close to a fire, then a message is sent to the brain via a pathway/wire (Figure 3.1). Descartes actually believed that nerves were hollow tubes through which spirits flowed in a mechanical manner. The message was sent to the brain, which was the center of all the senses. The injury to the foot, caused by the fire, had a mechanical input that resulted in the ringing of a bell at the other end of the pathway or tube in the brain, producing pain. This incorrect and overly simplistic view of pain leads to equally incorrect and overly simplistic treatment options.

Look at the Cartesian model and you'll see that to treat a patient in pain, several options become immediately apparent. First, the patient can take his or her foot out of the fire and then avoid the fire from thereon. Although this might seem logical and, likely, a good response in an acute, threatening scenario, it is less likely to help in the long run. In persistent pain states, the modern analogy of such an approach is the fear avoidance model, which has been shown to lead to increased pain and disability (Vlaeyen and Linton, 2000).

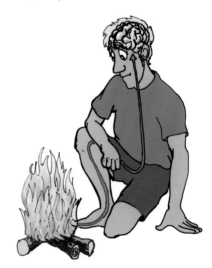

Figure 3.1: Updated image of the Cartesian model of pain (1664).

A second approach might be to douse the fire with a bucket of water. The modern medical analogy of a "water bucket" would be prescription medications or injections, which aim to 'put out the fires' of local inflammation. In Medicare in the US, there has been a 629% increase in expenditures in epidural steroid injections and a 423% increase in expenditures for LBP over the last five years (Deyo, Mirza et al., 2009), yet pain rates are increasing, not decreasing. Clearly, dousing the fire does not always work.

A third, and perhaps more drastic, approach to the Cartesian model of getting rid of pain is 'cutting the wire.' By cutting the wire, the message to the brain is severed; therefore, if the brain cannot receive 'pain messages,' no pain will be experienced. The modern analogy for this approach would be surgery. Continuing this line of thought, a body part that is injured sends "pain messages" to the brain and if the nerve (wire) is cut, pain will be abolished. If this Cartesian thinking actually worked then surgery would be 100% successful. This is, obviously, not the case as 20% of lumbar discectomy patients have the same or worse pain after surgery (Ostelo, Costa et al., 2004); lumbar fusions, in general, only have a 50% success rate in decreasing pain (Deyo, Nachemson et al., 2004; Deyo, Gray et al., 2005).

More than 350 years after his death, this model proposed by Descartes continues to exert undue influence on how therapists view pain. Specifically, there remain incorrect assumptions that

- There is a direct link between the amount of tissue damage and the level of pain experienced.
- All pain is caused by injury and increased pain means more damage.
- There is a division of mind and body where pain is either physical or psychological or mental illness versus physical illness. This may have fueled the social stigma of psychological issues or even psychological pain.
- In cases of chronic pain, according to the Cartesian model, tissues are not healing and damage is ongoing.
- Nociception and pain are synonymous.
- Pain is an input driven system.
- The nervous system is simply built for conduction (a wire).

Pain is actually much more complex, and therapists need to update their models to keep pace with the ever-increasing pain rates and subsequent challenges imposed on them. This includes the well-known pain gate. Originally developed by Ron Melzack and Patrick Wall more than 50 years ago, the pain gate served us well, but only up to a point. It does not help to explain the pain experienced in a phantom limb or pain in quadriplegics. Ron Melzack has urged healthcare providers to recognize the shortcomings of the pain gate and embrace the current, more updated view of pain, the brain and the neuromatrix (Melzack, 1996; Melzack, 1999; Melzack, 2001).

3.4: The Pain Neurophysiology Questionnaire (PNQ)

To help therapists develop a more updated view of pain, we will opt for a novel route: The Pain Neurophysiology Questionnaire (PNQ) (Moseley, 2003). The PNQ was designed around an updated view of pain science and neurobiology. It embraces the neuromatrix and has clinical application.

> *We will systematically pose each question of the PNQ and then explore the answers to the question as a means to develop a greater understanding of the modern view of pain science. We have changed the order of the questions in the PNQ so that answers build upon each other and our narrative on the updated view of pain science and neurobiology will have a better flow.*

3.4a: When part of your body is injured, special pain receptors convey the pain message to your brain (Q2)

Answer: False

In school, therapists are taught about various nerve fiber types, based upon size and speed of conduction – A, B and C fibers (Delcomyn, 1998; Barker and Barasi, 1999). These nerve fibers are also typically categorized as being responsible for things such as pain, light touch or pressure (Carter, 2009).

- **Type A-fibers** are the thickest and fastest conducting. They are myelinated, have a diameter of between 1.5-20 microns and their speed of conduction varies from 4-120 m/sec, which shows that they have a really fast conduction of impulse. Examples of type A-fibers are skeletomotor fibers and afferent fibers to the skin.

- **Type B-fibers** are medium in size, i.e., they are smaller than type A-fibers but larger than type-C. They are myelinated, have a diameter of 1.5-3.5 microns and their speed of conduction is 3-15 m/sec, which shows that they are slower than type A-fibers. Examples of type B-fibers are preganglionic autonomic efferents.

- **Type C-fibers** are the smallest and thinnest. They are non-myelinated, have a diameter of 0.1-2 microns and their speed of conduction is 0.5-4 m/sec, which shows that they have the slowest conduction. Examples of type C-fibers are postganglionic autonomic efferents and afferent fibers to skin. Many therapist are taught C-fibers are "pain fibers" and responsible, along with A-delta fibers, for 'conducting pain.'

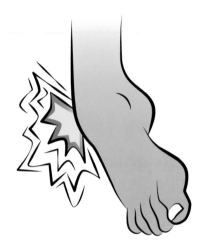

Figure 3.2: An ankle sprain would likely cause pain.

If C and A-delta fibers do 'conduct pain,' then all injuries would hurt and it could potentially endanger your life. For example, if you were to walk at work or home and sprain your ankle, it would likely cause pain (Figure 3.2). This is easy to understand and makes sense: tissue injury causes activation of the A-delta and C-fibers that send "pain messages" via sensory afferent nerves to the dorsal horn of the spinal cord. The "pain messages" are passed from the dorsal horn via second-order neurons to the brain to call upon action, such as walking funny, seeking medical help, canceling plans to run the local marathon tomorrow and more.

Now imagine that same ankle sprain but while crossing a busy street. As you walk across the street, you sprain your ankle, but out of the corner of your eye you see a speeding bus heading your way. Everyone will agree that, in this case, the ankle will not hurt, and you'll get out the way of the speeding bus to the sidewalk on the other side. Once on the other side, the ankle may actually start to hurt. What happened? If the injured ankle had sent "pain messages" to the brain, the pain could potentially have been so debilitating it would have caused you to fall down, grab the ankle and be run over by the bus. Why did it not hurt, then? The only thing the ankle can send the brain is a "danger message." The ankle contains various nociceptors, easily activated by inflammatory chemicals and mechanical input from the tissues. This nociception will then be passed onto the spinal cord and, ultimately, the brain via nociceptive fibers such as A-delta and C-fibers. Pain is, therefore, a brain construct. It is important that therapists designate these fibers as 'nociceptive fibers,' rather than 'pain fibers.'

Consider the following:

• The ear contains various 'vibration' and 'sound receptors.' Messages from these receptors are turned into 'hearing' by the brain.

• The eye contains 'light receptors' that send messages to the brain, which are processed by the brain to produce 'vision.'

• Joints and muscles contain 'nociceptors' and the brain may turn these nociceptive messages into 'pain.'

This redefinition is not merely a play on words or semantics, but rather an important shift in the language and concept of TNE.

Why did the ankle not hurt with the speeding bus bearing down on you? In response to the bigger threat of the bus, the brain determined that the bus was a larger threat to your survival and, therefore, no pain was produced to protect the ankle, allowing you to get out of the way. Once out of danger and on the sidewalk, the brain might produce pain in the ankle. Pain is a decision by the brain based on perception of threat (Melzack, 2001; Moseley, 2003). The brain constantly receives information from the environment as well as the body and determines the most appropriate response based on survival, experience and threat. There are numerous examples where people have significant injury, yet experience little to no pain. Tissues contain nociceptive or danger fibers, but it is the brain that decides if pain is needed to protect or not.

3.4b: Pain only occurs when you are injured (Q3)

Answer: False

Many patients (and even some therapists) believe that pain and injury are synonymous. Injury and disease states may or may not be experienced as pain. Many normative studies on asymptomatic subjects show the poor correlation between the health of the tissues and a pain experience:

- It is estimated that 40% of asymptomatic people have a bulging disc on MRI (Videman, Battie et al., 2003; Alyas, Turner et al., 2007).

- Lumbar spine degeneration starts in a person's early 20's and there is little correlation between arthritis and LBP (Taylor and Twomey, 1986; Twomey and Taylor, 1987; Kjaer, Leboeuf-Yde et al., 2005).

- In 40-year-old asymptomatic males and females, between 25-50% will demonstrate disc degeneration and signs of injury, endplate changes, foraminal stenosis and facet joint degeneration on spinal imaging (Kjaer, Leboeuf-Yde et al., 2005).

- After successful rotator cuff repairs and clinically sound examination, 90% of patients' imaging will indicate abnormal signaling with 16% partial tears, 20% complete tears, 33% sub-acromial effusion, 16% joint effusion and 20% bone marrow edema (Spielmann, Forster et al., 1999).

- Imaging of the asymptomatic general population shows a 35-40% prevalence of rotator cuff tears across all age groups (Sher, Uribe et al., 1995; Reilly, Macleod et al., 2006).

- In patients over the age of 70, two out of three will have an asymptomatic rotator cuff tear (Milgrom, Schaffler et al., 1995).

- In the general population, 25% of MRIs will show meniscus degeneration, and when re-scanned five years later > 90% remain unchanged (Munk, Lundorf et al., 2004).

- There is only a 50% correlation between knee pain and arthritis (Bedson and Croft, 2008).

- 35% of collegiate basketball players with no knee pain will have significant abnormalities on their MRI scans (Major and Helms, 2002).

Injury and/or degenerative processes can, therefore, be present, yet people may experience little to no pain. Furthermore, injuries heal. Even slow healing tissues, such as intervertebral discs, have been shown to heal over time (Komori, Shinomiya et al., 1996; Yukawa, Kato et al., 1996; Mochida, Komori et al., 1998; Masui, Yukawa et al., 2005; Autio, Karppinen et al., 2006). In the acute and sub-acute phase of injury and subsequent healing, it may be quite normal to think that pain and tissue injury are correlated. Even taking into consideration variables such as tissue type, general health, occupation, etc., tissues will undergo relatively predictable stages of healing as time progresses (Figure 3.3). In contrast, pain experience is poorly correlated to these stages of healing (Haldeman, 1990).

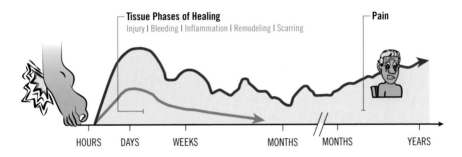

Figure 3.3: As time progresses, tissues demonstrate predictable stages of healing.

The opposite is also true. Many people suffer from significant pain, yet no injury has occurred and no disease process can be identified. The International Association for the Study of Pain (IASP) defines pain as an emotional experience (Merskey and Bogduk, 1994). In line with this definition and reflecting back on material covered in Chapter 1, where we discussed the fear avoidance model, there is compelling evidence that many pain patients develop pain due to an emotional overload (Knotkova, Crawford Clark et al., 2004; Huber, Suman et al., 2007). Many clinicians can attest to the fact that patients may present for therapy with significant pain yet recall no injury or accident. It is important to emphasize that this is not a psychosomatic issue. If we were to follow the classic Cartesian thinking, it would be easy to classify this pain as psychological. However, Cartesian thinking is outdated and wrong. It is now recognized that these patients experience pain and disability similar to patients who have had an injury event (Meeus and Nijs, 2007; Nijs, Van Houdenhove et al., 2010; Louw, Puentedura et al., 2011).

3.4c: The timing and intensity of pain matches the timing and number of signals in nociceptors (danger receptors) (Q4)

Answer: False

In mathematics, one plus one will equal two. In pain neuroscience, one plus one may end up being five. In an injury or degenerative process, nociceptive fibers send repeated messages to the dorsal horn of the spinal cord. In the spinal cord, repeated stimulation at constant strength of dorsal root afferents, including nociceptive C-fibers, can elicit a progressive increase in the number of action potentials generated by motoneurons and interneurons (IN) (Latremoliere and Woolf, 2009; Meeus, Vervisch et al., 2012). This process, referred to as action potential windup, is the consequence of a cumulative membrane depolarization, resulting from the temporal summation of slow synaptic potentials. Simply stated, with persistent input from the periphery, changes to the spinal cord second-order neurons and, ultimately, brain pathways lead to a heightened sensitization.

As an example, the medial aspect of your right knee contains various nociceptive fibers, including C-fibers and various A-fibers. With an immediate acute injury, A-delta fibers will send nociception to the spinal cord with the intent to pass the nociceptive message to the brain for action. For the medial aspect of the knee, the sensory afferent input will be received into the dorsal horn of the spinal cord (L3) from the affected side (i.e., right side) (Figure 3.4). The nociception from the A-delta fibers chemically activates AMPA receptors (α-amino-3-hydroxy-5-methyl-4-isoxazolepropionic acid receptor) on the second-order neurons via glutamate (Woolf and Mannion, 1999; Woolf and Salter, 2005). Second-order neurons will then relay messages from the spinal cord to the brain.

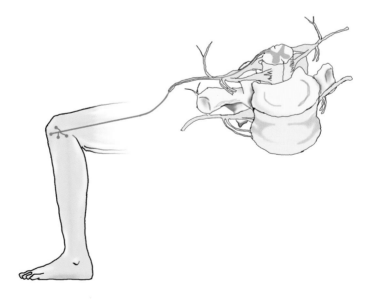

Figure 3.4: A-delta and C-fibers (red) send nociception to the spinal cord.

The nociception is passed onto the brain for interpretation and action. Although intense, pain will not usually last in this acute stage. Some of this is due to inhibition via the endogenous mechanisms of the brain, spinal cord and descending pathways. Descending pathways, usually from the periaqueductal gray area (PAG), produce serotonin, endorphins, opioids and enkephalins, which inhibit the nociception and, ultimately, the pain experience (Villaneuva and Fields, 2004). If stimulation of the medial knee persists (e.g., excessive valgus with prolonged walking, or sensitive nerves around the knee after surgery or injury) then nociceptive fibers will continue firing, in this case it's the longer lasting C-fibers.

From the same innervated area on the medial aspect of the knee, A-beta fibers constantly send nociception to the spinal cord for interpretation in the form of light touch. On a daily basis, as your pants touch the medial aspect of the knee, this nociception is also passed to the spinal cord via the L3 dorsal horn, hoping to inform the brain of the pants touching the medial aspect of the knee (Figure 3.5). In this case, the nociception is blocked at spinal cord level, partly due to actions of the interneuron. These interneurons are sometimes called relay neurons, association neurons, connector neurons or local circuit neurons and are best defined as a neuron that forms a connection between other neurons. Interneurons are neither motor nor sensory. The term is also applied to brain and spinal cord neurons whose axons connect only with nearby neurons, distinguishing them from "projection" neurons, whose axons (projection fibers) project to more distant regions of the brain or spinal cord. In the central nervous system, the term interneuron is used for small, locally projecting neurons, in contrast to larger projection neurons with long-distance connections. Central nervous system interneurons are typically inhibitory and use the neurotransmitter *gamma*-Aminobutyric Acid (GABA) or glycine. However, excitatory interneurons using glutamate also exist, as do interneurons that release neuromodulators like acetylcholine. Following input from A-beta fibers, the interneuron may block the message with a release of GABA. The message ends, the sensation of light touch from the pants is not registered cortically (Woolf, 2007) and you are, thus, not aware of the pants rubbing your leg.

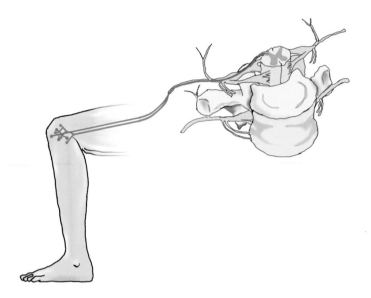

Figure 3.5: Along with the A-delta and C-fibers (red), there is constant sensory input from A-beta fibers (green) informing the brain of normally non-noxious stimuli, such as light touch from pants material.

Any nociception that passes the interneuron blockade needs to be sent onto the brain via second-order neurons (Figure 3.6). Basic neuroscience dictates that for a nerve impulse to continue, specific receptors are needed for specific neurotransmitters. If A-delta fibers release glutamate and there are no AMPA receptors available on the second-order neurons, the electrochemical message stops. This availability of receptors is part of the neuroplasticity of the nervous system and may therefore modulate a pain experience. Receptors are continually replaced and the expression of receptor types is variable. The ability to feel the pants touch the medial part of the knee is modulated by receptors on the second-order neurons and neurotransmitters. Although centrally mediated endogenous processes are important and well described in severe and acute injuries, the descending fibers from the brain are likely active in day-to-day stimuli, as well (Villaneuva and Fields, 2004).

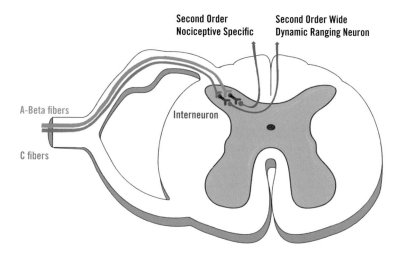

Second Order Nociceptive Specific

Second Order Wide Dynamic Ranging Neuron

A-Beta fibers

Interneuron

C fibers

Figure 3.6: Any nociception that passes the interneuron blockade must be sent on to the brain via second-order neurons such as the wide dynamic ranging and nociceptive specific neurons.

With persistent nociception via C-fibers from the knee, permanent neuroplastic changes are likely to occur. It is now well established that after constant barrage from the C-fibers, the interneuron may die, due to high levels of amino acids (Woolf and Doubell, 1994; Fukuoka, Tokunaga et al., 1998; Doubell, Mannion et al., 1999; Woolf, 2007). With a persistent toxic environment, it is unlikely the interneuron will regenerate. The end result is a decreased ability to modulate nociception and ultimately a pain experience. Second-order receptors change, as well. From a primitive survival viewpoint, the brain will want to know about danger in order to protect. Pain is there for protection. To facilitate this process, receptors in the second-order neurons are replaced with receptors that will facilitate an increase of danger messages to the brain for analysis. During day-to-day normal activity, receptors open and close in milliseconds (Devor, 2005). In response to this threat, receptors that usually open and close fast can be replaced with receptors that stay open longer, up to several minutes, such as the G-protein receptors, which are commonly found in the central nervous system. The end result is an open gate. The second-order neuron is therefore more easily stimulated and fires faster, creating increased sensitivity.

This "amplification" is often referred to as action potential windup. Windup is the consequence of a cumulative membrane depolarization resulting from the temporal summation of slow synaptic potentials. In the spinal cord, repeated stimulation (at constant strength) of dorsal root afferents including nociceptive C-fibers can elicit a progressive increase in the number of action potentials generated by motoneurons and interneurons (Latremoliere and Woolf, 2009; Meeus, Vervisch et al., 2012). This answers our PNQ question regarding the timing and intensity of pain matching the timing and number of signals in nociceptors (danger receptors), which is not correct (Woolf, 2007).

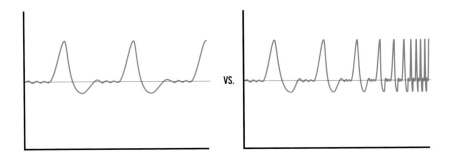

Figure 3.7: Amplification of signaling is referred to as action potential windup.

So far our description of what happens in the central nervous system has been necessarily quite basic. One nerve fiber brings a message to the dorsal horn of the spinal cord, which interacts with the interneuron, followed by the second-order neuron, and the message is sent to the brain. Obviously, the reality is a lot more complex (Figure 3.8) (Woolf and Mannion, 1999; Woolf, 2000; Woolf and Salter, 2005; Woolf, 2007):

- A-delta, A-beta, C-fibers and many more enter the dorsal horn.
- There are numerous interneurons.
- There are descending fibers from the brain supplying endogenous chemicals such as opioids, enkephalins, endorphins and serotonin, which allows for a cortical modulation of nociception and the pain experience.
- Convergence of adjacent spinal levels (L2 and L4) also accesses the L3 spinal level.
- Motor fibers are present.
- Input to the dorsal horn is also received from the other side of the body.
- There are numerous second-order neurons from the L3 spinal level aimed at relaying the nociceptive information to the brain for interpretation.

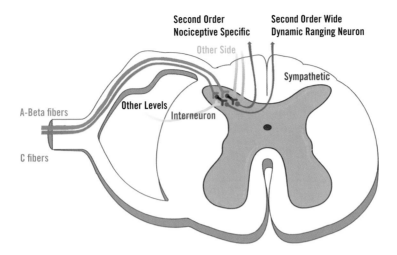

Second Order
Nociceptive Specific

Second Order Wide
Dynamic Ranging Neuron

Other Side

Sympathetic

A-Beta fibers

Other Levels

Interneuron

C fibers

Figure 3.8: Activity in the dorsal horn of the spinal cord is more complex.

Nociceptive processing, relay and ultimately the pain experience of a patient are very complex, and our description of events is basic at best. The aim is merely to provide for a clinical understanding of how nociceptive information from tissue is processed and how the central nervous system may increase its sensitization. Clinicians should also consider the devastating effect of persistent nociception where modulation of nociception is surely needed. Traditional therapy models, e.g., utilizing the pain gate, may be seen as a way to modulate the incoming nociception.

3.4d: Nerves have to connect a body part to your brain in order for that part to be in pain (Q5)

Answer: False

An easy way to answer this question is with a discussion of phantom limb pain. In phantom limb pain, patients describe pain in extremities that do not exist. They may even describe sensations of their amputated body part on another body part, e.g., feeling fingers on their shoulder or face, although the fingers on their extremity are not present. All body parts are represented in the brain, primarily within the somatosensory homunculus (SSH) (Figure 3.9) (Penfield and Boldrey, 1937; Moseley, 2005; Napadow, 2006; Stavrinou, Della Penna et al., 2007).

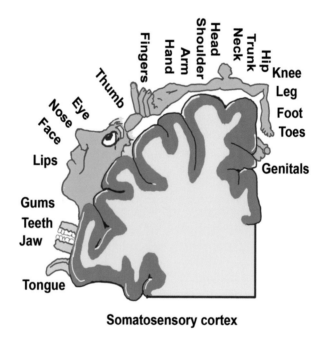

Figure 3.9: The Somatosensory Cortex (SSH) is a graphic representation or map of all body parts within the brain.

If you look at the SSH, you will see that the SSH resembles a person. The SSH is dynamically maintained, with the proverbial "use it or lose it" phenomenon applying in this case. The health of the SSH map is dependent on various issues, including use of the body part, pain, and immune responses in the body. The changes in representation of body parts within the SSH have been described extensively in chronic conditions, such as Complex Regional Pain Syndrome (CRPS) and chronic LBP (Flor, Braun et al., 1997; Flor, 2000; Maihofner, Handwerker et al., 2003). However, it is important to realize that such changes may occur in acute injury and pain experiences, with the changes happening in as little as 30 minutes (Stavrinou, Della Penna et al., 2007). Even though a body part may no longer be present (amputation), pain may be "felt" in the missing body part because that part is still present within the brain. It is now well established that patients with chronic pain have distorted views of body parts, and these distorted views may be strongly correlated to pain (Moseley, 2004; Moseley, Zalucki et al., 2008). Furthermore, the brain also struggles when identifying left and right body parts (left-right discrimination), and this has now been shown to be present in persistent pain states such as CRPS (Moseley, 2004; Moseley, Sim et al., 2005). Pain is a representation of threat to the body part. Thinking about moving a body part in pain evokes pain and swelling (Moseley, Zalucki et al., 2008). Altering the brain's view of the body part may alter the pain experience. Therefore, nerves do not have to connect a body part to the brain in order for that part to be in pain. Pain is also dependent on the health of the SSH and, more specifically, how the body part is represented within the SSH.

3.4e: In chronic pain, the central nervous system becomes more sensitive to nociception (danger messages) (Q6)

Answer: True

Review the answer to question 4 of the PNQ – The timing and intensity of pain matches the timing and number of signals in nociceptors (danger receptors). Consider the discussion regarding action potential windup (Latremoliere and Woolf, 2009; Meeus, Vervisch et al., 2012). The persistent input via C-fibers, interneuron changes, second-order neuron changes, sprouting and expansion of receptor fields all apply here. Light touch (Grade I mobilization) to the knee may now travel to the spinal cord via A-beta fibers, the interneuron does not stop the incoming message, the second-order neuron receptors are open and the area, in general, is being bombarded with input from the levels above and below, the other side of the body and other fibers. This hyper-stimulates the central nervous system.

With persistent input from the periphery, there is likely to be a change in the descending modulation of the brain and the endogenous chemical release of opioids, enkephalins, endorphins and serotonin (Basbaum and Fields, 1978; ter Riet, de Craen et al., 1998). This endogenous process is very powerful and essential for survival and placebo (Bialosky, Bishop et al., 2011). Endogenous chemicals, which are needed to modulate the incoming nociception and ultimately the pain experience, are reduced in chronic pain states (Figure 3.10) (Basbaum and Fields, 1978; Larsson, Cai et al., 1995; ter Riet, de Craen et al., 1998). In chronic pain, from an evolutionary survival perspective, the brain needs more information from the tissues (nociception). By reducing the normal endogenous chemicals, the brain allows more information to ascend for further interpretation.

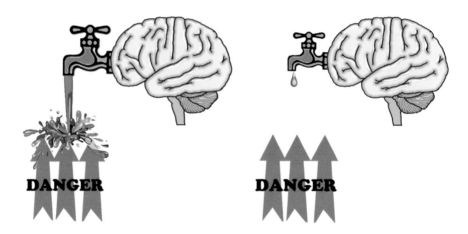

Figure 3.10: Endogenous chemicals, which are needed to modulate the incoming nociception and ultimately the pain experience, are reduced in chronic pain states. This drying up of the flow of descending modulation is sometimes referred to as a 'dry brain.'

3.4f: The body tells the brain when it is in pain (Q7)

Answer: False

Our answer to question 2 of the PNQ – When part of your body is injured, special pain receptors convey the pain message to your brain – established that the body only contains nociceptive fibers, not "pain fibers." Tissues, or the body, can only send danger messages to the brain. Ultimately, pain is a brain construct (Moseley, 2007). In the example of the ankle sprain and bus, even if the tissues are sending nociception (ankle sprain), the brain will likely not produce pain since a bigger threat (the bus) is coming. How the brain processes that nociception is important to understanding the modern neuroscience view of the pain experience.

Nociception from the tissues is mainly received by the thalamus (Dostrovsky, 1999; Brisby and Hammar 2007). In acute, immediate injury states, the lower centers of the brain usually activate, process the threat and produce immediate, protective responses, such as reflexive movement, adrenaline response, etc. (Figure 3.11 a) (Dostrovsky, 1999; Brisby and Hammar, 2007). Once the immediate threat is processed, the information about the threat is passed onto higher cognitive areas that deal more with thoughts, planning, memory, etc. (Figure 3.11 b) (Catani, 2006; Doidge, 2007).

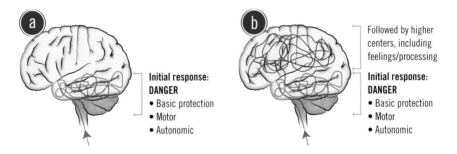

Figure 3.11: Initial protective responses to nociception are processed in lower centers of the brain (a) whereas thoughts, planning, memory, etc. will involve higher cognitive areas (b).

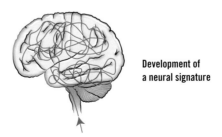

Figure 3.12: The combination of activity in lower and higher centers of the brain will lead to the development of a specific neural signature for a person's pain experience. This is referred to as a pain neurotag or pain neuromatrix.

To understand the brain's processing of this nociceptive information and, ultimately, a pain experience, we need to dispel the belief that there is a specific 'pain area' within the brain, e.g., when you hit your thumb with a hammer, this area will activate so that you will experience pain (Melzack, 2001). This single "pain area" notion was dispelled by observations of patients following cerebral lobotomy and even cerebral hemispherectomy (Bear, Connors et al., 1996; Juan, 2006). Multiple studies involving functional brain scanning have now shown that many different brain areas are active during a painful experience, and these areas have now been more comprehensively described (Table 3.1) (Flor, 2000; Melzack, 2001; Flor, 2003; Moseley, 2003).

Table 3.1: Areas of the brain involved in processing a painful experience

Area	Functions	Location

1. Amygdala	• Almond-shaped group of nuclei located deep within the medial temporal lobes of the brain
	• Part of the limbic system
	• Processing and memory of emotional reactions
	  ○ Fear
	  ○ Addictions
	• One of the most active areas during a pain experience	

2. Primary Somatosensory Cortex	• Somatic sensation • Visual stimuli • Movement planning	
3. Hippocampus	• Part of the limbic system • Consolidation of information from short-term to long-term memory • Spatial navigation	

4. Anterior Cingulate Cortex	• Plays a role in a wide variety of autonomic functions, such as regulating
	  ○ Blood pressure
	  ○ Heart rate
	• Plays a role in rational cognitive functions:
	  ○ Reward anticipation
	  ○ Decision making
	  ○ Empathy
	  ○ Emotion
	• Concentration
	• Focus	

Area	Functions	Location
5. Primary Motor Cortex	• Works in association with other motor areas including premotor cortex, the supplementary motor area, posterior parietal cortex, and several subcortical brain regions, to plan and execute movements	

6. Hypothalamus	• Below the thalamus and above the brain stem
	• Links to the nervous system via the endocrine system via the pituitary gland
	• Autonomic nervous system
	• Controls
	  o Body temperature
	  o Hunger and thirst
	  o Fatigue and sleep	

7. Thalamus	• Relaying sensory and motor signals to the cerebral cortex • Consciousness • Sleep • Alertness	
8. Prefrontal cortex	• Planning complex cognitive behavior • Personality expression • Decision making • Moderating social behavior	
9. Cerebellum	• Movement • Balance, proprioception • Fear • Coordination	

The end-result of a pain experience is a neural signature or map within the brain, which is referred to as a neurotag or neuromatrix (Figure 3.13) (Melzack, 2001; Moseley, 2003; Puentedura and Louw, 2012). This neural signature illustrates that pain is quite complex and involves various areas.

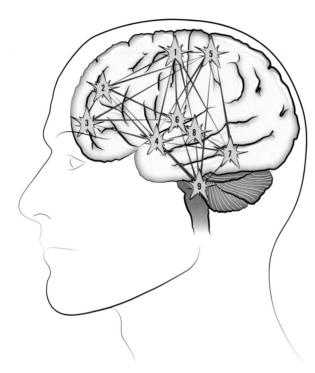

A Typical Pain Neurotag

1. PREMOTOR/MOTOR CORTEX
   organize and prepare movements

2. CINGULATE CORTEX
   concentration, focusing

3. PREFRONTAL CORTEX
   problem solving, memory

4. AMYGDALA
   fear, fear conditioning, addiction

5. SENSORY CORTEX
   sensory discrimination

6. HYPOTHALAMUS/THALAMUS
   stress responses, autonomic regulation, motivation

7. CEREBELLUM
   movement and cognition

8. HIPPOCAMPUS
   memory, spatial recognition, fear conditioning

9. SPINAL CORD
   gating from the periphery

Figure 3.13: A typical pain neurotag involves activity from many brain areas (redrawn from Butler and Moseley, 2003).

Further examination of a typical pain neurotag reveals two key clinical issues for therapists treating patients with chronic pain. First, if during a painful experience an area of the brain is activated that is typically designated to perform another task, e.g., motor control in transversus abdominus contraction in the therapeutic application of spinal stabilization exercises, the pain processing is likely to influence the motor control. Several studies have shown that cognitions such as fear and catastrophizing can impact motor control significantly (Moseley and Hodges, 2002; Moseley, Brhyn et al., 2003; Moseley, 2004). Secondly, each person's map is different and individualized (Moseley, 2003). This underscores the clinical notion that treatment should be individualized for the patient and may be a reason why one-on-one education produces superior results to group education (Moseley, 2003; Louw, Diener et al., 2011).

The neuromatrix is even more complex. Given the enormous complexity of neuronal activation, synaptic activity, neurotransmitters and modulators, the primary "pain map" can also be influenced by neighboring neural circuits, which will likely influence the pain experience (Figure 3.14) (Puentedura and Louw, 2012).

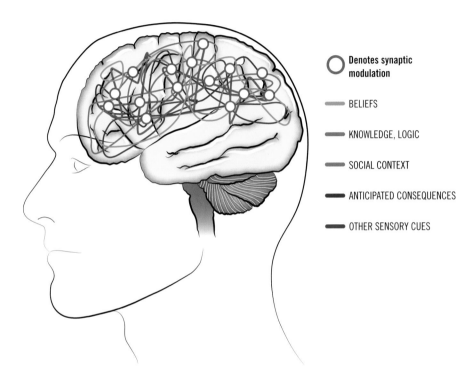

Denotes synaptic modulation

BELIEFS

KNOWLEDGE, LOGIC

SOCIAL CONTEXT

ANTICIPATED CONSEQUENCES

OTHER SENSORY CUES

Figure 3.14: The primary "pain map" (in red) can also be influenced by neighboring neural circuits.

Our current understanding of the neuromatrix is largely derived from the results of studies utilizing newer imaging techniques, such as functional magnetic resonance imaging (fMRI). MRI uses a very strong magnetic field to align our body's molecules and then uses a second magnetic pulse to invert (or 'flip') them (Lotze, Erb et al., 2000; Moseley, 2008). Because each type of molecule has a unique rate at which it reverts or 'relaxes' back to the magnetically imposed alignment, it is possible to 'tune' a radio frequency receiver within the MRI machine to detect particular types of molecules. The molecules to which the MRI are 'tuned' determines, after sophisticated data processing, the resultant image. Tuning it to water provides a structural image because water content varies between tissues. Tuning it to oxygenated hemoglobin provides a functional image (fMRI) because neuronal activity causes an increase in oxygenated hemoglobin. Functional MRI can provide very precise information about where neuronal activity occurs (spatial resolution) but not about when it occurs (temporal resolution) (Flor, 2000; Lotze, Erb et al., 2000; Moseley, 2008). New fMRI technology called diffusion tensor imaging (DTI) can reveal abnormalities in white matter fiber structure and provide models of brain connectivity. It's suggested that with fMRI images of neuronal activation in the brain, a pain signature can be visualized (Catani, 2006; Catani and Thiebaut de Schotten, 2008).

To obtain a "pain signature," a protocol typically involves having a patient in the MRI complete a non-noxious task, such as watching a movie or listening to music. This allows the MRI to detect "normal" brain activity. After this task (usually five minutes), the image provided represents baseline activity within the brain, and the activity noted in image can be "wiped clean" or set to zero, giving scientists a blank canvas to observe and record brain activation above baseline levels during a painful task (Louw, A et al., – submitted for publication).

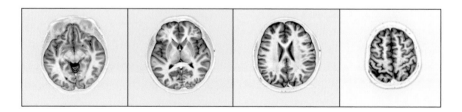

Figure 3.15: Functional MRI scans showing baseline activity to form a 'blank canvas' to map increase in neural activity associated with a pain provoking task. (Image from the authors).

Once the blank canvas has been developed, a patient may be asked to perform a pain-provoking task that, theoretically, would activate various brain areas; this is then recorded. In the scan shown in Figure 3.16, a patient with a L5/S1 disc lesion facing lumbar surgery performs supine anterior tilts of the spine (extension) for five minutes going through cycles of 30 seconds of painful stimulus and 30 seconds "off." Thus, a pain neural signature is developed (Moseley, 2005; Louw, Puentedura et al., 2013 – submitted for publication).

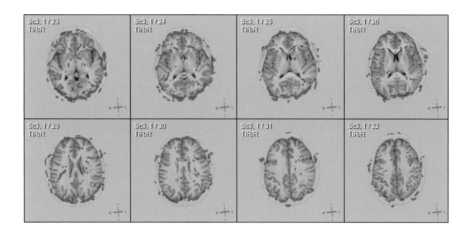

Figure 3.16: Areas of increased activity within the brain during a pain-provoking task. (Image from the authors).

Adding to the complexity of the neuromatrix and adjacent maps is the Hebbian Theory, which proposes that "neurons that fire together, wire together" (Amit, Brunel et al., 1994). This is a scientific theory in biological neuroscience that explains the adaptation of neurons in the brain during the learning process. It describes a basic mechanism for synaptic plasticity wherein an increase in synaptic efficacy arises from the presynaptic cell's repeated and persistent stimulation of the postsynaptic cell. The theory suggests that "when an axon of cell A is near enough to excite a cell B and repeatedly or persistently takes part in firing it, some growth process or metabolic change takes place in one or both cells such that A's efficiency, as one of the cells firing B, is increased" (Doidge, 2007).

It is believed that the neurotransmitter dopamine, which plays a major role in reward-driven learning, may play a significant role in wiring pathways together. Every type of reward that has been studied increases the level of dopamine transmission in the brain. A variety of highly addictive drugs, including the stimulants cocaine and methamphetamine, act directly on the dopamine system. Put simply, dopamine 'seals' pathways allowing for faster neuronal pathways. The clinical importance of this kind of plasticity may be appreciated in the case outlined in Table 3.2, where a patient suffering from LBP might try to do a simple task such as walking (Girault and Greengard, 2004).

Table 3.2: A demonstration of neural circuitry developing greater efficiency through repeated activation.

Stimulus	Experience	Neural Signature
1. Walk **30 minutes**	• After sufficient nociceptive stimulation and brain activation, the pain neural signature is developed and pain is produced to protect. Walking stops at 30 minutes. Too much pain.	Development of a neural signature
2. Walk **15 minutes**	• Since the circuitry of the neural signature of pain is activated over-and-over as the patient tries to walk, the neuronal firing occurs faster and easier. This way, it takes less activation (15 minutes) to develop a pain experience.	Living your pain *"Nerves that fire together wire together"*
3. Walk **5 minutes**	• The circuitry's firing speed and efficiency increases and less of a stimulus is needed to develop the pain response.	Living your pain *"Nerves that fire together wire together"*

Remember that tissues only contain nociceptors, not pain receptors; tissues can only inform the brain of danger. Pain must, therefore, be a brain construct based on whatever information the brain has available. It would also be timely to consider the definition of pain. The traditional and most used definition of pain is that of the IASP:

> "Pain is an unpleasant sensory and emotional experience which follows actual or potential tissue damage or is described in terms of such damage"
>
> (Merskey and Bogduk, 1994).

Our answers to the PNQ so far have highlighted the fact that the brain must process nociceptive information. It provides us with an opportunity to also consider a more updated view of pain, from a brain processing perspective.

The following definition is paraphrasing the material we have covered thus far:

Pain is produced by the brain after a person's neural signature has been activated and it is concluded that the body is in danger and action is required

(Moseley, 2003; Moseley, 2007).

This definition of pain provides us with a rather reductionist view of the brain's processing of nociceptive information, but it would seem to be logical from the survival perspective. Upon receiving a message about a threat, the brain processes the information regarding that threat. If the conclusion is that there is danger and action is required, pain will be produced to protect. This decision, that there is indeed danger, will increase activity along facilitatory pathways in the central nervous system to send additional information to the brain (Figure 3.17 a) (Woolf, 2007). If the end result of the neuronal circuitry is that there is no real threat, pain will not be produced to protect and descending pathways will modulate the threat messages (Figure 3.17 b) (Moseley, 2003; Moseley, 2007).

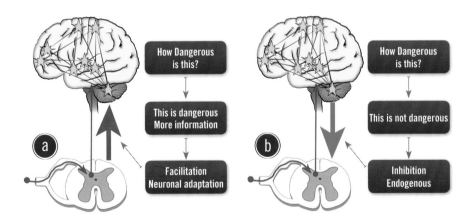

Figure 3.17: Danger messages from the body are received by the brain. If the brain concludes that the danger is real, facilitation will be unregulated to provide more information about the threat (a). If the brain concludes that there is no danger, inhibitory activity will modulate the danger messages (b).

Pain is a response by the brain based on threat. Webster's dictionary defines 'threat' as an "expression of intention to inflict evil, injury, or damage." As it pertains to pain, it could be argued that people may have different threats, based on various factors. For example, in a whiplash study comparing medical doctor's illness and care-seeking behaviors for whiplash-associated disorders, compared to those of non-medically trained personnel, a significant difference was observed (Virani, Ferrari et al., 2001). Both groups sustained similar injuries; however, the perception of the injury and recovery was seen as a major difference in the ensuing care seeking behaviors between the groups. Pain is based on perception of threat, since perceptions include the individualistic nature of pain (Moseley, 2007).

This inclusion of 'perception of threat' can easily be understood by clinicians. Patients exposed to provocative medical terminology proposed to be associated with pain, such as "degenerative disc disease," "bulging discs" and "wear and tear," show heightened levels of fear and anxiety (Sloan and Walsh, 2010). How patients perceive the health of their tissues (correctly or incorrectly) will determine to what extent the brain will produce pain to protect (Moseley, 2007). It is also interesting to note how fast the brain can make such decisions, even when it is presented with limited information. A simple way to examine how the brain makes decisions is a study of visual illusions. The following illusion (Figure 3.18) from scientist Edward Adelson asks, "Which block is darker: A or B?"

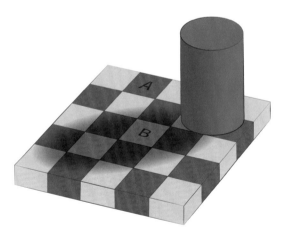

Figure 3.18: Image with permission from Edward H Adelson (1995).

If we could place two gray lines across the image, block A and block B are actually the exact same shade of gray. When the brain is confronted with a visual illusion, the brain makes the most logical choice. This is based on everything the brain knows about colors, lighting, shades, experience, logic and so forth. The brain decides block A is darker than block B. It is the most logical choice, even though it is factually incorrect. The brain makes the same decisions when it comes to interpreting the health of body tissues.

Another simple example is the illusion below: Which line is longer – line a or line b (Figure 3.19)? Again, it may seem that line b is longer than line a, but they are actually of equal length.

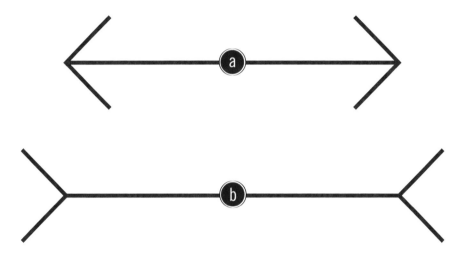

Figure 3.19: Visual illusion where arrowheads give the impression that line b is longer than line a.

This refinement of the definition of pain (perception of threat) is a key point in the treatment of pain. It is believed that TNE directly targets the perception of threat, and the cortical reorganization of perception of threat is likely a significant contributor to the effectiveness of TNE (Moseley, Hodges et al., 2004; Louw, Diener et al., 2011).

3.4g: The brain sends messages down your spinal cord that can increase the nociception (danger message) going up your spinal cord (Q8)

Answer: True

The previous answers to questions of the PNQ have already discussed the answer to this question. The process of facilitation (Q8) and action potential windup (Q4) describe changes in the central nervous system allowing for increased information to the brain for processing (Woolf, 1994; Woolf, 2007). Reflect on receptor changes in the second-order neurons (G-proteins staying open longer), decreased inhibition (dis-inhibition), and death of inhibitory neurons, which modulate the pain experience.

3.4h: Nerves adapt by increasing their resting level of excitement (Q10)

Answer: True

Neurons send messages electrochemically where the chemicals in/around neurons cause electrical impulses. Chemicals in the body are "electrically-charged" (ions), with the most important ones being sodium, potassium, calcium and chloride. Neurons contain semi-permeable membranes that regulate ions. When a neuron is not sending a signal, it is "at rest." When a neuron is at rest, the inside of the neuron is negative relative to the outside. Although the concentrations of the different ions attempt to balance out on both sides of the membrane, they cannot. When all these forces balance out and the difference in the voltage between the inside and outside of the neuron is measured, you have the resting potential. The resting membrane potential of a neuron is about -70 mV, which means that the inside of the neuron is 70 mV less than the outside. At rest, there are relatively more sodium ions outside the neuron and more potassium ions inside that neuron.

When an action potential occurs, the neuron sends information down an axon and away from the cell body. The action potential is an explosion of electrical activity that is created by a depolarizing current. This means that some event, a stimulus, causes the resting potential to move toward 0 mV. When the depolarization reaches about -55 mV, a neuron will fire an action potential. This is the threshold (Figure 3.20). If the neuron does not reach this critical threshold level, then no action potential will fire. Also, when the threshold level is reached, an action potential of a fixed size will always fire. For any given neuron, the size of the action potential is always the same. There are no big or small action potentials in one nerve cell; all action potentials are the same size. Therefore, the neuron either does not reach the threshold or a full action potential is fired. This is the "ALL OR NONE" principle.

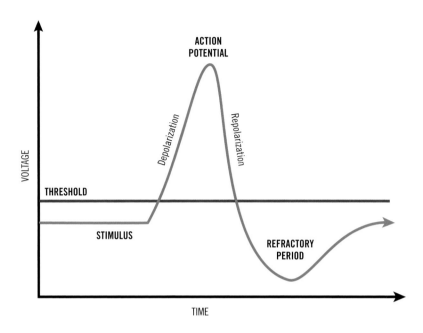

Figure 3.20: An action potential occurs when depolarization of the axon cell membrane reaches the critical threshold level.

The previous section described how a nerve has a resting membrane potential of -70 mV. It is also important to realize a nerve can have a resting membrane potential of -60mV. There is, however, a very definite threshold of -55 mV. Once -55 mV is reached, the action potential occurs. The gateway between the "outside" and "inside" of a nerve is an ion channel (Figure 3.21). Ion channels are proteins, clumped together to form a passage in the membrane of the nerve that allows ions to move in or out (Devor, 2005; Devor, 2006).

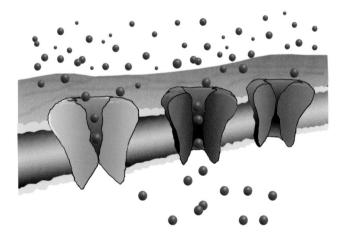

Figure 3.21: Ion channels in the axon cell membrane (axolemma) are gates or sensors that can open in response to various stimuli and allow passage of ions from outside the axon to alter the voltage across the axolemma.

Ion channels regulate the flow of ions across the membrane in all cells, and the opening and closing of the ion channels are governed by various signals:

- **Voltage channels** – Mainly open/close due to electrical activity of the ions
- **Chemical channels** – Open the channel with circulating fluid in the area, such as adrenaline
- **Temperature channels** – Open and close with changes in temperature
- **Mechanical channels** – Open due to mechanical stimuli, such as pressure or tension
- **Immune channels** – Open due to immune molecules, such as cytokines
- **Spontaneous channels** – Some TRP channels seem to open for no reason
- **Hydrogen channels** – Voltage-gated proton channels open with depolarization, but in a strongly pH-sensitive manner
- **Light-gated channels** – Open with changes in light

There are a variety of ion channels in axons and, to date, several hundred have been identified. From a survival perspective, it is logical to consider ion channel expression from a homeostatic perspective. When all is well and the organism is facing no threat, there is likely a need for a relatively equal expression of each type of ion channel in order to sense environmental stimuli, such as changes in temperature, changes in circulating immune molecules in the body, levels of circulating stress chemicals, etc. Within this homeostatic view of ion channel expression exists a very important neuroplastic event, which is important to consider in patients experiencing pain. Ion channel expression continually changes. It has been reported that the half-life of a typical ion channel is approximately 48 hours, thus allowing for a continued neuroplastic change in the sensitivity of the nervous system (Devor, Govrin-Lippmann et al., 1993; Devor, 2005).

Ion channel production does have a genetic/biological premise based on DNA coding. DNA provides the script for the development of proteins and, since DNA cannot escape the cell nucleus, messenger RNA (mRNA) transcribes the message and instructs the cell to build certain proteins. Depending on the type of proteins clumped together, different kinds of channels are genetically fabricated (Devor, 2005; Devor, 2006). This inherent genetic coding does ensure some predetermined ion channel expression, but it is believed that the more potent influences on ion channel expression may be from the brain's interpretation of the environment. When facing a specific threat, ion channels, acting as sensors, will be needed for that threat. For example, it is now well established that following a motor vehicle accident (MVA), patients develop immediate hypersensitivity of the nervous system (Sterling, Jull et al., 2003; Jull, Sterling et al., 2007). Given the high levels of stress and anxiety in and around the MVA and the uncertainty of the future in regards to recovery, pain and movement, higher numbers of movement-sensitive ion channels may be produced.

This causes a widespread sensitization of movement of the nervous system after the accident (Sterling, Jull et al., 2003; Sterling, Jull et al., 2005; Sterling and Kenardy, 2008). This increase of mechanosensitive ion channels in response to the threat of movement in the face of high levels of pain may well explain a patient with whiplash-associated disorders demonstrating increased sensitivity and decreased movement with neurodynamic tests, such as the upper limb neurodynamic tests and slump test (Yeung, Jones et al., 1997; Sterling, Treleaven et al., 2002). This continual change in ion channel expression is important:

1. It provides a biological explanation for "odd" pains reported by patients during the course of physical therapy, e.g., pain when a weather-related cold front nears or when faced with increased stress and adrenaline levels during a preoperative period.

2. The ion channel neuroplasticity provides hope for chronic pain patients. The fact that sensitivity is continually changing implies that with proper therapy, sensitivity can be reduced to allow for decreased pain and disability.

While we are discussing ion channel expression, the non-uniform distribution of ion channels warrants further investigation. Considering that ion channels are gateways between the inside of the axon and the outside, they need to be placed in the membrane of an axon. Myelinated nerves, however, would have a natural barrier to ion channel insertion with the presence of the myelin sheath. Therefore, it is well documented that ion channels typically are found in higher concentrations in areas where there is less myelin (Figure 3.22) (Devor, 2005; Devor, 2006).

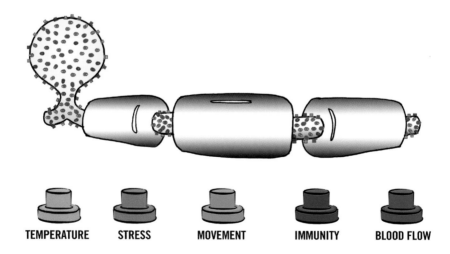

TEMPERATURE   STRESS   MOVEMENT   IMMUNITY   BLOOD FLOW

Figure 3.22: Ion channels are found in the dorsal root ganglion, Nodes of Ranvier and wherever myelin has been stripped from the axon.

One such area is the dorsal root ganglion (DRG). The DRG is non-myelinated and is an ideal locus for ion channel insertion. As well as being an easy target for ion channel expression, the DRG is also reported to have a specific affinity for adrenaline and mechanical ion channels (Howe, Loeser et al., 1977; Amir, Michaelis et al., 1999; Devor, 1999). A second target area for ion channel insertion can be found at the Nodes of Ranvier. The Nodes of Ranvier are normal, non-myelinated sections of the axons between the myelin sheets. These nodes also have high concentrations of ion channels, which is important in the electrochemical conduction of impulses. The third target area for ion channel insertion is any area along the nerve fiber where injury or a disease state has resulted in a loss of myelin (Black, Felts et al., 1991; Redford, Hall et al., 1995).

Wherever the myelin sheath is removed from the axon, ion channels will insert into the newly exposed axolemma. Myelin is actually quite fragile and is typically removed from a nerve by

- **Mechanical force:** Myelin can be physically "peeled" away from an axon. During an injury, such as an inversion ankle sprain, axons may actually have myelin removed via the sudden inversion sprain.

- **Immune processes:** There are several immune-based disease states that demyelinate axons, such as HIV (Louw, Peltzer et al., 2012).

- **Chemical:** Inflammatory substances released at the time of an injury may actually dissolve the myelin surrounding the axon. Various inflammatory and immune cells are known to be part of this "chemical stripping" of the axon, for example, phospholipase-A2 in a disc herniation is a chemical released by the disc, which can denervate the adjacent axon (Franson, Saal et al., 1992; Chen, Cavanaugh et al., 1997; Miyamoto, Doita et al., 2006).

The demyelination of axons and resultant upregulation of ion channels into the bare axolemma can help clinicians explain some of the pain patients experience after surgery or injury. For example, in a knee arthroscopy, the portholes inserted into the medial aspect of a patient's knee may in fact cut through the infrapatellar branches of the saphenous nerve (Wijdicks, Westerhaus et al., 2009). This mechanical invasion is likely to not only sever the small nerve fibers but also remove myelin. The resultant nerve sprouting, as the nerve regenerates to reconnect with its distal segments, leaves a series of un-myelinated axons with a resulting upregulation of ion channels (Portland, Martin et al., 2005, Papastergiou, Voulgaropoulos et al., 2006; Luo, Yu et al., 2007; Figueroa, Calvo et al., 2008; Kachar, Williams et al., 2008). Clinically, if a patient experiences disproportionate pain following a knee arthroscopy, even though ROM or stability appears to be unaffected, it may be more to do with nerve sensitivity than actual structural issues around the knee.

3.4i: Chronic pain means that an injury hasn't healed properly (Q11)

Answer: False

The answer to this question can be found in the discussion of the answers for previous PNQ questions. Injury and pain are not synonymous. Nociception is neither necessary nor sufficient for pain. Many patients have chronic pain yet no history of injury. Many patients have pain in joint regions well past the healing time for tissues.

3.4j: Receptors on nerves work by opening ion channels (gates) in the wall of the nerve (Q1)

Answer: True

The discussion of question 10 of the PNQ - Nerves adapt by increasing their resting level of excitement – and the answer provide with respect to nerve sensitization and ion channel expression provides the appropriate answer to this particular question.

Ion channels are pores in the axolemma allowing ions to flow between the intra- and extra-cellular environments, resulting in electrical activity of the axon. Ion channel expression is based on a combination of genetic coding as well as the brain's expression of the survival needs of the individual. Increased expression of a certain type of ion channel may result in a patient developing sensitivity to the stimulus known to activate the ion channel, e.g., adrenaline channels opening due to high levels of stress or anxiety. Ion channel expression is constantly changing, allowing a neuroplastic view of nerve sensitization.

3.4k: The brain decides when you will experience pain (Q9)

Answer: True

Pain is a brain construct, based on perception of threat. Nociception is received from the tissues by the brain via the dorsal horn and ascending second-order neurons for interpretation by the brain. Since we have been discussing the brain and its complex processing of nociception, how it utilizes various brain areas, and how changes in chemicals within the brain and activation patterns in the brain will occur with injury, it would be appropriate to reflect on the amazing brain (Carter, 1998; Juan, 2006; Doidge, 2007; Carter, 2009):

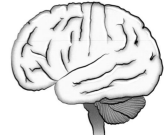

- The weight of the human brain is about 3 lbs.
- The cerebrum is the largest part of the brain and makes up 85% of the brain's weight.
- The brain is made up of about 75% water.
- Your brain consists of about 100 billion neurons.
- There is a network of approximately 125,000 miles of neurons in the brain.
- There are anywhere from 1,000 to 10,000 synapses for each neuron.
- There are no pain receptors in the brain, so the brain can feel no pain. (We left the term "pain receptors," but as per our neuroscience education, there are no "pain receptors" in the body.)
- The human brain is 2% of total body weight.
- There are 100,000 miles of blood vessels in the brain.
- The human brain is the fattest organ in the body and consists of at least 60% fat.
- Neurons develop at the rate of 250,000 neurons per minute during early pregnancy.
- A newborn baby's brain grows about three times its size in the first year.
- Humans continue to make new neurons throughout life in response to mental activity.
- Your brain uses 20% of the total oxygen in your body.
- As with oxygen, your brain uses 20% of the blood circulating in your body.
- If your brain loses blood for 8 to 10 seconds, you will lose consciousness.
- While awake, your brain generates between 10 and 23 watts of power – or enough energy to power a light bulb.
- The brain can live for 4 to 6 minutes without oxygen, and then it begins to die. No oxygen for 5 to 10 minutes will result in permanent brain damage.
- Laughing at a joke is no simple task as it requires activity in five different areas of the brain.
- The average number of thoughts that humans are believed to experience each day is 70,000.

3.4l: Worse injuries always result in worse pain (Q13)

Answer: False

This belief that worse injuries result in worse pain might appear to make sense, but it's amazing how often the opposite occurs. Many unfortunate souls have arrived in hospital emergency departments impaled or severely injured following some gruesome accident, yet they may report experiencing little or no pain (Ahmad and Busuttil, 1993; Guneren, Birinci et al., 2000; Nicolaisen, Ahmed et al., 2012). So many examples exist where injury is apparent and there is little to no resultant pain. Examples include soldiers being shot and not being aware of it, or athletes competing despite significant tissue damage or injury. Conversely, small and seemingly insignificant injuries, such as paper cuts or cutting a nail too close to the nail bed, may result in marked pain experiences.

3.4m: When you are injured, the environment that you are in will not have an effect on the amount of pain you experience (Q16)

Answer: False

All injuries occur in some kind of environment. Ankle sprains, whiplash injuries and back pain do not occur without some influence from the environment. Environmental issues such as work, stress and anxiety, financial concerns, beliefs and fears can significantly impact how a patient may experience the injury (Kendall and Watson, 2000; Watson and Kendall, 2000). The environmental influences can be seen as having either a positive (lessening the pain experience) or negative (increasing the pain experience) influence.

Negative

It has been shown that injuries occurring in high-stress environments, such as car accidents, injury at a stressful job, etc., have a much higher chance of producing persistent pain (Figure 3.23) (Sterling, Jull et al., 2006; Walton, Pretty et al., 2009). It is reported that injuries sustained in high-stress environments are seven to eight times more likely to result in chronic pain (Hellsing, Linton et al., 1994).

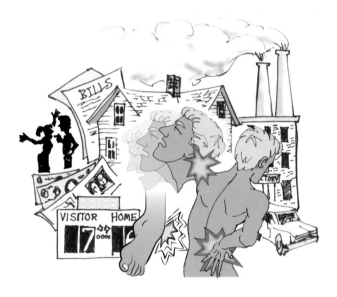

Figure 3.23: Injuries sustained in high-stress environments may have a negative influence and result in an increased pain experience.

Positive

Kids that play contact sports early in life are likely to have a lower chance of developing chronic pain (Raudenbush, Canter et al., 2012). Demolition derby drivers experience an average of 1500+ motor vehicle collisions during their career yet less than 10% develop chronic neck pain. Compare this to the general population involved in motor vehicle accidents where 33% will develop chronic pain (Simotas and Shen, 2005).

3.4n: It is possible to have pain and not know about it (Q17)

Answer: False

The answer to this question is intertwined with the discussion of consciousness. It is now becoming more and more accepted that pain is an output of the brain in response to threat and that the decision to produce pain is a conscious decision by the brain. In an immediate threat response, e.g., stepping onto a nail, the lower centers of the brain produce an immediate protective strategy such as reflexive withdrawal, adrenaline and pupil dilation. The neuronal activation is then processed by the higher, cortical centers of the brain that deal with conscious decisions. This current view of a conscious decision of the brain producing pain helps us to understand how general anesthesia works (Figure 3.24).

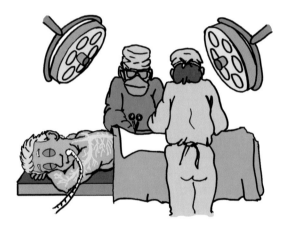

Figure 3.24: During anesthesia, controlled loss of consciousness results in no pain being experienced by the patient.

It is believed that anesthesia given during surgery removes the conscious experience associated with the surgery (Carter, 2009). Surely there would still be nociceptive bombardment of the central nervous system during the surgical intervention, yet no pain will be experienced (Woolf, 2007). Anesthetics can be categorized into two classes: general anesthetics, which cause a reversible loss of consciousness; and local anesthetics, which cause a reversible loss of sensation for a limited region of the body while maintaining consciousness. Combinations of anesthetics are sometimes used for their synergistic and additive therapeutic effects. It is postulated that anesthetic agents act on neurons in the reticular activating system, suppressing alertness and awareness. Additionally neurons in the hippocampus are affected by temporarily wiping out memory, and nuclei in the thalamus are affected to alter sensory information from the tissues.

3.4o: Nerves can adapt by making more ion channels (gates) (Q12)

Answer: True

Refer to answers provided for questions 9 and 11 of the PNQ.

3.4p: Second-order nociceptor (messenger nerve) post-synaptic membrane potential is dependent on descending modulation (Q15)

Answer: True

Second-order neurons are responsible for taking the incoming nociception from the dorsal horn of the spinal cord to the brain for processing. There are various types of second-order neurons with the two most commonly reported ones being the wide dynamic ranging neurons (WDR) and nociceptive specific (NS) neurons. Review the answer to question 4 of the PNQ. Activation of the second-order neurons is dependent on the following (Woolf and Salter, 2005; Woolf, 2007):

• Amount of nociception from the tissues
• Interneuron activity
• Competing information from the contralateral side of the body as well as spinal levels above and below (convergence)
• Ion channel available in the second-order neurons
• Availability of neurotransmitters
• Descending modulation

The brain can modulate the ascending information by descending modulation via endogenous mechanisms (Nijs, Kosek et al., 2012; Van Oosterwijck, Nijs et al., 2012). This descending modulation highlights a common misbelief regarding a common therapeutic effect called 'placebo.' Webster's defines 'placebo' as "a pharmacologically inert preparation prescribed more for the mental relief of the patient than for its actual effect on a disorder." Obviously, placebo does not only pertain to medications, but also therapeutic interventions. Unfortunately, placebo is often viewed as a "fake" or sham treatment. Placebo should be seen more as the endogenous mechanisms of pain experience modulation. Beliefs are at the heart of this. Believing a treatment will work allows for an enhanced endogenous mechanism and, even if the actual, physical treatment is supposed to "do nothing," it is hard to consider the treatment fake (Moseley, 2008). Patients attending therapy carry expectation and beliefs in them, which can modulate their pain experiences (Bialosky, Bishop et al., 2010; Bishop, Bialosky et al., 2011; Puentedura, Cleland et al., 2012).

It is also noteworthy to consider the power of placebo. Placebo, or enhancing the brain's ability to modulate pain through beliefs, is likely a significant future source of treatment for patients with chronic pain. Although care should be taken when interpreting a low number of studies, a recent systematic review of sham surgery for orthopedics (Louw, et al., 2013 – submitted for publication), demonstrated that placebo surgery was just as effective in reducing pain and disability as actual surgery for compression fractures of the spine and knee arthroscopies (Moseley, 2002; Buchbinder, Osborne et al., 2009; Kallmes, Comstock et al., 2009).

3.4q: Nerves adapt by making ion channels (gates) stay open longer (Q14)

Answer: True

Refer to questions 4, 9 and 11 of the PNQ and the discussion about the answers. Most ion channels open for milliseconds, allowing ions to polarize or depolarize the membrane. Some channels, such as G-protein channels, can remain open for minutes. With persistent pain, especially in the dorsal horn, second-order neurons may have higher concentrations of G-proteins. From an evolutionary biological perspective, these higher G-protein concentrations would seem logical as the pathways would then be able to enhance nociceptive information to the brain, such as action potential windup.

3.4r: When you are injured, chemicals in your tissue can make nerves more sensitive (Q18)

Answer: True

Refer again to questions 9 and 11 of the PNQ. The answers and discussion of ion channels was covered at length. Various chemicals can influence electrical activity in axons by opening or closing ion channels specific to that chemical. The chemical response to threat is a major contributor to pain, specifically adrenaline and cortisol. For therapists treating pain, it is important to develop an understanding of stress responses and the resulting chemical changes in the body and brain, and how they are linked to a pain experience.

3.4s: In chronic pain, chemicals associated with stress can directly activate nociception pathways (danger messenger nerves) (Q19)

Answer: True

To better understand why this is true, we should spend some time covering the stress response.

The Stress Response (Sapolsky, 1998)

The basic threat response, often assigned to the sympathetic nervous system, is the fight and flight response. The stress response during an immediate threat, however, is significantly more complex and involves various other bodily systems. An example we like to use in patient education about the stress response is the scenario of a big, roaring African lion entering the room (Figure 3.25).

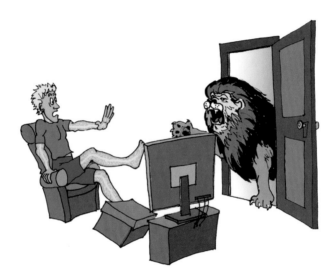

Figure 3.25: Most would agree that a large, roaring African lion entering the room would elicit an immediate stress response.

To deal with this immediate threat, the body reacts with various systems:

- **Adrenaline**—Adrenaline is a centrally acting excitatory neurotransmitter and a hormone that affects just about all body tissues, but it is best known to regulate heart rate, blood vessel and air passage diameters, and metabolic shifts (Sapolsky, 1998). The action varies depending on the tissues and adrenergic receptors, for example, high levels of adrenaline cause smooth muscle relaxation in the airways but cause contraction of the smooth muscle that lines most arterioles. Adrenaline works via the sympathetic nervous system. In response to perceived threat, heart rate increases rapidly to pump blood though the body to areas needing blood and oxygen. Adrenaline causes hyper vigilance. If a lion enters the room, it is not time for a nap (Riva, Mork et al., 2012).

- **Muscles**—In an immediate threat response, large muscles capable of evading or facing the threat are needed. Big, strong leg muscles activate to run away. Arm muscles activate to 'punch the lion.' Smaller muscles are not needed, such as postural muscles or even stabilizing muscles (Larsson, Cai et al., 1995; Hodges and Richardson, 1998; Moseley, 2004). Deactivating these muscles for the immediate threat seems like a good strategy, and they should be switched back on when the threat has been removed.

- **Language**—When startled with a threat such as the lion, you will likely say a few choice words in a loud, short, sharp and abrasive voice (Stephens, Atkins et al., 2009).

- **Breathing**—With the impending threat, breathing becomes faster and shallower.

- **GI System**—Digestion of food is slowed down or even put on hold, allowing for all possible energy and blood flow to be allocated to the immediate, much needed systems.

- **Other**—There are other responses such as reproduction, pain, motivation, memory, etc.

Once the lion is captured by a game keeper or animal control officer (Figure 3.26), the stress response dissipates and homeostasis allows the systems to normalize and prepare for the next stress response (Sapolsky, 1998). This process occurs daily as people are faced with differing stressors. The system, however, is designed to elevate and then calm down, not continue to run at elevated levels for prolonged periods.

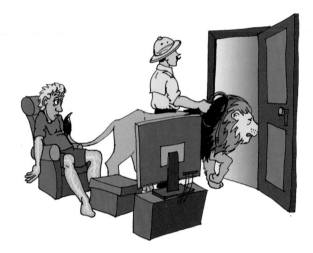

Figure 3.26: Once the lion (threat) is removed, the stress response dissipates and homeostasis allows systems to normalize.

Pain is a reaction to threat. Apart from the daily pain, various psychosocial issues have been correlated to a persistent pain experience (Kendall and Watson, 2000; Watson and Kendall, 2000). Chapter 1 of this textbook described various yellow flags and it is believed that the presence of these biopsychosocial yellow flags will, over time, result in a stress response. Put together, the lion is a metaphorical description of these yellow flags along with the daily pain. (Figure 3.27)

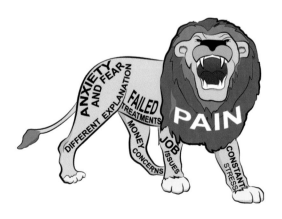

Figure 3.27: The lion as a metaphor for stressors associated with a persistent pain state.

During this acute stress response, adrenaline levels are increased. It is thought that adrenosensitive ion channels open, allowing for an easier depolarization of the nervous system and resultant pain response. Clinically, the patient may experience pain due to stress, anxiety or fear, not just injured or damaged tissues. This pain response may explain increased pain experiences reported during high stress scenarios, such as spinal surgery, litigation or whiplash injuries. In chronic pain, the stress response is protracted.

If the stressors and biopsychosocial factors (lion) remain in place for months, or years, the resultant chemical activation will have significant repercussions for the nervous system, tissues and brain. The stress biology analogy would be the lion following a patient for months (Figure 3.28). The stress response is primarily executed by adrenaline, initially, followed by cortisol changes in the body.

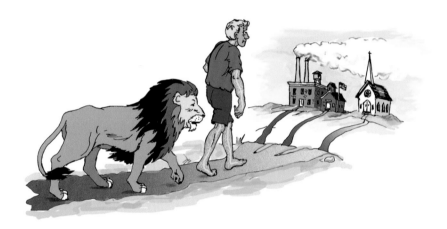

Figure 3.28: Patients with chronic pain are thought to have persistent stressors and biopsychosocial factors (metaphorically speaking, a lion) following them for months or years.

Adrenaline is a fast-acting neurotransmitter and likely very effective in the immediate stress response, which should last no longer than several minutes. Cortisol is a more potent and longer lasting chemical, similar in effect to adrenaline but produced to deal with longer lasting threats (Sapolsky, 1998). Cortisol is a glucocorticoid steroid hormone produced by the adrenal gland and more formally known as hydrocortisone (Sapolsky, 1998). Cortisol's primary function is to increase blood sugar, suppress the immune system and aid in fat, protein and carbohydrate metabolism (Segal, Hindmarsh et al., 2005; Riva, Mork et al., 2012). The release of cortisol from the adrenal gland is controlled by the hypothalamus. The secretion of corticotropin-releasing hormone (CRH) by the hypothalamus triggers anterior pituitary secretion of adrenocorticotropic hormone (ACTH). ACTH is carried by the cells to the vascular cortex, where it triggers blood secretion (Figure 3.29) (Geiss, Rohleder et al., 2005; Van Houdenhove, Van Den Eede et al., 2009).

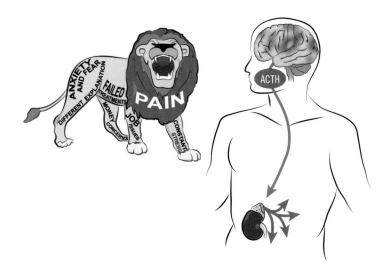

Figure 3.29: Release of cortisol from the adrenal gland in response to threat is controlled by the hypothalamus via corticotropin-releasing hormone (CRH), which triggers secretion of adrenocorticotropic hormone (ACTH) from the anterior pituitary gland. The ACTH triggers release of cortisol into the blood stream.

Cortisol prevents the release of substances in the body that cause inflammation. This is why cortisol is used to treat conditions resulting from over activity of the B-cell mediated antibody response, such as inflammatory and rheumatoid diseases and allergies. Low-potency hydrocortisone is used to treat skin problems, such as rashes, eczema and others. Elevated levels of cortisol, if prolonged, can lead to proteolysis and muscle wasting. Cortisol has a daily pattern, typically peaking around 8 am and reaching its low point between midnight and 4 am, or 3-5 hours after sleep initiation (Chervin, Teodorescu et al., 2009; Fabian, McGuire et al., 2009).

Cortisol levels are affected by changes in ACTH, depression, psychological stress and physiological stressors, such as illness, surgery, fear, injury and pain. Change in cortisol levels have been linked to reduction in bone formation and thought to be responsible for the mechanism behind stress dwarfism (van de Ven, Andressoo et al., 2006). Cortisol works along with adrenaline to create short-term memories. Long-term exposure to cortisol damages hippocampus cells, limiting learning and altering memory (Mohs, Mease et al., 2012). Cortisol dysregulation increases blood pressure, shuts down the reproductive system, and is associated with weight gain, appetite changes and obesity.

A more significant effect of cortisol change is on the immune system, specifically pro-inflammatory cytokines. Cytokines are immune molecules, and they impact tissue healing significantly (Dinarello, 1999). During infections or trauma/injury, cytokines such as interleukin 6 (IL-6) increase 1000-fold, thus allowing for more ion channels specific to cytokines to open up, potentially resulting in increased sensitivity. This is the process that is seen to occur during a bout of the flu. A major stimulus for the production of cytokines is cortisol. With increased cytokines, there is further possibility to increase inflammatory processes all over the body, including keeping tissues inflamed.

Inflammation is a normal biological process aimed at protecting the body tissues and signaling the start of the healing and repair process. During an injury, tissues cause the release of inflammatory substances, such as prostaglandins and bradykinins. Local C-fibers, via retrograde depolarization (nerves firing the other way), will also contribute to the inflammatory process by releasing substance P, which results in a vasodilatation and mast cell release of histamine (Ikawa, Atsuta et al., 2005; Marinus, Moseley et al., 2011). During a painful experience filled with many stressors (fear and anxiety), cortisol levels will be increased, resulting in increased cytokines, which may keep an injured body part swollen for a longer period.

All the discussion so far on the stress response should allow therapists to appreciate how various chemicals contribute to a pain experience.

3.5: Putting It All in Perspective

The 19 PNQ questions discussed in this chapter provide a terrific introduction into the neuroscience of pain. This processing of information by the central nervous system, particularly the brain, and its response is central to the definition of pain (Moseley, 2003):

Pain is a multiple system output activated by an individual's specific pain neural signature. The neural signature is activated whenever the brain concludes that body tissues are in danger and action is required.

This chapter's discussion of the questions and answers to the PNQ is also conceptually described in the pain mechanism model, as set forth by Gifford (1998) (Figure 3.30).

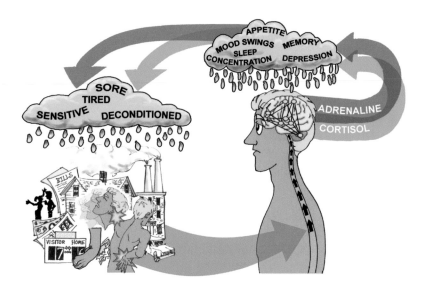

Figure 3.30: The pain mechanism model based on the mature organism model by Gifford (1998).

The pain mechanism model provides a bigger picture of pain. It de-emphasizes a joint, muscle or ligament as the sole source of pain and instead teaches a broader view of pain processing, which is in line with the current content of TNE (Louw, Diener et al., 2011). The pain mechanism model also allows therapists to view pain as an input-dominant, processing-dominant or output-dominant mechanism. This distinction is very important in the clinical presentation and resulting treatment planning (Smart and Doody, 2007; Smart, Blake et al., 2009; Smart, Blake et al., 2012; Smart, Blake et al., 2012; Smart, Blake et al., 2012; Smart, Blake et al., 2012).

Input
Three sources of input mechanisms can be identified. The first source is from the tissues. Tissues do get injured or undergo disease processes and can send nociceptive information to the spinal cord and, ultimately, the brain. Pain as a result of nociception from tissues is often referred to as 'nociceptive pain.' The tissue issues are well understood by therapists and signs and symptoms are easily recognized. Recent symptom and exam clusters studies indicate individuals that have certain clinical features are 100 times more likely to accurately predict a clinical classification of nociceptive pain (Smart, Blake et al., 2012).

The symptom and exam clusters are as follows:

- Proportionate pain
- Aggravating and easing factors
- Intermittent sharp, dull ache or throb at rest
- No night pain, dysesthesia, burning, shooting or electric symptoms

A second source of input can be based upon a consideration of the environmental issues surrounding a pain experience. As described in the answer to PNQ question 13, environmental issues can influence the pain experience considerably. The third source of input is from peripheral neuropathic pain mechanisms. Peripheral neuropathic mechanisms include the peripheral nervous system processes distal to the dorsal horn. The sensitization of the peripheral nervous system is dependent on changes to blood supply to the nervous system, altered ion channel expression, chemical influences on the peripheral nervous system, demyelination and more. Patients are 150 times more likely to have a peripheral neuropathic pain state if the following clinical symptoms and signs are present (Smart, Blake et al., 2012):

- Pain in dermatomal or cutaneous distribution
- Positive neurodynamic & palpation (mechanical tests)
- History of nerve pathology or compromise

Processing

Pain mechanisms due to processing issues, commonly referred to as 'central sensitization,' occur due to neuroplastic changes in the dorsal horn of the spinal cord, inappropriate synapsing, neuronal death, sprouting, receptor field expansion, activation of the neuromatrix, changes in neurotransmitters and ion channels in the CNS and brain, and loss of gray matter. In central sensitization, pain is due more to abnormal processing of the nociception by the spinal cord, brainstem and cerebral hemispheres. Similarly, as with nociceptive and neuropathic mechanisms, symptom and sign clustering studies have been conducted, indicating patients are 486 times more likely to have a central sensitization pain state if they present with the following (Smart, Blake et al., 2012):

- Disproportionate pain
- Disproportionate aggravating and easing factors
- Diffuse palpation tenderness
- Psychosocial issues

Output

Although not currently examined in symptoms and sign clustering studies, output mechanisms describe the resultant response to the input to the central nervous system and resultant processing. As outlined in the answer to PNQ question 19, various bodily systems activate to protect during a threat and resultant output may include pain, sympathetic nervous system changes, motor response, immune response, endocrine response and more.

3.6: Key Points from Chapter 3

- Pain is complex.
- Cartesian models are outdated and no longer helpful.
- There is ever-increasing knowledge of how pain works.
- Pain is a conscious decision by the brain based on threat and is only one of MANY defenders.

Answers to the Pain Neurophysiology Questionnaire (Moseley 2003)

Questions	True	False	Unsure
1. Receptors on nerves work by opening ion channels (gates) in the wall of the nerve.	X		
2. When part of your body is injured, special pain receptors convey the pain message to your brain.		X	
3. Pain only occurs when you are injured.		X	
4. The timing and intensity of pain matches the timing and number of signals in nociceptors (danger receptors).		X	
5. Nerves have to connect a body part to your brain in order for that body part to be in pain.		X	
6. In chronic pain, the central nervous system becomes more sensitive to nociception (danger messages).	X		
7. The body tells the brain when it is in pain.		X	
8. The brain sends messages down your spinal cord that can increase the nociception (danger message) going up your spinal cord.	X		
9. The brain decides when you will experience pain.	X		
10. Nerves adapt by increasing their resting level of excitement.	X		

Questions	True	False	Unsure
11. Chronic pain means that an injury hasn't healed properly.		X	
12. Nerves can adapt by making more ion channels (gates).	X		
13. Worse injuries always result in worse pain.		X	
14. Nerves adapt by making ion channels (gates) stay open longer.	X		
15. Second-order nociceptor (messenger nerve) post-synaptic membrane potential is dependent on descending modulation.	X		
16. When you are injured, the environment that you are in will not have an effect on the amount of pain you experience.		X	
17. It is possible to have pain and not know about it.		X	
18. When you are injured, chemicals in your tissue can make nerves more sensitive.	X		
19. In chronic pain, chemicals associated with stress can directly activate nociception pathways (danger messenger nerves).	X		

Chapter 3 References

Ahmad, N. and A. Busuttil (1993). Impaling-type head injury in a road traffic incident. *Medicine, Science, and the Law, 33*(3): 261-263.

Alyas, F., M. Turner and D. Connell (2007). MRI findings in the lumbar spines of asymptomatic, adolescent, elite tennis players. *Br J Sports Med, 41*(11): 836-841; discussion 841.

Amir, M., M. Michaelis and M. Devor (1999). Membrane potential oscillations in dorsal root ganglion neurons: role in normal electrogenesis and neuropathic pain. *Journal of Neuroscience, 19*: 8589-8596.

Amit, D. J., N. Brunel and M. V. Tsodyks (1994). Correlations of cortical Hebbian reverberations: theory versus experiment. *The Journal of Neuroscience: The Official Journal of the Society for Neuroscience, 14*(11 Pt 1): 6435-6445.

Autio, R. A., J. Karppinen, J. Niinimaki, R. Ojala, M. Kurunlahti, M. Haapea, H. Vanharanta and O. Tervonen (2006). Determinants of spontaneous resorption of intervertebral disc herniations. *Spine, 31*(11): 1247-1252.

Barker, R. A. and S. Barasi (1999). *Neuroscience at a Glance*. Oxford, Blackwell.

Basbaum, A. I. and H. L. Fields (1978). Endogenous pain control mechanisms. *Annals of Neurology, 4*: 451-462.

Bear, M. F., B. W. Connors and M. A. Paradiso (1996). *Neuroscience. Exploring the Brain*. Baltimore, Williams & Wilkins.

Bedson, J. and P. R. Croft (2008). The discordance between clinical and radiographic knee osteoarthritis: a systematic search and summary of the literature. *BMC Musculoskeletal Disorders, 9*: 116.

Bialosky, J. E., M. D. Bishop and J. A. Cleland (2010). Individual expectation: an overlooked, but pertinent, factor in the treatment of individuals experiencing musculoskeletal pain. *Physical Therapy, 90*(9): 1345-1355.

Bialosky, J. E., M. D. Bishop, S. Z. George and M. E. Robinson (2011). Placebo response to manual therapy: something out of nothing? *The Journal of Manual & Manipulative Therapy, 19*(1): 11-19.

Bishop, M. D., J. E. Bialosky and J. A. Cleland (2011). Patient expectations of benefit from common interventions for low back pain and effects on outcome: secondary analysis of a clinical trial of manual therapy interventions. *The Journal of Manual & Manipulative Therapy, 19*(1): 20-25.

Black, J. A., P. Felts, K. J. Smith, J. D. Knocsis and S. G. Waxman (1991). Distribution of sodium channels in chronically demyelinated spinal cord axons: Immuno-ultrastructural localization and electrophysiological observations. *Brain Research, 544*: 59-70.

Brisby, H. and I. Hammar (2007). Thalamic activation in a disc herniation model. *Spine, 32*(25): 2846-2852.

Buchbinder, R., R. H. Osborne, P. R. Ebeling, J. D. Wark, P. Mitchell, C. Wriedt, S. Graves, M. P. Staples and B. Murphy (2009). A randomized trial of vertebroplasty for painful osteoporotic vertebral fractures. *N Engl J Med, 361*(6): 557-568.

Carter, R. (1998). *Mapping the Mind*. London, Weidenfeld and Nicholson.

Carter, R. (2009). *The Human Brain Book*. New York, Dorling Kindersley Limited.

Catani, M. (2006). Diffusion tensor magnetic resonance imaging tractography in cognitive disorders. *Current Opinion in Neurology, 19*(6): 599-606.

Catani, M. and M. Thiebaut de Schotten (2008). A diffusion tensor imaging tractography atlas for virtual in vivo dissections. *Cortex; A Journal Devoted to the Study of the Nervous System and Behavior, 44*(8): 1105-1132.

Chen, C., J. M. Cavanaugh, A. C. Ozaktay, S. Kallakuri and A. I. King (1997). Effects of phospholipase A2 on lumbar nerve root structure and function. *Spine, 22*(10): 1057-1064.

Chervin, R. D., M. Teodorescu, R. Kushwaha, A. M. Deline, C. B. Brucksch, C. Ribbens-Grimm, D. L. Ruzicka, P. K. Stein, D. J. Clauw and L. J. Crofford (2009). Objective measures of disordered sleep in fibromyalgia. *The Journal of Rheumatology, 36*(9): 2009-2016.

Delcomyn, F. (1998). *Foundations of Neurobiology*. New York, W.H. Freeman.

Devor, M. (1999). Unexplained peculiarities of the dorsal root ganglion. *Pain, Supplement 6*: S27-S36.

Devor, M. (2005). Response of nerves to injury in relation to neuropathic pain. *Melzack and wall's Textbook of Pain*. S. McMahon and M. Koltzenburg. Edinburgh, Elsevier.

Devor, M. (2006). Sodium channels and mechanisms of neuropathic pain. *J Pain, 7*(1 Suppl 1): S3-S12.

Devor, M., R. Govrin-Lippmann and K. Angelides (1993). Na+ channel immunolocalization in peripheral mammalian axons and changes following nerve injury and neuroma formation. *Journal of Neuroscience, 13*: 1976-1992.

Deyo, R. A., D. T. Gray, W. Kreuter, S. Mirza and B. I. Martin (2005). United States trends in lumbar fusion surgery for degenerative conditions. *Spine, 30*(12): 1441-1445; discussion 1446-1447.

Deyo, R. A., S. K. Mirza, J. A. Turner and B. I. Martin (2009). Overtreating chronic back pain: time to back off? *J Am Board Fam Med, 22*(1): 62-68.

Deyo, R. A., A. Nachemson and S. K. Mirza (2004). Spinal-fusion surgery - the case for restraint. *N Engl J Med, 350*(7): 722-726.

Dinarello, C. A. (1999). Overview of cytokines and their role in pain. *Cytokines and Pain.* L. R. Watkins and S. F. Maier. Basel, Birkhauser.

Doidge, N. (2007). *The Brain That Changes Itself.* New York, Penguin Books.

Dostrovsky, J. O. (1999). Immediate and long-term plasticity in human somatosensory thalamus and its involvement in phantom limbs. *Pain Supplement, 6*: S37-S43.

Doubell, T. P., R. Mannion and C. J. Woolf (1999). The dorsal horn: state dependent sensory processing, plasticity and the generation of pain. *Textbook of Pain.* P. D. Wall and R. Melzack. Edinburgh, Churchill Livingstone.

Fabian, L. A., L. McGuire, G. G. Page, B. R. Goodin, R. R. Edwards and J. Haythornthwaite (2009). The association of the cortisol awakening response with experimental pain ratings. *Psychoneuroendocrinology, 34*(8): 1247-1251.

Figueroa, D., R. Calvo, A. Vaisman, M. Campero and C. Moraga (2008). Injury to the infrapatellar branch of the saphenous nerve in ACL reconstruction with the hamstrings technique: clinical and electrophysiological study. *Knee, 15*(5): 360-363.

Flor, H. (2000). The functional organization of the brain in chronic pain. *Prog Brain Res, 129*: 313-322.

Flor, H. (2003). *The image of pain.* Annual scientific meeting of The Pain Society (Britain), Glasgow, Scotland.

Flor, H., C. Braun, T. Elbert and N. Birbaumer (1997). Extensive reorganization of primary somatosensory cortex in chronic back pain patients. *Neurosci Lett, 224*(1): 5-8.

Franson, R. C., J. S. Saal and S. J.A. (1992). Human disc phospholipase A2 is inflammatory. *Spine, 17* (Suppl): S129-S132.

Fukuoka, T., A. Tokunaga, E. Kondo, K. Miki, T. Tachibana and K. Noguchi (1998). Change in mRNAs for neuropeptides and the GABA(A) receptor in dorsal root ganglion neurons in a rat experimental neuropathic pain model. *Pain, 78*(1): 13-26.

Geiss, A., N. Rohleder, C. Kirschbaum, K. Steinbach, H. W. Bauer and F. Anton (2005). Predicting the failure of disc surgery by a hypofunctional HPA axis: evidence from a prospective study on patients undergoing disc surgery. *Pain, 114*(1-2): 104-117.

Gifford, L. S. (1998). Pain, the tissues and the nervous system. *Physiotherapy, 84*: 27-33.

Girault, J. A. and P. Greengard (2004). The neurobiology of dopamine signaling. *Arch Neurol, 61*(5): 641-644.

Goldberg, J. S. (2008). Revisiting the Cartesian model of pain. *Medical Hypotheses, 70*(5): 1029-1033.

Guneren, E., H. Birinci, O. A. Uysal, L. Eroglu and P. M. Geary (2000). Facial impaling on a scythe. *British Journal of Plastic Surgery, 53*(3): 267-268.

Haldeman, S. (1990). Presidential address, North American Spine Society: failure of the pathology model to predict back pain. *Spine, 15*(7): 718-724.

Hellsing, A., S. J. Linton and M. Kalvemark (1994). A prospective study of patients with acute back and neck pain in Sweden. *Physical Therapy, 74*: 116-128.

Hodges, P. W. and C. A. Richardson (1998). Delayed postural contraction of transversus abdominis in low back pain associated with movement of the lower limb. *J Spinal Disord, 11*(1): 46-56.

Howe, J. F., J. D. Loeser and W. H. Calvin (1977). Mechanosensitivity of dorsal root ganglia and chronically injured axons: a physiological basis for the radicular pain of nerve root compression. *Pain, 3*(1): 25-41.

Huber, A., A. L. Suman, C. A. Rendo, G. Biasi, R. Marcolongo and G. Carli (2007). Dimensions of 'unidimensional' ratings of pain and emotions in patients with chronic musculoskeletal pain. *Pain, 130*(3): 216-224.

Ikawa, M., Y. Atsuta and H. Tsunekawa (2005). Ectopic firing due to artificial venous stasis in rat lumbar spinal canal stenosis model: a possible pathogenesis of neurogenic intermittent claudication. *Spine, 30*(21): 2393-2397.

Juan, S. (2006). *The Odd Brain: Mysteries of our Weird & Wonderful Brains Explained.* New York, MJF Books.

Jull, G., M. Sterling, J. Kenardy and E. Beller (2007). Does the presence of sensory hypersensitivity influence outcomes of physical rehabilitation for chronic whiplash?--A preliminary RCT. *Pain, 129*(1-2): 28-34.

Kachar, S. M., K. M. Williams and H. A. Finn (2008). Neuroma of the infrapatellar branch of the saphenous nerve a cause of reversible knee stiffness after total knee arthroplasty. *J Arthroplasty, 23*(6): 927-930.

Kallmes, D. F., B. A. Comstock, P. J. Heagerty, J. A. Turner, D. J. Wilson, T. H. Diamond, R. Edwards, L. A. Gray, L. Stout, S. Owen, W. Hollingworth, B. Ghdoke, D. J. Annesley-Williams, S. H. Ralston and J. G. Jarvik (2009). A randomized trial of vertebroplasty for osteoporotic spinal fractures. *N Engl J Med, 361*(6): 569-579.

Kendall, N. and P. Watson (2000). Identifying psychosocial yellow flags and modifying management. *Topical Issues in Pain 2.* L. S. Gifford. Falmouth, CNS Press.

Kjaer, P., C. Leboeuf-Yde, L. Korsholm, J. S. Sorensen and T. Bendix (2005). Magnetic resonance imaging and low back pain in adults: a diagnostic imaging study of 40-year-old men and women. *Spine, 30*(10): 1173-1180.

Knotkova, H., W. Crawford Clark, P. Mokrejs, F. Padour and J. Kuhl (2004). What do ratings on unidimensional pain and emotion scales really mean? A Multidimensional Affect and Pain Survey (MAPS) analysis of cancer patient responses. *Journal of Pain and Symptom Management, 28*(1): 19-27.

Komori, H., K. Shinomiya, O. Nakai, I. Yamaura, S. Takeda and K. Furuya (1996). The natural history of herniated nucleus pulposus with radiculopathy. *Spine, 21*(2): 225-229.

Larsson, S. E., H. Cai, Q. Zhang, R. Larsson and P. A. Oberg (1995). Microcirculation in the upper trapezius muscle during sustained shoulder load in healthy women--an endurance study using percutaneous laser-Doppler flowmetry and surface electromyography. *Eur J Appl Physiol Occup Physiol, 70*(5): 451-456.

Latremoliere, A. and C. J. Woolf (2009). Central sensitization: a generator of pain hypersensitivity by central neural plasticity. *The Journal of Pain: Official Journal of the American Pain Society, 10*(9): 895-926.

Lotze, M., M. Erb, H. Flor and E. Huelsman (2000). fMRI evaluation of somatotopic representation in human primary motor cortex. *Neuroimage, 5 Pt 1*: 473-481.

Louw, A. and D. S. Butler (2011). Chronic Pain. *Clinical Orthopaedic Rehabilitation.* B. S.B. and R. Manske. Philadelphia, PA, Elsevier.

Louw, A., I. Diener, D. S. Butler and E. J. Puentedura (2011). The effect of neuroscience education on pain, disability, anxiety, and stress in chronic musculoskeletal pain. *Archives of Physical Medicine and Rehabilitation, 92*(12): 2041-2056.

Louw, A., E. L. Puentedura and P. Mintken (2011). Use of an abbreviated neuroscience education approach in the treatment of chronic low back pain: A case report. *Physiotherapy Theory and Practice.*

Louw, J., K. Peltzer, P. Naidoo, G. Matseke, G. McHunu and B. Tutshana (2012). Quality of life among tuberculosis (TB), TB retreatment and/or TB-HIV co-infected primary public health care patients in three districts in South Africa. *Health and Quality of Life Outcomes, 10*(1): 77.

Luo, H., J. K. Yu, Y. F. Ao, C. L. Yu, L. B. Peng, C. Y. Lin, J. Y. Zhang and X. Fu (2007). Relationship between different skin incisions and the injury of the infrapatellar branch of the saphenous nerve during anterior cruciate ligament reconstruction. *Chin Med J (Engl), 120*(13): 1127-1130.

Maihofner, C., H. O. Handwerker, B. Neundorfer and F. Birklein (2003). Patterns of cortical reorganization in complex regional pain syndrome. *Neurology, 61*(12): 1707-1715.

Major, N. M. and C. A. Helms (2002). MR imaging of the knee: findings in asymptomatic collegiate basketball players. *AJR. American Journal of Roentgenology, 179*(3): 641-644.

Marinus, J., G. L. Moseley, F. Birklein, R. Baron, C. Maihofner, W. S. Kingery and J. J. van Hilten (2011). Clinical features and pathophysiology of complex regional pain syndrome. *Lancet Neurology, 10*(7): 637-648.

Masui, T., Y. Yukawa, S. Nakamura, G. Kajino, Y. Matsubara, F. Kato and N. Ishiguro (2005). Natural history of patients with lumbar disc herniation observed by magnetic resonance imaging for minimum 7 years. *J Spinal Disord Tech, 18*(2): 121-126.

Meeus, M. and J. Nijs (2007). Central sensitization: a biopsychosocial explanation for chronic widespread pain in patients with fibromyalgia and chronic fatigue syndrome. *Clinical Rheumatology, 26*(4): 465-473.

Meeus, M., S. Vervisch, L. S. De Clerck, G. Moorkens, G. Hans and J. Nijs (2012). Central sensitization in patients with rheumatoid arthritis: a systematic literature review. *Semin Arthritis Rheum, 41*(4): 556-567.

Melzack, R. (1996). Gate control theory: on the evolution of pain. *Pain Forum, 5*: 128-138.

Melzack, R. (1999). From the gate to the neuromatrix. *Pain, Suppl 6*: S121-126.

Melzack, R. (2001). Pain and the neuromatrix in the brain *Journal of Dental Education, 65*: 1378-1382.

Merskey, H. and N. Bogduk (1994). *Classification of Chronic Pain.* Seattle, IASP Press.

Milgrom, C., M. Schaffler, S. Gilbert and M. van Holsbeeck (1995). Rotator-cuff changes in asymptomatic adults. The effect of age, hand dominance and gender. *The Journal of Bone and Joint Surgery. British volume, 77*(2): 296-298.

Miyamoto, H., M. Doita, K. Nishida, T. Yamamoto, M. Sumi and M. Kurosaka (2006). Effects of cyclic mechanical stress on the production of inflammatory agents by nucleus pulposus and anulus fibrosus derived cells in vitro. *Spine, 31*(1): 4-9.

Mochida, K., H. Komori, A. Okawa, T. Muneta, H. Haro and K. Shinomiya (1998). Regression of cervical disc herniation observed on magnetic resonance images. *Spine, 23*(9): 990-995; discussion 996-997.

Mohs, R., P. Mease, L. M. Arnold, F. Wang, J. Ahl, P. J. Gaynor and M. M. Wohlreich (2012). The effect of duloxetine treatment on cognition in patients with fibromyalgia. *Psychosomatic Medicine, 74*(6): 628-634.

Moseley, G. L. (2003). A pain neuromatrix approach to patients with chronic pain. *Man Ther, 8*(3): 130-140.

Moseley, G. L. (2003). Unravelling the barriers to reconceptualisation of the problem in chronic pain: the actual and perceived ability of patients and health professionals to understand the neurophysiology. *J Pain, 4*(4): 184-189.

Moseley, G. L. (2004). Evidence for a direct relationship between cognitive and physical change during an education intervention in people with chronic low back pain. *Eur J Pain, 8*(1): 39-45.

Moseley, G. L. (2004). Why do people with complex regional pain syndrome take longer to recognize their affected hand? *Neurology, 62*(12): 2182-2186.

Moseley, G. L. (2005). Distorted body image in complex regional pain syndrome. *Neurology, 65*(5): 773.

Moseley, G. L. (2005). Widespread brain activity during an abdominal task markedly reduced after pain physiology education: fMRI evaluation of a single patient with chronic low back pain. *Aust J Physiother, 51*(1): 49-52.

Moseley, G. L. (2007). Reconceptualising pain according to modern pain sciences. *Physical Therapy Reviews, 12*: 169-178.

Moseley, G. L. (2008). Pain, brain imaging and physiotherapy--opportunity is knocking. *Manual Therapy, 13*(6): 475-477.

Moseley, G. L. (2008). Placebo effect: Reconceptualising placebo. *BMJ336* (7653):1086.

Moseley, G. L., L. Brhyn, M. Ilowiecki, K. Solstad and P. W. Hodges (2003). The threat of predictable and unpredictable pain: differential effects on central nervous system processing? *The Australian Journal of Physiotherapy, 49*(4): 263-267.

Moseley, G. L. and P. W. Hodges (2002). Chronic pain and motor control. *Grieves Modern Manual Therapy of the Vertebral column.* G. Jull and J. Boyling. Edinburgh, Churchill-Livingstone.

Moseley, G. L., P. W. Hodges and M. K. Nicholas (2004). A randomized controlled trial of intensive neurophysiology education in chronic low back pain. *Clinical Journal of Pain, 20*: 324-330.

Moseley, G. L., D. F. Sim, M. L. Henry and T. Souvlis (2005). Experimental hand pain delays recognition of the contralateral hand--evidence that acute and chronic pain have opposite effects on information processing? *Brain Res Cogn Brain Res, 25*(1): 188-194.

Moseley, G. L., N. Zalucki, F. Birklein, J. Marinus, J. J. van Hilten and H. Luomajoki (2008). Thinking about movement hurts: the effect of motor imagery on pain and swelling in people with chronic arm pain. *Arthritis and Rheumatism, 59*(5): 623-631.

Moseley, J. B. (2002). A controlled trial of arthroscopic surgery for osteoarthritis of the knee. *New Eng J Med, 347*: 81-88.

Moseley, L. (2003). Unraveling the barriers to reconceptualization of the problem in chronic pain: the actual and perceived ability of patients and health professionals to understand the neurophysiology. *The Journal of Pain: Official Journal of the American Pain Society, 4*(4): 184-189.

Munk, B., E. Lundorf and J. Jensen (2004). Long-term outcome of meniscal degeneration in the knee: poor association between MRI and symptoms in 45 patients followed more than 4 years. *Acta Orthopaedica Scandinavica, 75*(1): 89-92.

Napadow, V. (2006). Somatosensory cortical plasticity in carpal tunnel syndrome. *Neuroimage, 31*: 520-530.

Nicolaisen, N., A. Ahmed, T. Hancock and R. Ogren (2012). Field airway management of a construction worker with an impaling rebar injury to the neck and brain. *Prehospital Emergency Care: Official Journal of the National Association of EMS Physicians and the National Association of State EMS Directors, 16*(4): 548-552.

Nijs, J., E. Kosek, J. Van Oosterwijck and M. Meeus (2012). Dysfunctional endogenous analgesia during exercise in patients with chronic pain: to exercise or not to exercise? *Pain Physician, 15*(3 Suppl): ES205-213.

Nijs, J., B. Van Houdenhove and R. A. Oostendorp (2010). Recognition of central sensitization in patients with musculoskeletal pain: Application of pain neurophysiology in manual therapy practice. *Man Ther, 15*(2): 135-141.

Ostelo, R. W., L. O. Costa, C. G. Maher, H. C. de Vet and M. W. van Tulder (2004). Rehabilitation after lumbar disc surgery. *Cochrane Database Syst Rev* (4): CD003007.

Papastergiou, S. G., H. Voulgaropoulos, P. Mikalef, E. Ziogas, G. Pappis and I. Giannakopoulos (2006). Injuries to the infrapatellar branch(es) of the saphenous nerve in anterior cruciate ligament reconstruction with four-strand hamstring tendon autograft: vertical versus horizontal incision for harvest. *Knee Surg Sports Traumatol Arthrosc, 14*(8): 789-793.

Penfield, W. and E. Boldrey (1937). Somatic, motor and sensory representation in the cerebral cortex of man as studied by electrical stimulation. *Brain, 60*: 389-448.

Portland, G. H., D. Martin, G. Keene and T. Menz (2005). Injury to the infrapatellar branch of the saphenous nerve in anterior cruciate ligament reconstruction: comparison of horizontal versus vertical harvest site incisions. *Arthroscopy, 21*(3): 281-285.

Puentedura, E. J., J. A. Cleland, M. R. Landers, P. E. Mintken, A. Louw and C. Fernandez-de-Las-Penas (2012). Development of a clinical prediction rule to identify patients with neck pain likely to benefit from thrust joint manipulation to the cervical spine. *The Journal of Orthopaedic and Sports Physical Therapy, 42*(7): 577-592.

Puentedura, E. J. and A. Louw (2012). A neuroscience approach to managing athletes with low back pain. *Physical Therapy in Sport: Official Journal of the Association of Chartered Physiotherapists in Sports Medicine, 13*(3): 123-133.

Raudenbush, B., R. J. Canter, N. Corley, R. Grayhem, J. Koon, S. Lilley, B. Meyer and I. Wilson (2012). Pain threshold and tolerance differences among intercollegiate athletes: implication of past sports injuries and willingness to compete among sports teams. *North American Journal of Psychology Publisher, 14*(1).

Redford, E. J., S. M. Hall and K. J. Smith (1995). Vascular changes and demyelination induced by intraneural injection of tumour necrosis factor. *Brain, 118*: 869-878.

Reilly, P., I. Macleod, R. Macfarlane, J. Windley and R. J. Emery (2006). Dead men and radiologists don't lie: a review of cadaveric and radiological studies of rotator cuff tear prevalence. *Annals of the Royal College of Surgeons of England, 88*(2): 116-121.

Riva, R., P. J. Mork, R. H. Westgaard and U. Lundberg (2012). Comparison of the cortisol awakening response in women with shoulder and neck pain and women with fibromyalgia. *Psychoneuroendocrinology, 37*(2): 299-306.

Riva, R., P. J. Mork, R. H. Westgaard, T. Okkenhaug Johansen and U. Lundberg (2012). Catecholamines and heart rate in female fibromyalgia patients. *Journal of Psychosomatic Research, 72*(1): 51-57.

Sapolsky, R. M. (1998). *Why zebras don't get ulcers: an updated guide to stress, stress-related diseases, and coping*. New York, W.H. Freeman and Co.

Segal, T. Y., P. C. Hindmarsh and R. M. Viner (2005). Disturbed adrenal function in adolescents with chronic fatigue syndrome. *J Pediatr Endocrinol Metab, 18*(3): 295-301.

Sher, J. S., J. W. Uribe, A. Posada, B. J. Murphy and M. B. Zlatkin (1995). Abnormal findings on magnetic resonance images of asymptomatic shoulders. *The Journal of Bone and Joint Surgery. American volume, 77*(1): 10-15.

Simotas, A. C. and T. Shen (2005). Neck pain in demolition derby drivers. *Arch Phys Med Rehabil, 86*(4): 693-696.

Sloan, T. J. and D. A. Walsh (2010). Explanatory and diagnostic labels and perceived prognosis in chronic low back pain. *Spine, 35*(21): E1120-1125.

Smart, K. and C. Doody (2007). The clinical reasoning of pain by experienced musculoskleletal physiotherapists. *Man Ther, 12*: 40-49.

Smart, K. M., C. Blake, A. Staines and C. Doody (2009). Clinical indicators of 'nociceptive', 'peripheral neuropathic' and 'central' mechanisms of musculoskeletal pain. A Delphi survey of expert clinicians. *Man Ther, 15*(1): 80-87.

Smart, K. M., C. Blake, A. Staines and C. Doody (2012). Self-reported pain severity, quality of life, disability, anxiety and depression in patients classified with 'nociceptive', 'peripheral neuropathic' and 'central sensitisation' pain. The discriminant validity of mechanisms-based classifications of low back (+/-leg) pain. *Man Ther, 17*(2): 119-125.

Smart, K. M., C. Blake, A. Staines, M. Thacker and C. Doody (2012). Mechanisms-based classifications of musculoskeletal pain: Part 1 of 3: Symptoms and signs of central sensitisation in patients with low back (+/-leg) pain. *Man Ther, 17*(4): 336-344.

Smart, K. M., C. Blake, A. Staines, M. Thacker and C. Doody (2012). Mechanisms-based classifications of musculoskeletal pain: Part 2 of 3: Symptoms and signs of peripheral neuropathic pain in patients with low back (+/-leg) pain. *Man Ther, 17*(4): 345-351.

Smart, K. M., C. Blake, A. Staines, M. Thacker and C. Doody (2012). Mechanisms-based classifications of musculoskeletal pain: Part 3 of 3: Symptoms and signs of nociceptive pain in patients with low back (+/-leg) pain. *Man Ther, 17*(4): 352-357.

Spielmann, A. L., B. B. Forster, P. Kokan, R. H. Hawkins and D. L. Janzen (1999). Shoulder after rotator cuff repair: MR imaging findings in asymptomatic individuals--initial experience. *Radiology, 213*(3): 705-708.

Stavrinou, M. L., S. Della Penna, V. Pizzella, K. Torquati, F. Cianflone, R. Franciotti, A. Bezerianos, G. L. Romani and P. M. Rossini (2007). Temporal dynamics of plastic changes in human primary somatosensory cortex after finger webbing. *Cereb Cortex, 17*(9): 2134-2142.

Stephens, R., J. Atkins and A. Kingston (2009). Swearing as a response to pain. *Neuroreport, 20*(12): 1056-1060.

Sterling, M., G. Jull and J. Kenardy (2006). Physical and psychological factors maintain long-term predictive capacity post-whiplash injury. *Pain, 122*(1-2): 102-108.

Sterling, M., G. Jull, B. Vicenzino and J. Kenardy (2003). Sensory hypersensitivity occurs soon after whiplash injury and is associated with poor recovery. *Pain, 104*(3): 509-517.

Sterling, M., G. Jull, B. Vicenzino, J. Kenardy and R. Darnell (2005). Physical and psychological factors predict outcome following whiplash injury. *Pain, 114*(1-2): 141-148.

Sterling, M. and J. Kenardy (2008). Physical and psychological aspects of whiplash. Important considerations for primary care assessment *Man Ther, 13*: 93-102.

Sterling, M., J. Treleaven and G. Jull (2002). Responses to a clinical test of mechanical provocation of nerve tissue in whiplash associated disorder. *Man Ther, 7*(2): 89-94.

Taylor, J. R. and L. T. Twomey (1986). Age changes in lumbar zygapophyseal joints. Observations on structure and function. *Spine (Phila Pa 1976), 11*(7): 739-745.

ter Riet, G., A. J. de Craen, A. de Boer and A. G. Kessels (1998). Is placebo analgesia mediated by endogenous opioids? A systematic review. *Pain, 76*(3): 273-275.

Twomey, L. T. and J. R. Taylor (1987). Age changes in lumbar vertebrae and intervertebral discs. *Clin Orthop Relat Res (224)*: 97-104.

van de Ven, M., J. O. Andressoo, V. B. Holcomb, M. von Lindern, W. M. Jong, C. I. De Zeeuw, Y. Suh, P. Hasty, J. H. Hoeijmakers, G. T. van der Horst and J. R. Mitchell (2006). Adaptive stress response in segmental progeria resembles long-lived dwarfism and calorie restriction in mice. *PLOS Genetics, 2*(12): e192.

Van Houdenhove, B., F. Van Den Eede and P. Luyten (2009). Does hypothalamic-pituitary-adrenal axis hypofunction in chronic fatigue syndrome reflect a 'crash' in the stress system? *Med Hypotheses, 72*(6): 701-705.

Van Oosterwijck, J., J. Nijs, M. Meeus, M. Van Loo and L. Paul (2012). Lack of endogenous pain inhibition during exercise in people with chronic whiplash associated disorders: an experimental study. *The Journal of Pain: Official Journal of the American Pain Society, 13*(3): 242-254.

Videman, T., M. C. Battie, L. E. Gibbons, K. Maravilla, H. Manninen and J. Kaprio (2003). Associations between back pain history and lumbar MRI findings. *Spine, 28*(6): 582-588.

Villaneuva, L. and H. L. Fields (2004). Endogenous Central mechanisms of Pain Modulation. *The Pain System in Normal and Pathological States*. L. Villaneuva, A. Dickenson and H. Ollat. Seattle, IASP Press.

Virani, S. N., R. Ferrari and A. S. Russell (2001). Physician resistance to the late whiplash syndrome. *J Rheumatol, 28*(9): 2096-2099.

Vlaeyen, J. W. and S. J. Linton (2000). Fear-avoidance and its consequences in chronic musculoskeletal pain: a state of the art. *Pain, 85*(3): 317-332.

Wade, D. (2006). Why physical medicine, physical disability and physical rehabilitation? We should abandon Cartesian dualism. *Clin Rehab, 20*: 85-90.

Walton, D. M., J. Pretty, J. C. MacDermid and R. W. Teasell (2009). Risk factors for persistent problems following whiplash injury: results of a systematic review and meta-analysis. *The Journal of Orthopaedic and Sports Physical Therapy, 39*(5): 334-350.

Watson, P. and N. Kendall (2000). Assessing psychosocial yellow flags. *Topical Issues in Pain 2*. L. S. Gifford. Falmouth, CNS Press.

Wijdicks, C. A., B. D. Westerhaus, E. J. Brand, S. Johansen, L. Engebretsen and R. F. Laprade (2009). Sartorial branch of the saphenous nerve in relation to a medial knee ligament repair or reconstruction. *Knee Surg Sports Traumatol Arthrosc.*

Woolf, C. J. (1994). The dorsal horn: state dependent sensory processing and the generation of pain. *Textbook of Pain*. P. D. Wall and R. Melzack. Edinburgh, Churchill Livingstone.

Woolf, C. J. (2000). Pain. *Neurobiol Dis, 7*(5): 504-510.

Woolf, C. J. (2007). Central sensitization: uncovering the relation between pain and plasticity. *Anesthesiology, 106*(4): 864-867.

Woolf, C. J. and T. P. Doubell (1994). The pathophysiology of chronic pain - increased sensitivity to low threshold A beta fibre inputs. *Current Opinion in Neurobiology, 4*: 525-534.

Woolf, C. J. and R. J. Mannion (1999). Neuropathic pain: aetiology, symptoms, mechanisms, and management. *Lancet, 353*(9168): 1959-1964.

Woolf , C. J. and M. W. Salter (2005). Plasticity and pain: the role of the dorsal horn. *Wall and Melzack's Textbook of Pain*. S. McMahon and M. Koltzenburg. Edinburgh, Elsevier.

Yeung, E., M. Jones and B. Hall (1997). The response to the slump test in a group of female whiplash patients. *Aust J Physiother, 43*(4): 245-252.

Yukawa, Y., F. Kato, Y. Matsubara, G. Kajino, S. Nakamura and H. Nitta (1996). Serial magnetic resonance imaging follow-up study of lumbar disc herniation conservatively treated for average 30 months: relation between reduction of herniation and degeneration of disc. *J Spinal Disord, 9*(3): 251-256.

Chapter 4

Neuroscience Education for Patients

4.1: Neuroscience Education for Patients

In Chapter 2, we pointed out that biomedical education models have not been found to be helpful and might actually make patients' pain worse. We also pointed out that there is recent and compelling evidence for a therapeutic neuroscience education (TNE) approach. To follow the evidence and incorporate TNE into their clinical approach therapists will need to be able to explain various aspects of neuroscience (Moseley, Hodges et al., 2004; Louw, Diener et al., 2011). Chapter 3 presented the current best understanding of the neuroscience of pain by using the revised Pain Neuroscience Questionnaire (R-PNQ). The challenge now is to present this information to the patient in an easy-to-understand format.

Patients want to know more about their pain (Louw, Louw et al., 2009), and healthcare providers consistently underestimate their ability to understand the neuroscience of pain (Moseley, 2003). Clinicians will need to carefully consider the language and terminology that they use with their patients. Too often, healthcare information provided by a therapist is seen as a proud display of knowledge or it is presented in such a complex manner that it sounds like a foreign language to the patient. For it to be effective, educational material must be understood and the patient must see how it applies to their specific situation. It has been shown that patients relate more readily to metaphors, examples, pictures and drawings (Louw, Diener et al., 2011; Gallagher, McAuley et al., 2013). The material presented in Chapters 2 and 3 and, more specifically, a recent systematic review on TNE appears to have set the script that therapists should follow in their TNE sessions. TNE should include discussion of nociceptive pathways, neurons, synapses, action potentials, spinal inhibition and facilitation, peripheral and central sensitization, and plasticity of the nervous system (Louw, Diener et al., 2011).

In the next chapter of this book, we will provide guidelines for clinical application of TNE. Given the complexity and individual nature of pain, the precise starting point will vary from patient to patient and clinical scenario to clinical scenario. In this chapter, we aim to utilize the newfound understanding of the neuroscience of pain and develop "patient language" to help educate the patient. Each topic will feature the following:

- A therapist introductory section describing the general goal of the section.

- A patient section, utilizing patient language to show an example of how to educate a patient regarding the particular topic. The patient section will also feature prepared pictures used in TNE studies and clinical practice.

- An image section. Images are powerful; a list is provided at the conclusion of each section, based on the section's information. We propose that therapists should gather such images to develop a clinical tool for educating patients.

4.2: Alarm Systems, Nails in the Foot and Christmas Trees

THERAPIST

The aim of this topic is to educate patients about nerves. It has been proposed that patients have poor beliefs regarding nerves and often equate nerves with pain (Coppieters, Ryan et al., 2005).

PATIENT

In your body, and in all people, there are over 400 individual nerves or, better yet, 45 miles of nerves traveling through the body, connecting all body parts. These nerves are all connected like a road/highway system. Nerves work like an alarm system. At all times, nerves have a little bit of electricity traveling through them, which is normal and shows you're alive. Depending on many different factors, such as stress, movement, temperature, etc., the electrical activity in nerves can go up or down.

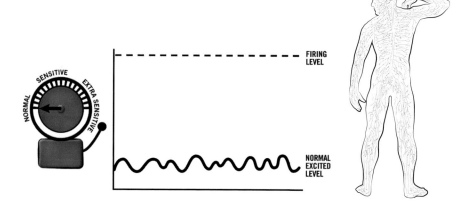

However, nerves have thresholds. When nerves get excited enough to reach the threshold, the message from the area will be sent on to your brain for analysis and, possibly, appropriate action.

If you step on a rusted nail, do you want to know about it? The answer is obviously yes, in order to get a tetanus shot, take the nail out, walk funny and get some help. In this case, the alarm system goes off.

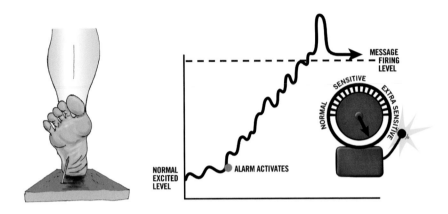

As soon as the alarm system goes off and sends the message, the alarm system will return to its resting level, ready to warn of additional danger.

Another way to think of this is a Christmas tree. It is already established that if you step on a rusted nail, you'd like to know about it. When you step on a nail, the nerves in your foot light up like a Christmas tree, sending alarm signals to the spinal cord and, ultimately, the brain for action to be taken.

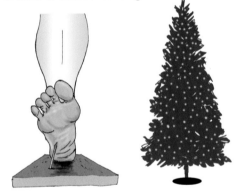

Once the message has been received, it is reasonable to turn the Christmas tree lights down. The brain ultimately makes the decision, once the message has been received, that it's OK to turn the Christmas tree lights down. Think of it this way: Dad walks down the stairs, sees the Christmas tree lights have been on for a while and asks, "Who's paying for that?" He tells you to turn the Christmas tree lights down. After a few days of this, the message has been received (Christmas is over), and it's OK to turn them down, pack them into the box and store for the next time their needed.

IMAGES
Images pertaining to this section would include action potentials, a foot stepping onto a rusted nail, a Christmas tree and a full body nervous system.

4.3: Waking Up the Alarm System

THERAPIST

Section 4.2 describes the normal electrical activity of the nervous system and how the nervous system acts like an alarm system (Louw, Puentedura et al., 2011; Louw, 2012). It is proposed that a major goal of TNE is for patients to understand that their pain is not related to the health of their tissues but rather to increased nerve sensitivity (Moseley, 2007; Louw, Diener et al., 2011). This section may be powerful enough to change pain behaviors in many patients, even though it is still a rather peripheralistic view of pain (Louw, Puentedura et al., 2011). The main goal of this next section is to have patients develop a deeper understanding that injured tissues will heal, and a persistent pain experience may have more to do with heightened sensitivity in their nervous system (Tifford, Spero et al., 2000; Sterling, Jull et al., 2003; Louw, Puentedura et al., 2011).

PATIENT

Recap of section 4.2

Nerves work like an alarm system. At all times, nerves have a little bit of electricity traveling through them, which is normal and shows you're alive. Depending on many different factors, such as stress, movement, temperature, etc., the activity can go up or down. However, nerves have thresholds. When nerves get excited enough to reach the threshold, the message from the area will be sent on to your brain for analysis and, possibly, appropriate action. If you step on a rusted nail, do you want to know about it? The answer is obviously yes, in order to get a tetanus shot, take the nail out, walk funny and get some help. As soon as the alarm system goes off and sends the message, the alarm system will return to its resting level, ready to warn of additional danger.

We now know that in approximately one in four people, the alarm system gets activated following a threat, but the alarm system rests just slightly below firing level instead of returning to its resting level. The nerve is thereby "extra sensitive."

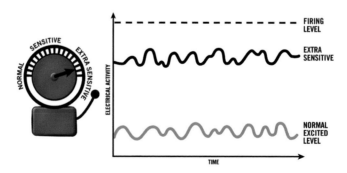

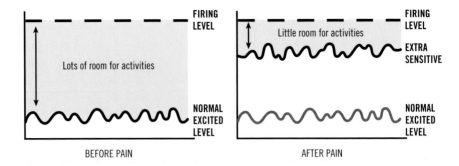

BEFORE PAIN

This is not that uncommon and actually quite normal, but it impedes movement and function quite a bit. In the following graphs, you can clearly see how the sensitivity of the alarm system has impacted your activities. Before you developed pain, you were able to do a lot of activities with no problem, for example, drive and sit two hours in a car. After sitting so long and driving, tissues get sore and tired (as expected) and start sending messages to your brain saying: "stop, get out, take a break and move a little to get some blood flowing again." In this scenario, the nerves will calm down to their resting level, allowing for another two-hour stint of driving.

Since you developed pain, you may have noticed, and likely told many doctors and therapists, it takes only five minutes of the same activity, e.g., driving, to cause the same pain. Tissues heal and we now know that the longer pain lasts, the more likely it is due to extra-sensitive nerves in the area. Now that your nerves are 'extra sensitive,' it does not take much to reach the alarm level. No wonder you think something must be wrong.

Another way to view this 'extra-sensitive' alarm system is to think of a house alarm. An alarm system is set up at your home. Normal day-to-day activities do not set off the alarm. It's set to be sensitive to big issues, e.g., breaking a window. Since you have developed pain, your alarm system is so sensitive (i.e., your nerves are so sensitive) that when a leaf blows by the house, it sets off the alarm. The system needs to be changed to decrease its sensitivity.

In describing this extra-sensitive alarm setting, we have encountered three typical questions patients such as you commonly ask and thought it may be good to answer these to help you develop a greater understanding of extra-sensitive nerves:

1. How do healthcare providers know the alarm system is extra sensitive?

2. Why did your nerves stay so extra sensitive and not calm down to their normal resting level?

3. What can be done to calm the extra-sensitive nerves down to the normal resting level?

4.3a: How do healthcare providers know the alarm system is extra sensitive?

This is a common question, especially if medical tests show up as normal, including nerve conduction tests. Unfortunately, there are no medical tests that are able to detect 'extra-sensitive' nerves at this time. The good news is that current medical tests are designed to detect big, threatening issues, and people with persistent pain are tested extensively, which typically clears major issues. If you listen to your own story, you will find that you instinctively know something has slowed you down. It does not take a lot of activity or emotion to experience pain. You may even experience being extra sensitive to certain movements, pressure against body parts or certain activities. Healthcare providers can detect extra-sensitive nerves as they test you, especially using physical movement tests. You may even notice sensitivity away from the area you have most of your pain. If you remember, you have a network of 45 miles of nerves and they are all connected, allowing a pathway to spread sensitivity. Finally, physicians often indirectly inform other healthcare providers, such as therapists, of the extra-sensitive nerves by the medication they prescribe. Membrane stabilizers and anti-depressants are designed to calm the nervous system down. A quick scan of your medicine list shows that your physician may think your nerves are extra sensitive and is trying to help with the medicine he or she is prescribing.

4.3b: Why did your nerves stay so extra sensitive and not calm down to their normal resting level?

This is a common question, especially if a seemingly similar situation, e.g., injury from a car accident or surgery, occurred to a family member, friend or neighbor and they are fine. First of all, the extra-sensitive nerves are normal and occur in everyone. In some people, the nerves calm down quickly and in others, a little more slowly. It is now well established that the sensitivity of your alarm system will be determined by various factors going on in your life at the time of the pain, including failed treatments, family issues, levels of fear, concerns about your job, and even having been given different explanations for your pain.

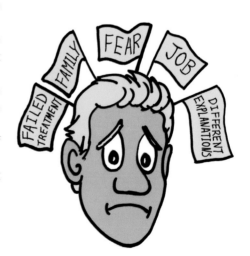

If pain persists, you will undoubtedly have seen numerous healthcare providers. Every time you hoped that it would work but, after a while, it has not. Every time a treatment does not work, you get a little more worried. What is going on? This should be better by now. In this scenario your brain, which determines the sensitivity level of your nerves, has little incentive to decrease the sensitivity of the alarm system, leaving it extra sensitive. Additionally, each person trying to help may have a different opinion. Surely not all of them can be right. The list keeps growing, which ends up making you more confused. As long as the cause for your persistent pain is unknown or poorly answered, the brain might as well keep the defenses up, so the alarm system is kept at the extra-sensitive level. Although we believe pain is normal, living in pain daily is not normal. This can add more stress, worry and a need to keep the alarm system elevated. The list can go on and on, including various concerns about your job, family issues and finances. Simply stated, all the concerns surrounding a pain experience can keep the alarm system elevated. Again, this is a normal process, and understanding how various factors can keep the alarm system elevated is a key factor in treating your pain.

4.3c: What can be done to calm the extra-sensitive nerves down to the normal resting level?

Most people want to know about this one right off the bat. It is important to have a good understanding of why your nerves have remained extra sensitive, because that alone can actually help decrease the sensitivity of the alarm system. Calming the nervous system down closer to the resting level requires education, blood flow, oxygen and medication. The good news is that if you understand this concept of nerve sensitivity and an 'extra-sensitive' level, you are already in the process of decreasing the sensitivity. Exciting new research has shown that if people understand more about their pain, the alarm system immediately starts turning down its sensitivity. This makes sense. The alarm system is kept on high alert when there are more questions than answers. By understanding that your pain is likely due to sensitive nerves rather than injured tissues, which heal, fear is reduced, which in turn calms the nerves.

As for blood flow and oxygen, research has shown that aerobic exercise aimed at increasing blood flow and oxygen in your body has a significant calming effect on your nerves. No need to run marathons or climb mountains! Studies show that a brisk walk, a swim or a bike ride resulting in a little sweat is more than enough.

The final strategy involves medicine. Drug companies have developed a series of drugs to calm nerves down. Any questions related to your medication should be directed to your physician. There is, however, another drug cabinet we can utilize in the brain. The brain produces the most potent pain medicine on the planet, helping people survive severe injuries while experiencing little or no pain. The brain produces these "happy chemicals" that have a calming effect on the alarm system. We can describe this scenario as a 'wet brain:' a brain that is juicy – full of good, healthy medicine and able to release them to help you when you are in pain. We now know that people with persistent pain have 'dry brains' where the healthy medicine has dried up, making them more sensitive to protect. Interestingly, aerobic exercise also helps release these happy chemicals. Understanding more about your pain helps open up a dry brain, to become a wet brain.

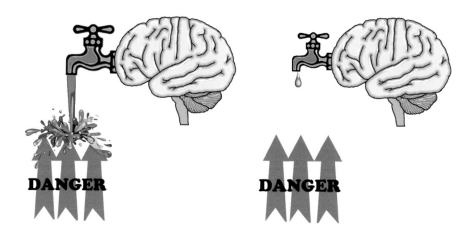

IMAGES

Images that therapists may consider using in describing an extra-sensitive nervous system may include an action potential, an action potential allowing space to show or draw extra-sensitive nerves and a brain with blank flags allowing a patient to reflect and fill in their own flags that are keeping their alarm system extra sensitive.

4.4: Nerve Sensors

THERAPIST

Apart from nerves becoming extra sensitive, nerves also have the biological capacity to develop sensitivity to various non-traditional stimuli (Devor, 2006; Louw and Butler, 2011). Pain is based on the perception of threat. A patient experiencing increased pain when faced with a stressful situation or pain that seems to increase with cold weather are examples of non-traditional stimuli enhancing nerve sensitization and, ultimately, a pain experience. It is proposed that explaining the biological process of ion channels in an easy-to-understand way may indeed help decrease a pain experience.

PATIENT

Your alarm system is even more complicated. You may have noticed that beyond the "normal" sensitivity described, you may have become sensitive to other things, such as cold temperature or stress. Inside your nerves, there are various sensors also designed to protect and inform you of any changes in your life. Many different kinds of sensors have been identified, but the following may be of particular interest to you:

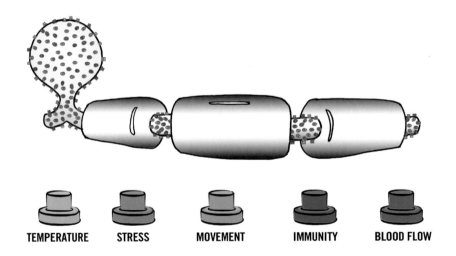

TEMPERATURE   STRESS   MOVEMENT   IMMUNITY   BLOOD FLOW

- **Temperature**—There are sensors in nerves that tell you if there is a change in temperature. It's not uncommon to become sensitive to cold temperature and feel more aches and pains in the affected area when it gets cold outside.

- **Stress**–There are sensors in nerves that are sensitive to stress chemicals flowing in your blood. The more stressed, anxious, nervous or upset you are, the more you will experience aches and pains. The more stress chemicals that run through your body, the more likely additional stress sensors will be activated.

- **Blood flow**–There are sensors in your nerves that are sensitive to the amount of blood around your tissues. When blood flow slows down slightly, for example, after sitting too long, these sensors "wake up" and make the nerve sensitive.

- **Movement and pressure**–There are sensors in your nerves that are sensitive to movement and pressure around them. For example, movement after injury may activate a few more sensors and make the movement more sensitive for a little while.

- **Immunity**–When you're sick with the flu, there are many immune molecules floating through your body helping you deal with the illness. This is the same following injury or surgery. Recent research shows that when you are really worried or have an inflamed body part, you'll have an immune response. Nerves have sensors telling them of the increased immune molecules, and the immune chemicals produced can make you ache.

Knowing more about your nerve sensors can help you understand more about your pain. When you developed pain, your nerves increased their sensitivity to protect you. This is a normal response and happens in every human being. These sensors are constantly updated based on your environment. Your sensitive nerves can therefore be changed for the better.

Another way to view these sensors is to think of your car. Modern cars have sensors all over them to alert you of any issues, such as oil pressure, low fuel or an engine problem. Any of these issues could cause a dashboard light to switch on. Our body dashboard may thus light up with any of the sensors being activated. This is normal and does not necessarily signal injury or disease, but rather sensitivity.

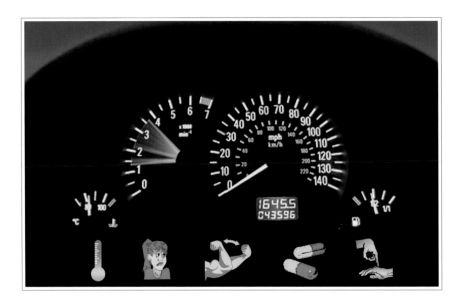

As mentioned before, some people's nerves are slow to calm down. Why is this? In some people, there may be so many issues surrounding the injury that the brain decides it's best to keep the alarm system elevated. These factors have already been discussed and include multiple explanations for your pain, failed treatments, worries about job, family and money, and many more.

At this point, you may ask what can be done. The good news is that nerve sensors change all the time. Most sensors change over every 2-3 days, which is heavily influenced by your understanding of your pain. Also think of what stimulus is activating the sensor and, more importantly, what you can do to take the stimulus away from the sensor. This may include gentle movement allowing more blood and oxygen in the area that calms nerves down. Meditation, relaxation or just some nice cleansing deep breaths may help.

The key, however, appears to be knowledge. The next time you're outside and a bit of cold air comes across the arm in which you recently had surgery or an injury, it will most definitely activate the nerve sensors, and the sensors will activate the alarm system to let you, your brain, know there is an issue in the arm. With your newfound knowledge of nerve sensors and alarm systems, your new, well-educated brain will likely realize: "It's just cold out and my alarm system is telling me it is cold; nothing is really wrong." In this scenario, there is no need to make the alarm system extra sensitive. The alarm system will steadily, over time, be turned down and less pain will be experienced.

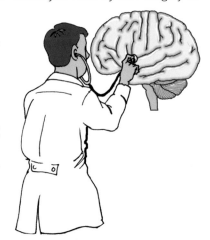

IMAGES

To educate patients on the complexities of ion channel expression and a pain experience, therapists may consider showing a picture of a car dashboard with various sensors and equate it to ion channel expression.

4.5: Speeding Buses Hurt More than Ankle Sprains

THERAPIST

Patients often equate pain with injury and injury with pain. In this section, we aim to have patients develop an understanding that injury and pain are not synonymous (Moseley, 2007). Additionally, it is very important to shift patients to the realization that pain is an output from the brain, rather than an input to the brain (Moseley, 2003). Many patients incorrectly believe that pain is an input, where injuries and diseased tissues send "pain signals into the spinal cord to the brain" and that is why they are experiencing pain.

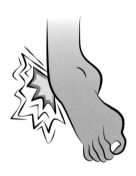

PATIENT

If you sprained your ankle right now, would it hurt? Probably everyone would answer yes. Ankle injury is associated with pain. Now, what happens if you sprain your ankle, but it happens while you're crossing a busy road? As you roll your ankle, out of the corner of your eye you see a speeding bus coming straight for you. It's not stopping. Does the ankle still hurt? Of course the ankle doesn't hurt! In this case, it isn't logical for the brain to produce pain in the ankle. Pain in the ankle would cause you to fall down, grab the ankle and leave you with no effective way of dealing with the speeding bus. If you could listen in on the brain during such decision-making situations, the brain would undoubtedly have to decide which is more dangerous, a speeding bus or an ankle sprain?

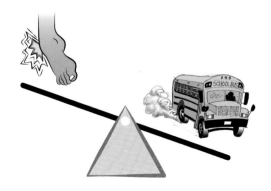

Have you ever been out in the yard raking leaves and, when you sat down to have something to drink, you noticed blood on your leg? In this case, there was tissue injury, i.e., a scrape on the leg, but no pain. Maybe your brain got the danger messages from the scrape, but it's a nice day outside, working and having fun was more important, so the brain decided not to produce pain. Can you remember such a time?

There are many examples of people having tissue injury, but no pain. Look at the X-ray of a man's head with a nail in it. He went to his doctor for a headache. Can you imagine the doctor's face when he saw the X-ray? When the doctor asked the man about it, he said he thought it may have happened four years ago! Could it be that he worked at a busy, noisy construction site and, perhaps, was so focused on his work he didn't realize a nail went into his head? Do you have examples you can think of? Have you ever heard of athletes competing despite injury or soldiers having been shot during battle but were not aware of it?

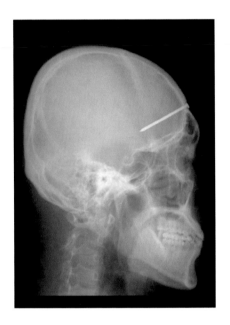

Many people with pain claim they have no tissue issues or have never had an injury, and all tests came back negative. So why do they hurt? Tissues do not have to be injured for pain to be experienced. As the brain evaluates all threats, such as stress, anxiety or tissue injury, it may decide to defend you by producing pain. Many patients in pain tell us they just started developing pain without an injury. Pain can easily be developed due to emotional overload or stress.

IMAGES
To educate patients about tissues and pain, therapists may wish to use images of an ankle sprain, a speeding bus, and a scale to weigh the relative importance of the bus and ankle. It may also be helpful to have pictures of 'amazing x-rays' such as the nail in the head.

4.6: CEO Making Big Decisions

THERAPIST

The goal of this session is to explain to patients the concept of central sensitization along with an increase in widespread sensitization and action potential windup. This session also discusses plasticity of the central nervous system, which is important for patients as "an ability to change" provides hope.

PATIENT

All the areas in which you experience pain have extra-sensitive nerves. They need to send information somewhere, so something can be done. Nerves pass information on to the spinal cord, which passes it on to the brain. This allows your brain to process the information and take action, such as stopping movement of a painful body part and going to see the doctor. When pain persists and there are many worries, the brain will analyze the incoming messages of danger very closely. A good way to think of this is when you press an 'X' on your computer keyboard and 'XXXX' shows up on your screen, instead. It's not the information you sent. Somehow, your computer overanalyzed your input on the computer keyboard. This response does not seem fair, but it's normal and essential to your survival. The danger messages from your already overactive nerves are amplified as they reach your brain. The best way to understand why this occurs is to see your brain as the body's Chief Executive Officer (CEO).

Think of a large office building or organization. At the top floor is the CEO, running the organization. It's customary for each division of the company to provide the CEO with monthly reports. Monthly reports, however, follow a line of command. The department manager develops the report and then passes it on to the director who analyzes it and makes a few corrections if needed. Then he passes his version of the report on to the vice president. The vice president also checks the report, makes changes as needed, and finally passes it on to the CEO. What happens when there's a problem in a division? When a division of a company is under-performing, it's customary for a CEO to become worried. The CEO now asks for weekly reports to find out what the issues are and to keep an eye on the department. To ensure timely reports from the problem division, the CEO also informs the department manager to send the message straight to him/her, bypassing the director and vice president, to speed up the communication process and allow for faster action. Once enough information is gathered by the CEO, action is taken to correct the problem.

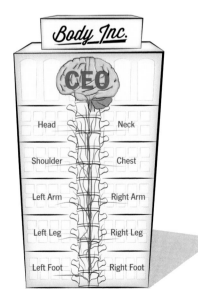

Each of your body parts, such as your shoulders and hips, are divisions in the larger company called Body, Inc.

Your body parts constantly send information to the brain to inform them of how they're doing.

The information is sent to the brain, the CEO, via the nervous system and various checkpoints along the way, similar to how CEOs receive messages from managers, directors and vice presidents. En route, the message can become altered.

If there's persistent pain in an area, the organizational process described previously is likely to occur. As a result, more information will be sent to the brain. When pain persists, extra-sensitive nerves send increased messages to the spinal cord and, ultimately, to the brain to analyze. This is no fun, but again, a normal, protective process to help you deal with the pain. In the process, the messages to the brain will be less altered, and the brain will become more aware of the painful body part.

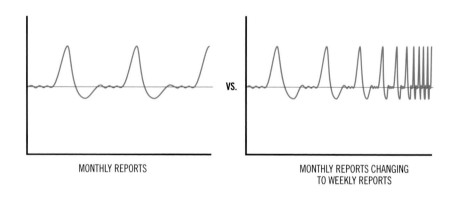

MONTHLY REPORTS   VS.   MONTHLY REPORTS CHANGING
                                      TO WEEKLY REPORTS

A VERY IMPORTANT next step follows. When the report finally arrives at the CEO's desk, it would make sense to carefully analyze all the data, as if using a magnifying glass. This magnification performs a protective task, which is normal. To add to the complexity, we need to remember that most CEOs are paranoid. Once the CEO is dealing with the troubled section, for example, the lower back, the CEO may start worrying about other divisions: snooping around and asking for more reports from them. Now the organization, Body, Inc. (you), becomes aware of all these areas. Experiencing pain in other adjacent areas could be seen

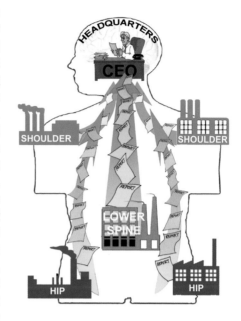

as normal and part of this survival process. It's not an indication of injury but rather of sensitive nerves in the area and a CEO snooping around to make sure everything at Body, Inc. is OK.

IMAGES

Therapists aiming to educate patients more about central sensitization may consider finding an image of a large office building to describe the CEO phenomenon. Clinically, a commonly used body chart may also suffice to show how various body parts inform the body's CEO, the brain, of their status. Additionally, therapists should also practice drawing the action potential windup to show how, especially during persistent pain, there is an amplification of information.

4.7: Nosy Neighbors

THERAPIST

When pain is experienced in areas remote from the originating site, it is likely to induce fear and anxiety. By explaining how a sensitive nervous system develops spreading sensitization, a patient's fear can be allayed, thus helping the pain experience. A key part of this description is for patients to develop an understanding that pain in other areas is more a result of spreading sensitization rather than spreading injury.

PATIENT

When you develop pain in an area of your body and the nerves in the area "wake up," there are usually some interested neighbors. Remember that your nervous system is connected, and the nervous system works like an alarm system. If the alarm in your house were to go off, it would probably wake the neighbors right next to you. They would be curious and concerned about you. If the alarm kept going, some neighbors down the street might also wake up. Nerves work in the same way. The areas where you are experiencing pain have the alarm system going off all the time, and the tissue's neighbors have been awakened. It is not uncommon to experience some sensitivity, such as aches and pains in areas adjacent to the involved areas, or to sense a spreading pain.

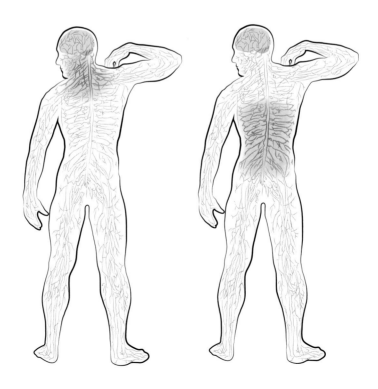

To add to this already irritable neighbor situation, the police are called to inspect the neighborhood. Your body contains various immune molecules traveling through your body to make sure you stay healthy. Think of immune molecules as police officers, checking out the neighborhood. With the alarms going off, the police are called to check if everything is OK. The police then go door-to-door, checking on all the neighbors. This in itself will make the situation a little testier. While the police, or your immune molecules, are checking in on the neighborhood, adjacent neighborhoods are also checked on, thus waking the other neighborhoods, as well. This process is normal and expected. Agitated nerves may be felt as aches, but they do not indicate injury. It's important to note that 'previous crime areas' in your body, such as old surgeries, scars and previously injured areas, will definitely be checked out by the police. Remember: there are nerve sensors that will sense the immune molecules, and old aches and pains may show up again. It is important to realize that this is simply due to sensitivity – not injury.

IMAGES
As with the description of the CEO and central sensitization, therapists may use a simple blank body chart to describe and/or draw spreading pain. To further enhance this, therapists may even consider using blank pages of a whole body nervous system to drive home the fact that the nervous system is connected and, thus, a likely conduit for spreading sensitization. The immune response and potential additional wake-up of the nervous system can be portrayed with a picture of police knocking at the door.

4.8: Little People in Your Head

THERAPIST
The goal of this section is to explain the somatosensory cortex to patients and how pain is allocated to body parts. This section will cover the "use it or lose it" phenomenon, encouraging patients to move and use body parts during exercise. The education session also explains increased pain in body parts that have misrepresentation such as Complex Regional Pain Syndrome (CRPS) (Maihofner, Handwerker et al., 2003; Moseley, 2004; Marinus, Moseley et al., 2011) and when body parts are not present, e.g., phantom limb pain (Flor, Elbert et al., 1995; Moseley and Flor, 2012).

PATIENT

Have you ever wondered how people experience pain in a body part that does not even exist? In phantom limb pain, people often describe significant pain in their foot or hand, but the foot or hand has been amputated. Not only is this an interesting question but it is also very important to understanding your pain experience.

Several years ago, scientists were able to record brain activity while carefully stimulating various body parts in animals and later in human beings. The end result of these experiments is that we now know there are body maps in your brain where each part of your body, hands, feet, etc., is represented in your head. Do a simple little experiment. Close your eyes and think of your right hand. Now, while your eyes are closed, touch your nose and return to the starting point. All of this is done quite easily without your eyes to guide you. This "knowing" where your hand is, your left versus right, and where your nose is, is based on the map in your head.

In healthy people, these maps are clear, well-defined or 'sharply focused.' When pain affects a body part, for example, your right hand, the map is a little messed up; it's "fuzzy," as if the sharp lines are blurred or it's 'out of focus.' Unfortunately, we now also know that the more a body part is out of focus, the more pain is present. Due to pain, the hand (or affected body part) is not used as much and it's thought that using the hand (or body part) is essential to keep the body maps healthy and sharply focused. Movement is therefore a key component in recovery. Regular use of a body part allows for the constant training and recognition of the body part and is vital for recovery. Gentle, easy, repetitive movement and understanding pain is helpful in defining body parts in this body map in the brain.

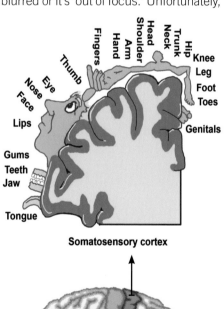

Somatosensory cortex

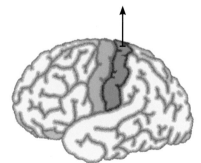

In scenarios where it is too painful to move a body part, it may be helpful to close your eyes and imagine where the body part is or imagine gentle easy movements, without actually moving. This will help keep the map healthy, the body part well represented and ease some pain, eventually allowing for healthy movement to further recover the map. Understanding that these maps are, in a sense, "fed" by movement should help you understand why movement is essential and that exercise, even though seemingly mundane and boring, helps keep the maps healthy and directly helps ease pain. Another way to think of this is how athletes repeatedly practice the same tasks over and over, for example, basketball free throws, golf swing, etc. As a result, they become really good at the task.

If you happen to have pain in a body part that is not there anymore, say after an amputation, the same process applies. Even though the hand or foot is not there, the map is still in the brain. Since the map is not getting much of a workout, the body part is likely "fuzzy" or even missing. The most potent defender the brain has available for protection is pain. Quite simply, pain is produced by the brain; as long as the brain is confused, more pain will be produced. Understanding why there is still pain helps ease stress and anxiety and calms the brain and nervous system down, thus easing some pain. Exercising the maps in the brain is very important. Visualization, recognizing left and right body parts, mirrors and watching other people move can help restore these maps and ease pain.

IMAGES

The most powerful image to use in body map recognition and pain is the somatosensory homunculus. This image will help patients realize there are body maps and, with additional instruction, as above, help solidify the importance of keeping these maps healthy. Mirror box images can further help patients delve into the complexities of body part recognition, making them understand how changing what the brain sees can alter the pain experience. Therapists may also wish to show patients the case series of visual illusions used by Moseley to help paraplegics reconceptualize their legs and, thus, alter their pain experience (Moseley, 2007).

4.9: Airlines are Flying Through Your Head

THERAPIST

The goal of this section is to explain that multiple brain areas are involved in processing nociception and, ultimately, a potential pain neural signature. Additionally, therapists can help patients understand how various aspects associated with pain can increase pain or start a pain experience, e.g., memory, words and visions. Finally, patients need to understand how the pain neural signature impacts the function of other brain areas that are called upon during normal functioning, e.g., motor control, focus, concentration and memory.

PATIENT

The brain's processing of danger messages from the tissues is important in understanding your pain. For years, it was generally believed that there was a single pain area in the brain. When you stub your toe, the light bulb flashes on and there it is – pain. If pain were so simple, it would be easy to cut this area out of the brain, and all pain would be gone. When you have a pain experience, it is now well established by scientists that various areas of your brain are involved in processing this pain experience. These areas then connect and form a pain map. This happens for any and all kinds of pain. Patients diagnosed with low back pain, neck pain, fibromyalgia and chronic fatigue syndrome have very similar brain areas that light up during a pain experience.

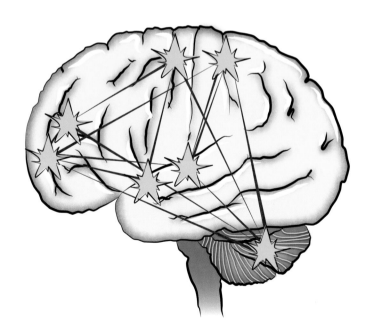

These areas that light up in a pain experience also deal with the following:

Sensation–Each body part, such as your back, neck, shoulder, hand or foot, is represented in the brain. Your brain tells you where you are experiencing sensations in your body, including pain.

Movement–The areas that plan, coordinate and execute your movements are also busy protecting you. Maybe some muscles needed to protect you will stiffen up and not allow you to bend as far forward.

Focus and concentration–The areas dealing with focus and concentration are also busy dealing with your pain experience.

Fear–The emotional areas of the brain dealing with fear, such as fear of injury, re-injury or even fear of movement, are called upon, especially when pain is poorly understood.

Memory–The areas of the brain dealing with memory are busy. They remember previous similar experiences and call on those strategies to help.

Motivation–The area dealing with motivation is now used to process pain instead of motivating.

Stress responses–There are specialized areas in the brain that deal with stress. These centers control the release of various stress chemicals, such as adrenaline and cortisol, into the body to help protect you. These centers also control sleep, appetite, body weight, and body temperature.

The key issue here is that many brain areas are involved in all pain experiences. These areas then communicate with each other to "discuss" the appropriate action. Think of it as a board meeting in your brain. When danger messages are received from the tissues, the brain calls a board meeting to discuss these danger messages. If the board believes there is a threat and action is required, it produces pain to protect you.

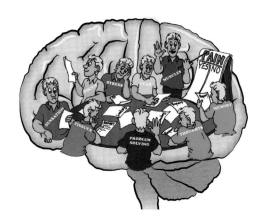

Another way to think of it is an airline map. If you page through any airline magazine, you will notice the map showing where the airline flies. With all the areas in your brain processing danger messages, you have developed something similar to an airline map in the brain. In addition, it's important for you to know that just as in real life, people fly different airlines. Each person that experiences pain uses similar areas of the brain, but the pathways are different. Pain is individualized, which makes it so hard to treat. You need treatment tailored to your pain.

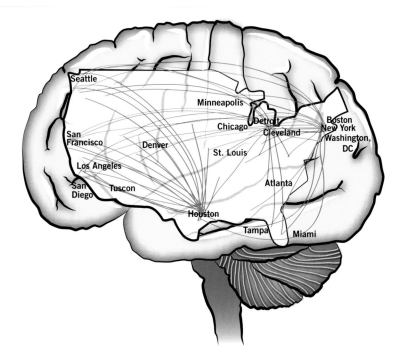

A common but unfortunate saying is that 'pain is in your head.' The saying implies that it's not real; it is fabricated. This is not true. Yes, pain is located in your head within your brain. When you have pain, the brain is very active processing it. How your brain processes information determines the pain you experience. So, yes, your pain experience is 'in your head,' but it is very real. It can be measured, and it can be changed for the better.

IMAGES

An easy way for therapists to educate patients on the pain neuromatrix is a blank, black and white picture of a brain. This allows the ability to highlight areas specific to the patient, connect them and personalize their pain experience. Airline maps provide a good metaphor and visual expression, especially when two different airlines are contrasted to show they service the same cities, but the pathways are different. With the emerging neuroscience of pain, actual images of the pain neuromatrix and even fMRI images can be found and used to educate patients.

4.10: Driving the Same Road Over and Over and Over and…

THERAPIST

The goal of this section is to have patients develop a greater understanding of the brain's processing of pain and how living in pain strengthens pathways and heightens sensitivity. This section also aims to explain why previous tasks that were not painful may now be very painful and why it does not take a lot to activate pain.

PATIENT

Various areas of the brain are activated during a pain experience, thus involving the whole brain, similar to a board meeting. These areas communicate with each other and develop a pain map, which is individualized for each person. When you develop pain, for instance, after an injury, the map is activated. As tissues heal over time, stress and anxieties ease and progress is made, causing the map to slowly fade away. When pain lasts longer than it should, the map is used a lot and changes are bound to happen. For example, every day you drive the same road to work. You live in a rural area and drive a single-lane dirt road to work. It is a single-lane dirt road, so you drive a little slower and carefully. This is similar to the process in your brain when you first develop pain. For example, you bend forward and your back sends danger messages to the brain, activating your pain map. In this case, the danger messages are new and travel a simple, easy dirt road to communicate the information between the various brain areas.

Returning to the story of a daily commute to work, the county is studying traffic patterns to determine the needs of the community. The county assessor counts the number of trips taken on this particular dirt road. This single-lane dirt road (pain map) is travelled a lot lately. Based on the increased use of this road, the assessor determines the road needs to be widened to a two-lane dirt road. This results in faster speeds. The same process occurs in pain. If you experience pain for a while, the circuitry (road) gets travelled a lot more, the pathways are widened and speeds increase. After a while, if pain persists as well as anxiety and fear, the road is constantly utilized, leaving the county assessor to determine that the road needs to be paved due to the volume of traffic. This once again allows for more traffic and higher speeds. The trend continues, potentially expanding the double-lane paved road to a four-lane freeway, etc.

What does this have to do with pain? If you live in pain every day and constantly use these paths in the brain, they change. They run easier and faster and, in essence, get you to experience pain faster and easier. You may have noticed in the past it took 30 minutes of doing laundry to produce pain and now it takes barely five minutes. Another part of your increased sensitivity is due to the efficiency of the road system and the continuous driving of the same path over and over. Reflect on this as well: the same thing happens in professional athletes but on a more positive note. Constant repetition of tasks (driving the road a lot) makes seemingly difficult athletic tasks look quite simple.

A key message here is that the pain you experience is not necessarily an indication of bad or injured tissues. The nervous system has just become more sophisticated in processing your pain, which makes tasks seem more painful. There is a saying that 'nerves that fire together, wire together,' and this helps us understand the ability of the nervous system to create faster pathways (four-lane freeways). It is currently believed that this increased sensitivity of the nervous system is the key process behind most persistent pain. The good news is there are many strategies to calm the nervous system down, including understanding more about your pain, aerobic exercise, relaxation, breathing, medicine and lots more.

IMAGES
As with section 4.8, all the images helping patients understand the neuromatrix would be helpful to educate them on the multiple brain areas and pathways. The blank brain with drawn areas activated and connected can be used powerfully here with the ability to go over the pathways with markers showing how the paths expand their width.

4.11: Believing Everything You See

THERAPIST
The current definition of pain leads us to believe pain is a response based on perception of threat. The key word here is 'perception.' Many patients in pain have deep-rooted beliefs regarding bulging discs, arthritis and more. By showing a patient how 'perceptions' are not necessarily reality, specifically how tissue findings may not correlate to pain, it may open a window for TNE to become effective. By discussing a simple sense such as vision and then relating it to pain, patients often have the "ah-hah" moments.

PATIENT

'Pain is the process whereby your brain, based on everything it knows about your current situation, makes a conscious decision to defend you.' To understand this statement, look at the process whereby your brain processes information. First, some clarification is needed. This does not mean there's something going on in your head that isn't real. It's important that you see how the brain processes information in all people. A fun way to start viewing how the brain works would be to look at other body senses, such as vision, using a visual illusion. Look at the two lines below. Which one is longer?

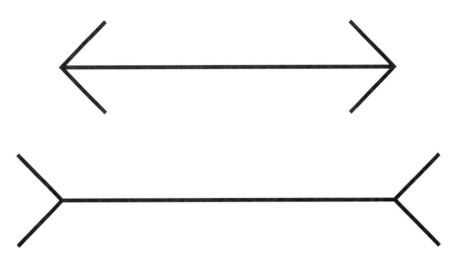

The interesting fact is that they are the same length. When the brain is confronted with a visual illusion, the brain makes its most logical choice based on everything the brain knows about shapes, sizes, measurements, experience and logic. It makes you believe that one line is longer than the other. Why is your brain doing this? It's the most logical choice, even though it's wrong. The interesting thing is that the brain makes the same decisions when it comes to interpreting the health of your tissues.

For example, you may have developed low back pain. In the meantime, your experience with low back pain has led you to see many healthcare providers, you have been given many ideas and thoughts, and you may even have taken a look on the Internet. If you are not well schooled on what all the medical tests and findings mean, it is likely that your perception of your low back situation may indeed be bleak. This will likely result in increased stress and anxiety, which will further increase your pain

IMAGES

There is a plethora of visual illusions that can be used to have patients realize how quickly decisions are made and how incorrect decisions are also made.

4.12: Wet and Dry Brains

THERAPIST

The goal of this section is to have patients understand how the brain can modulate pain. With descending inhibition calming danger messages from the tissues and with facilitation, a heightened sensitivity of the nervous system, such as central sensitization, may occur. Furthermore, this session aims to educate patients on strategies that may help engage the endogenous mechanisms and, thus, help modulate the pain experience.

PATIENT

When you stub your toe it really hurts, right? How long does it hurt badly? A few seconds and then it seem to "ease." What happens here? We now know that the brain has the most advanced drug cabinet known to man. The brain produces chemicals, which it uses to ease the danger messages. This is normal and part of survival. This ability to ease pain is helpful in survival situations. Often, a person will be badly injured yet experience little to no pain. In actual fact, emergency room physicians have a common saying: 'the worse the injury, the less the pain.' There are also numerous stories of soldiers wounded in the battlefield who felt no pain or were even unaware they were shot. This is truly amazing and exciting. Pain experiences can be altered.

This process of helping during the pain is often referred to as a wet brain. The brain is full of chemicals, ready to flush down and ease the pain. In a wet brain, the faucet is open and chemicals flush down to ease the pain experience. Unfortunately, people who have struggled with pain for a long time will have this drug cabinet affected in a negative way. As the brain becomes more worried and interested in what exactly is going on in the painful part, it takes the numbing medicine out of the body, making you more sensitive to protect yourself. This is one reason why you have developed some increased sensitivity for tasks that used to not be painful. In a dry brain, the faucet is closed and chemicals are not flushed down to ease the pain experience.

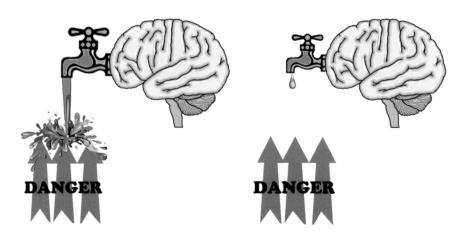

We have thus established that in persistent pain, your brain produces less of the medicine helping you to deal with pain on a daily basis. Is this permanent? Can it be changed? The answer is 'yes,' it can be changed with the following:

Knowledge–We have a lot of research that shows increased knowledge of your pain experience allows for greater understanding and less fear. With less fear and a greater realistic understanding of a pain experience, the brain will once again produce increased numbing medicine to help.

Aerobic exercise–You have probably heard of the "runner's-high." This is a known medical fact. After approximately 10 minutes of moderate aerobic exercise, the brain produces more of a calming effect on nerves, pumping blood and oxygen around nerves to calm them down.

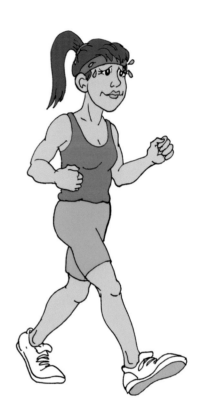

Medicine–Most patients with persistent pain are prescribed anti-depressant medications. Many patients may mistakenly believe their physician thinks they are depressed; in fact, anti-depressants are able to gently open this medicine cabinet in the brain.

Foods–The topic of food is a loaded one. In general, foods high in carbohydrates (bread, pasta) help produce a calming effect. Carbohydrates, along with turkey, contain tryptophan, which is turned into calming medicine in the brain. Think how calm you feel after eating a little too much Thanksgiving turkey and stuffing.

IMAGES

Therapists aiming to discuss the 'wet' and 'dry' brain may choose to simply use a black and white brain image and draw a faucet. A series of amazing X-ray images, easily found on the Internet, would allow for a discussion of significant injury with little or no pain and, thus, would be an easy way to explain to a patient the endogenous mechanisms of the brain.

4.13: Injuries Occur in a Vacuum, Right?

THERAPIST

The goal of this section is to help patients understand how environmental issues may influence pain in either a positive or negative way.

PATIENT

Have you ever wondered why people might experience very similar injuries to their tissues, e.g., an ankle sprain or car accident, yet recovery can be so different and varied? There are countless reasons for these seemingly different experiences. However, you need to realize injuries occur in various environments. Ankle sprains may occur during stressful times, happy times, being employed, being unemployed, wife happy and even wife mad. Scientists have now shown that the environment surrounding a tissue injury can determine, to a large degree, how much pain may be experienced.

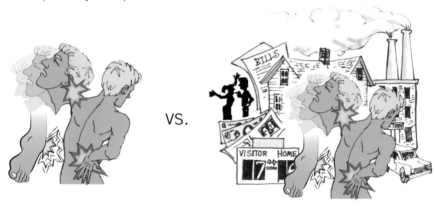

A good start is to realize that if you hurt yourself in a stressful environment, there are likely to be a lot of stress chemicals floating through your body; it will cause your nerves to wake up, get extra-sensitive and take a long time to calm. Stressful environments include car accidents, injury at work, medical tests and surgery. It

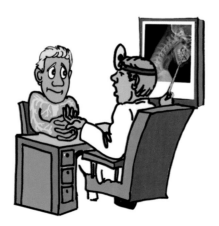

is always helpful to reflect upon the time period in which you developed your pain and all the issues going on in your life at that time, which have likely contributed to your pain experience.

The environment surrounding an injury can also yield a positive experience and actually help you experience less pain. For example, it has been shown that kids who play contact sports early in life tend to have less pain later in life. These kids learn that not all pain is bad. Pain may be felt, and injury seen, as a bruise on the body after playing football. However, these 'injuries' are seen as part of being on the team and sometimes as badges of honor. "Hey dude, check out the bruise I got from that tackle in the second quarter!" "Cool! Check out my bruise. It's way bigger than yours!"

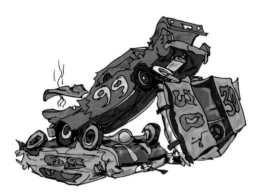

Another neat example involves demolition derby drivers. It is now widely known that one in three people develop some lasting pain from injuries sustained in car accidents. In a recent study of demolition derby drivers, who crash their cars purposefully until the "last man standing," showed that they experience 52 collisions during an event, on average. Each driver surveyed participated in an average of 30 events. You guessed it – that's a lot of crashing and whipping their necks around. The interesting part is that less than 10% of the demolition derby drivers experienced long lasting pain. More than 90% were doing great despite the vast number of crashes, often measured at 45 miles/hour (70 km/h). Scientists analyzing this firmly believe that the accidents and tissue injury, which are all real, occur in a much less stressed environment. Drivers put their immediate neck pain into context, accept it and move on as they prepare the next car for the next event.

So what? As you journey through this deeper understanding of pain, it is important to develop a greater understanding that tissue injury and pain are not one and the same, and various other issues will determine how much pain you experience.

IMAGES

Many images are available to educate patients on the influence of the environment on a pain experience. They may include pictures of demolition derby drivers, kids playing contact sports and surgery environments. Other good examples may be to discuss how athletes have performed brilliantly despite injury when it was 'all on the line,' e.g., Olympic gymnast Kerri Strugg vaulting and sticking a landing on her injured ankle, or US Olympic Marathon runner Alan Culpepper qualifying under pressure for the Olympics while running on a broken toe.

4.14: Inflammatory Soup

THERAPIST

The goal of this section is to explain persistent inflammation to patients, including antidromic impulses (retrograde depolarization) as well as thoughts contributing to inflammation and nerve sensitization. The information in this section is likely more important for peripheral joint issues and especially post-surgery patients.

PATIENT

When you sprain your ankle, you have seen the ankle turn all purple. The ankle becomes swollen in order to protect you and to stop you from running or even walking on it until it has healed. For the ankle to swell and turn purple, however, a few things need to happen. You will likely damage some of the tissues, such as the ankle ligaments, which in turn release some chemicals into the ankle, making it sore, stiff and

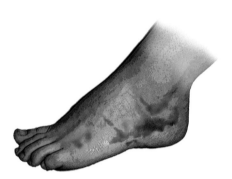

swollen. This is part of an immediate protection response. It is normal; it protects and starts the healing process. Scientists now also know that nerves in the area will release some chemicals to aid in this defense. This is normal and, again, aims to start the healing process. All of these chemicals (they have long, fancy names) make blood vessels open up, allowing for swelling, warmth and redness. Finally, immune molecules (remember the police in Nosy Neighbors?) will also send a series of molecules to the area to investigate (making it more swollen and crowded) and signaling for help to clear up the ankle. A good way to view this is a 'soup.' Various tissues in and around the ankle produce these chemicals after the injury, resulting in an 'inflammatory soup.'

It is believed that after the initial injury, extra-sensitive nerves are a major cause for persistent inflammation and swelling. Additionally, if we remember that thoughts are nerve impulses, worrying about injuries may in fact cause the ankle to stay a little more swollen. Nerves send messages both ways: up to the spinal cord and brain, signaling danger; and also down to the tissues, which signals release of chemicals, if needed.

So what? What you think can determine your pain and even tissue swelling. As you recover physically after an injury or surgery, make sure you keep your spirits up. Think happy, positive thoughts to help healing.

IMAGES

To help patients understand neurogenic inflammation, therapists may choose to show patients a swollen, purple ankle to help explain the inflammatory soup. Additionally, therapists may need to show specific nerves to a patient in the affected area. For example, if a patient has undergone knee arthroscopy and has persistent swelling, showing them anatomical pictures of the infrapatellar nerves and then explaining antidromic impulses may help them to understand why the knee has stayed swollen. The superficial fibular nerve around the ankle can help explain persistent ankle swelling, and the tibial and plantar nerves may help educate patients on persistent plantar fasciitis.

4.15: When Lions Attack

THERAPIST

The goal of this section is to help your patient understand the basic stress response and the various protective systems, with pain being only one defense mechanism. Additionally, this section helps patients develop a biological understanding of issues such as problems with sleeping, mood swings and fatigue. This section also helps patients develop a broader understanding of medical diagnoses such as fibromyalgia, chronic fatigue syndrome, irritable bowel syndrome, etc.

PATIENT

If a big, roaring African lion jumped in this room right now, what would you do? Is it time to take a nap? Is it time to focus on your posture or conserve energy? Of course not!

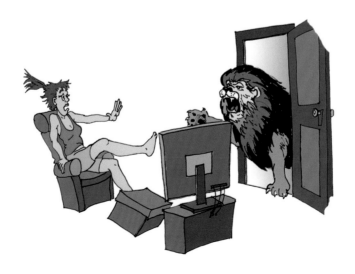

You have some key systems in place that will help you develop an appropriate stress response to ensure your survival. For example, adrenaline is a stress chemical that controls heart rate, breathing, moving blood to where you need it, your level of alertness, etc. In response to the threat imposed by the lion, your heart rate increases rapidly to pump blood though the body to areas needing blood and oxygen. Adrenaline also causes hypervigilance. No time for a nap right now! In an immediate threat response, large muscles that are capable of evading or facing the threat are needed. Big, strong leg muscles activate to run away. Arm muscles activate to push away or punch the lion. Smaller muscles, such as postural muscles, are not needed right now. Those small abdominal (core) muscles you've been working on in therapy the past few weeks to improve your back pain are not important right now.

When startled with a threat such as the lion, you will probably say a few choice words in a loud voice. With the impending threat, breathing becomes faster and shallower. Digestion of food is slowed down or even put on hold, allowing for all possible energy and blood flow to be allocated to the systems that are in immediate need. There are other responses, of course, such as pain, motivation and memory.

How does this relate to you and your pain? Everything in your life associated with the struggle of your pain can be bundled together to represent a 'lion' or a constant threat in your life. In order to defend you, your body or, more correctly, your brain, will make survival decisions and engage systems for your protection, just as if a huge lion was attacking you.

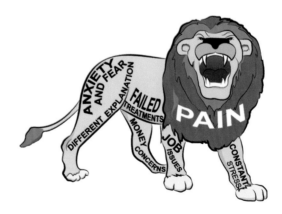

The list of 'threats' is long: no one knows what is causing you pain, life is miserable, job issues, failed treatment, exercise and movement hurt, nothing helps, there is no hope, family issues, different explanations, what does the future hold?, no one wants to help, constant pain, money issues and fear it will get worse.

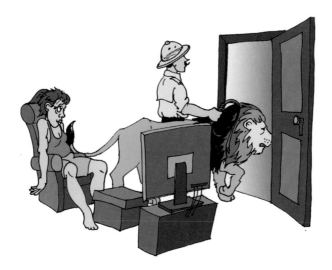

Returning to the lion story, what happens if the lion is captured by a game keeper and the threat is removed? When the lion is removed, balance is restored, allowing bodily systems to return to a normal, resting level. Wow; what an experience! You find yourself exhausted, yet relieved, and sink into your chair. You're glad this threat is gone. By the way, your systems calm down, ready for the next lion to enter the room. This process occurs in us daily as we are faced with stressors.

What a great system for our survival! The system, however, is designed to elevate temporarily and then calm down again, not run at elevated levels for prolonged periods. What happens if that lion stays with you for days, weeks, months or even years?

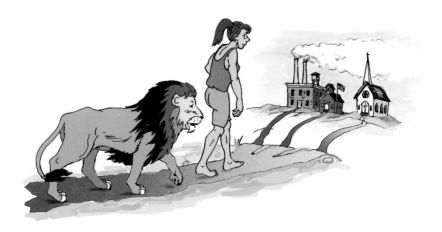

Metaphorically, patients who live in pain every day have a massive, roaring African lion following them around each day. The lion is a metaphor for the constant stress they experience associated with issues such as pain, fear, anxiety, worries about their job, worries about money, failed treatments, different explanations for their pain, etc. Clumped together, all these issues are a threat similar to an African lion. As you can see, there is a widespread reaction to threat and the various bodily systems trying to protect you. If these systems have been activated for months or years, you will probably be able to identify the various symptoms from your persistent pain:

Sore muscles—When you're under threat and blood is shifted to big, strong muscles to protect you, other smaller, but still important, muscles will have less blood supply and oxygen. This will leave them sore and sensitive.

Mood swings—With increased stress, the body produces more stress chemicals. Cortisol is one such chemical. It is now known that if cortisol levels are raised long enough, mood swings occur.

Appetite changes—Cortisol also changes appetite and food intake. Additionally, remember that many different areas of the brain are involved in processing pain. We know a key area, the hypothalamus, regulates hunger and affects food intake and changes in taste. It's also a key area for regulating body temperature.

Weight gain—High levels of cortisol are associated with increased weight gain. The hypothalamus, which regulates appetite, hunger and a sense of being full, is altered. Patients in pain also move and exercise less. All of this ties into difficulty losing weight.

Sensitive nerves—While under threat, the alarm system will stay sensitive. Decreased oxygen and blood around nerves will also contribute to increased pain. Nerve sensors that are sensitive to stress chemicals, such as adrenaline, can increase nerve sensitivity.

Sleep disturbance—Stress equals stress chemicals, which makes sleeping very difficult. Brain areas associated with sleep, especially deep restorative sleep, are busy processing pain. Body temperature is altered. The digestive system is altered. Sensitive tissues can cause problematic positioning while trying to sleep.

Posture issues—Strong, big muscles dominate. Remember, there's a lion in the room. Smaller muscles dealing with posture have less blood supply and oxygen. The brain may also question the importance of correct posture in a 'survival situation.'

Irritable bowel—When under stress, blood is pulled away from the digestive system to big muscles that can protect us through the fight or flight response. This leaves the GI system to work double time and can make it irritable.

Low libido–You probably won't be thinking about sex when a lion enters the room. Over time, libido and the hormones associated with libido, such as testosterone and estrogen, are altered. People in pain are less interested in sex with their partners. Depression feeds into this as well.

Fatigue–With stress and stress chemicals burning calories fast and furious, fatigue sets in.

Problems with focus and concentration–Several studies have shown that cortisol alteration leads to problems with focus and concentration, especially for prolonged periods.

Depression–It is well established that altered cortisol is a leading cause of depression, which is very prevalent in patients dealing with pain for prolonged periods.

A very common message reported from people with persistent pain is the soreness or tenderness of their muscles. This includes poking and pushing on them as well as using them. This is to be expected, but there is a neuroscience explanation for this. The good news is that tissues can be made to be a lot less sensitive. Consider the fact that your tissues heal, but nerves can remain sensitive. When tissues get injured, they go through phases of healing. These phases are predictable. Muscles, due to their large blood supply, heal quickly – taking only days and weeks. When pain persists for months and years, it is not because the muscles have failed to heal but rather that adjacent nerves have remained sensitive. Additionally, your muscles and body have become deconditioned because of the relative inactivity brought on by the persistent pain. The months and years of ever-decreasing activity have taken their toll, as your muscles and tendons have been exposed to less stress due to less work and exercise. It's not surprising that they get sore easily, even with a small amount of activity. Also, remember that the nerves around your muscles have become more sensitive. Underneath, alongside and over these sore muscles, you have extra-sensitive nerves. Your whole nervous system has "awakened" and no matter where you poke, push or prod, you will probably run into some tenderness. A key issue is to realize that the whole body or large areas spanning several muscles are sore. It is not a specific, single muscle that is at fault for the soreness.

You also need to consider some issues related to your posture. Certainly, posture is not that important when a lion jumps into a room. Blood is diverted from these muscles to more important, bigger muscles so you can run away. By having less blood, these muscles, especially in the upper body, get very sore and tired. They run out of fuel. So how does this pertain to you? You live with a huge, roaring lion in your life every minute of every day, diverting blood to big muscles, not posture muscles.

Many patients in persistent pain also struggle with "core muscles" and have been told their core is weak. The abdominal muscles allow us to stay upright and protect our joints. The most famous ones would be the deep abdominal and back muscles used as part of your abdominal-bracing or core exercises. In healthy, pain-free people, they work by protecting your spine when you move, perform activities or lift weights. When pain sets in, we know there is an interference of these muscles, and they cannot adequately do their job. As long as you're in 'survival mode' with a lion in your life, your brain has little interest in spending time and energy getting these core muscles to work. The immediate threat of the lion requires the brain to allocate all the available energy to the larger muscles.

The take home message is this: many body systems are used to protect you. This explains why you have so many different issues going on, as well as why you're dealing with increased fatigue, sensitivity and weakness.

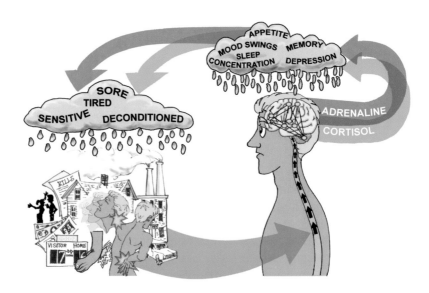

Here is one additional, important lion issue. Review the stress response about the lion jumping in the room. What would you do if, while watching TV and relaxing, a lion cub enters the room? Unless you have a major fear of lions, you'd be OK with it. You'd likely go to the lion cub and pet it. In this example lies an important statement. If the threat is perceived as small, as in the lion cub, there is no need to get all of your defense systems up and running. The more you know about your pain and treatment options, the smaller the threat. Consider the lion cub versus a massive African lion! There is hope. You have the opportunity to take control and get your life back.

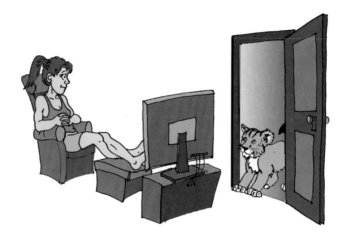

IMAGES

To help patients understand the multiple systems used to protect, images of lions or threatening situations can be appropriate. An image of the body with plenty of space around it to draw and discuss the output mechanisms can be useful. Therapists can systematically go through each of the relevant output mechanisms associated with a threat response and highlight the important fact that these are meant to operate for only a short time until the threat dissipates. Once this occurs, all of these multiple output systems should return to homeostasis. Emphasize that with persistent pain, those systems have remained active and how over-activity in each system can explain what they may currently feel as a result of their persistent pain, e.g., tired, sore, poor memory, low libido, depressed, etc.

Chapter 4 References

Coppieters, M. W., L. Ryan, et al. (2005). *Do patients' beliefs based on widespread medical information hinder accurate diagnosis?* 11th World Congress on Pain, Sydney.

Devor, M. (2006). Sodium channels and mechanisms of neuropathic pain. *J Pain, 7*(1 Suppl 1): S3-S12.

Flor, H., T. Elbert, et al. (1995). Phantom limb pain as a perceptual correlate of cortical reorganisation following arm amputation. *Nature, 375*: 482-484.

Gallagher, L., J. McAuley, et al. (2013). A randomized-controlled trial of using a book of metaphors to reconceptualize pain and decrease catastrophizing in people with chronic pain. *The Clinical Journal of Pain, 29*(1): 20-25.

Louw, A. (2012). *Your Nerves Are Having Back Surgery.* Minneapolis, OPTP.

Louw, A. and D. S. Butler (2011). Chronic Pain. *Clinical Orthopaedic Rehabilitation.* B. S.B. and R. Manske. Philadelphia, PA, Elsevier.

Louw, A., I. Diener, et al. (2011). The effect of neuroscience education on pain, disability, anxiety, and stress in chronic musculoskeletal pain. *Archives of Physical Medicine and Rehabilitation, 92*(12): 2041-2056.

Louw, A., Q. Louw, et al. (2009). Preoperative Education for Lumbar Surgery for Radiculopathy. *South African Journal of Physiotherapy, 65*(2): 3-8.

Louw, A., E. L. Puentedura, et al. (2011). Use of an abbreviated neuroscience education approach in the treatment of chronic low back pain: A case report. *Physiotherapy Theory and Practice.*

Maihofner, C., H. O. Handwerker, et al. (2003). Patterns of cortical reorganization in complex regional pain syndrome. *Neurology, 61*(12): 1707-1715.

Marinus, J., G. L. Moseley, et al. (2011). Clinical features and pathophysiology of complex regional pain syndrome. *Lancet Neurology, 10*(7): 637-648.

Moseley, G. L. (2003). A pain neuromatrix approach to patients with chronic pain. *Man Ther, 8*(3): 130-140.

Moseley, G. L. (2003). Unravelling the barriers to reconceptualisation of the problem in chronic pain: the actual and perceived ability of patients and health professionals to understand the neurophysiology. *J Pain, 4*(4): 184-189.

Moseley, G. L. (2004). Why do people with complex regional pain syndrome take longer to recognize their affected hand? *Neurology, 62*(12): 2182-2186.

Moseley, G. L. (2007). Reconceptualising pain according to modern pain sciences. *Physical Therapy Reviews, 12*: 169-178.

Moseley, G. L. (2007). Using visual illusion to reduce at-level neuropathic pain in paraplegia. *Pain, 130*(3): 294-298.

Moseley, G. L. and H. Flor (2012). Targeting cortical representations in the treatment of chronic pain: a review. *Neurorehabilitation and Neural Repair, 26*(6): 646-652.

Moseley, G. L., P. W. Hodges, et al. (2004). A randomized controlled trial of intensive neurophysiology education in chronic low back pain. *Clinical Journal of Pain, 20*: 324-330.

Sterling, M., G. Jull, et al. (2003). Sensory hypersensitivity occurs soon after whiplash injury and is associated with poor recovery. *Pain, 104*(3): 509-517.

Tifford, C. D., L. Spero, et al. (2000). The relationship of the infrapatellar branches of the saphenous nerve to arthroscopy portals and incisions for anterior cruciate ligament surgery. An anatomic study. *The American Journal of Sports Medicine, 28*(4): 562-567.

Chapter 5

Clinical Application Guidelines for Therapeutic Neuroscience Education

5.1: Introduction

In the preceding chapters, we outlined the importance of cognitions and pain then followed this with a review of educational strategies that can be employed by therapists to address possible faulty cognitions in order to alter their patient's pain experience. We introduced therapeutic neuroscience education (TNE) as a means to help patients reconceptualize their pain according to the updated neuroscience model of pain. This reconceptualization has been correlated to patients experiencing decreased pain, improved function, decreased catastrophization and improved physical movements (Moseley, 2002; Moseley, Hodges et al., 2004; Moseley, 2007; Louw, Diener et al., 2011). We then introduced a systematic method of bringing about this reconceptualization of pain by utilizing the pain neurophysiology questionnaire (PNQ) (Moseley, 2003) and followed this up with clinical examples using metaphors, pictures and examples to help patients develop a deeper understanding of their pain.

The TNE information is based on the latest evidence (Louw, Diener et al., 2011); however, it is likely clinicians will have many "real life" questions regarding its clinical application. Many of the studies on the effectiveness of TNE incorporated extensive education sessions lasting hours (Moseley, 2002; Moseley, 2005), which from a clinical perspective, would make it impractical for clinicians to implement as they face significant time constraints. It is highly unlikely that clinicians will be able to spend over three hours at a time providing a comprehensive TNE program for each of their patients with persistent pain.

This chapter will discuss various clinical aspects regarding the clinical application of TNE. The information in this chapter is based on our experience through trial and error, and years of testing various aspects of TNE application. Our message to you is that you should review the suggestions and apply them where appropriate. Not all of the strategies will work for you. Not all of the strategies can be absorbed by healthcare systems, and every therapist will likely have their own unique clinical environment.

5.2: Time

Conceptual change is complex, and it could be argued that one of the most important components involves time. The greater the time that can be devoted to TNE, the greater the chances for success. TNE is usually started as soon as the evaluation is completed on the first visit, which is commonly scheduled to allow for extra time (Louw, Puentedura et al., 2012). After a thorough subjective and objective examination, education should be started. Therapists may also choose to schedule specific times for patients who are likely to require the TNE approach. In a busy clinical practice, specific time slots can be allocated for patients requiring TNE to allow for longer sessions, especially for the more involved patients. The remaining clinical time may well represent typical clinical practice, accommodating higher volumes for patients not in need of extensive TNE.

Clinical experience would suggest scheduling such TNE-specific sessions in the late mornings as the last appointment before lunch or immediately after lunch. The fact that there is a break before other patients will arrive, i.e., being the last patient before lunch, may alleviate stress on the therapist and provide a potential extra few minutes (if needed) to drive a very important issue home. Furthermore, appointments around lunch time could potentially alleviate stress on patients. Many patients are concerned about work issues, especially time missed at work, which adds to their stress. By scheduling the TNE session in the middle of the day, patients may be able to attend TNE while missing minimal work, which will help alleviate stress. Patients may even be advised to designate such lunch-time therapy sessions as days to bring lunch with them, considering therapy will utilize most of the available time needed for treatment.

Another strategy worth reserving for TNE is to designate a specific day of the week for such patients. Many clinicians may notice that some days of their workweek are slower than others. It may be well worth it to designate one day, or a half-day, as a TNE pain clinic day. On those days, appointment times should be of longer duration to allow adequate time for one-on-one education. It will provide a once-a-week schedule for that particular patient and allow the clinic to remain more productive (from the business point of view) on the remaining clinical days.

To effectively provide TNE and achieve success, it is vital that clinics develop a team approach to patient care. Implementing TNE in clinical practice will necessarily require a little more time and flexibility to go 'overtime' with patients who need it. Having a team to support the therapist providing TNE to their patient can be invaluable. A good example might be a situation where a therapist is working in a TNE session trying to help a more complex patient with fibromyalgia. The therapist runs over their allotted time with that complex patient and the next patient on their schedule arrives. If the next scheduled patient is a less complicated follow-up session, perhaps continued rehabilitation of a high school student with an ankle sprain, then it would be helpful if a team member in the clinic could begin treatment of that next patient with the ankle sprain. This would allow the therapist performing the TNE to complete their session and not have to cut it short at a perhaps pivotal moment for that complex patient with fibromyalgia.

The more recent studies of TNE provided it in 30-minute sessions, spread over time (Meeus, Nijs et al., 2010; Van Oosterwijck, Nijs et al., 2011). Once the evaluation is completed, a therapist may review the case and make a list of 6-8 main issues he/she would like to educate the patient about to coincide with the proposed schedule, for example, 2x/week for four weeks. At each session, 15-20 minutes may be devoted to the TNE, followed by the adjunct therapy (Nijs, Paul van Wilgen et al., 2011). A good clinical strategy may also involve the revised PNQ as a guide for education (Moseley, 2003). Therapists may choose to read, answer and discuss 2-3 questions per session, thus pacing the education over time.

An important aspect of creating time for TNE is screening patients in advance to ensure they are appropriate for that approach. The last thing a busy clinician would need is for a new patient with low back pain to suddenly develop into a more complex patient with central sensitization issues five minutes into their typical "orthopedic" examination. It is recommended that front office staff be trained to ask appropriate questions to determine if a patient needs to be directed to the longer TNE examination and treatment sessions. Screening strategies may include a list of diagnoses that may need TNE. The list may include fibromyalgia and chronic disorders such as chronic LBP or whiplash, etc. A list of referring physicians who specialize in more chronic or complex disorders may be used as a guide, especially if a therapist has marketed TNE as a treatment to a specific referral source. It is also highly recommended that paperwork be sent to patients in advance to help decide if a TNE session may be appropriate. In this digital age of e-mails and online forms, many facilities have patients complete intake information prior to attending their first appointment. A quick screen of the FABQ, description of the issues, main complaint, and/or duration of symptoms can be used to flag appropriate patients.

5.3: Cost-Effectiveness

The issues raised in the previous section should be considered in any discussion of cost-effectiveness. Suggestions in that section provide strategies to balance intense TNE sessions, which are more time consuming, with day-to-day busy clinical practice, which allows for a more fiscally responsible approach. In future proposed payment systems, it is possible that third party payers may allow for increased reimbursements for more complex patients. In that case, TNE may likely be more cost-effective. Researchers should also further examine the efficacy of more cost-effective TNE programs such as group therapy (Moseley, 2003). Therapists should also realize that not all TNE sessions should be extensive, stand-alone counseling sessions. In fact, it is argued that TNE is likely more effective when administered in the context of physical therapy, including exercise and manual therapy (Louw, Diener et al., 2011; Louw, Puentedura et al., 2011; Nijs, Paul van Wilgen et al., 2011).

The evidence currently suggests one-on-one offers superior outcomes to group therapy, but group therapy sessions do result in a more cost-effective strategy (Moseley, 2003; Louw, Diener et al., 2011). The evidence for superiority of outcomes for the one-on-one approach should not be surprising considering that pain is based on an individual's specific pain neuromatrix; thus each person's pain experience will be individualized. The one-on-one approach allows TNE to be individualized.

It could also be argued that group sessions present limitations on patients expressing very personal issues and limit a deeper learning process. In contrast to this potential limitation of sharing personal information, it is important to realize group sessions may, indeed, create an opportunity for sharing experiences that have shown benefit in spine surgery patients after lumbar fusion (Christensen, Laurberg et al., 2003). In the TNE study utilizing group therapy, groups of 7-10 patients were instructed using a single four-hour session (Moseley, 2003). It is highly recommended that clinicians and researchers explore future group designs to optimize outcomes and provide the most cost effective approach. For the moment, we would recommend that groups be limited to 4-10 patients. An additional strategy to consider in regards to cost-effectiveness is homework. Providing written material and self-study has been shown to enhance the learning experience (Moseley, 2002; Louw, 2013).

5.4: Billing for TNE

Billing for services is a complex issue and all clinicians are encouraged to consult with their respective billing departments to gain clarification and also keep updated on the ever-changing world of insurance reimbursement. Despite this, it is important to consider appropriate billing strategies for TNE.

There is good evidence for TNE; even more compelling, there is evidence for its use in treating some of the most challenging patients therapists may ever encounter – patients in chronic pain (Louw, Diener et al., 2011). Therapists should therefore be reimbursed accordingly. In chapter 1, we strongly advocated for the concept that TNE should be seen as part of therapy and not as a separate psychological intervention. Changing beliefs and cognitions directly impact movement, function and motor control. It is therefore suggested that TNE be billed under appropriate codes such as 'neuromuscular reeducation.' Considering there is ample biological evidence that TNE changes brain activity (Moseley, 2005), neurodynamic testing (Moseley, 2004; Moseley, Hodges et al., 2004; Van Oosterwijck, Nijs et al., 2011), and nerve sensitivity via pressure pain threshold testing (Louw A, et al., – submitted for publication), we argue that TNE affects the nervous system and 'neuromuscular reeducation' would be an appropriate billing code in the current therapy environment. Therapists may also wish to consider billing for TNE under codes for 'therapeutic exercise' or 'therapeutic activities.' There is evidence that a multimodal approach to therapy provides superior outcomes to single intervention approaches, and our clinical experience suggests that TNE should be woven into the fabric of therapy and provided during the performance of therapeutic exercises and activities.

As with all therapeutic interventions, documentation of the TNE sessions should address two important factors. First, the documentation should validate the billing; second, it should provide for clinical consistency. If a therapist wishes to bill for TNE under 'neuromuscular education,' then the documentation should support such billing. For example, a therapist may decide to discuss nerve sensitivity in the session and cover nerve sensitization, as outlined in chapter 4, sections 4.1 and 4.2. Such a discussion may last 15 minutes, and documentation should include discussion of normal nerve electrical activity, action potentials, extra-sensitive nerves, yellow flags associated with the extra-sensitive nerves and how the extra-sensitive nerves correlate to specific personal functional and physical limitations of the patient (Louw, Puentedura et al., 2011). To ensure clinical consistency in any patient's care, the documentation should convey to a colleague what he or she did, allowing them to reproduce, adjust or progress the treatment in the event he or she sees this particular patient (Maitland, 1986). This underscores the need to develop a standard TNE language; given the infancy of TNE, it is highly recommended that clinicians and researchers start this process early to avoid later pitfalls (Mintken, DeRosa et al., 2008).

5.5: Training Staff

The medical profession, in general, remains grounded in a biomedical approach focusing on anatomy, pathoanatomy and biomechanics (Houben, Ostelo et al., 2005; Henrotin, Cedraschi et al., 2006). Therapists who have received some training in TNE, e.g., a weekend seminar, are likely to face a significant challenge when returning to the clinic. Several hard-fought TNE sessions can be easily undone with some seemingly simple words from a 'biomedically focused' colleague: "*Has anyone checked your SI joint?*"

For a clinic to practice and utilize a true biopsychosocial approach, we propose that all staff members need some form of TNE education, ranging from a short in-service to a more comprehensive two-day TNE class. In an ideal world, all clinicians will have been trained in the TNE approach. A typical weekend class on TNE has been shown to change therapists' views on pain drastically (Latimer, Maher et al., 2004).

In some clinics, depending on a therapist's aptitude for TNE, clinicians may take on the role of a 'pain specialist' and thus have all patients in need of TNE directed to the specific care of this one therapist. This may be common practice as it pertains to other specializations. If a therapist happens to demonstrate greater skill rehabilitating shoulder pain or treating neck pain, it is more likely that patients with those conditions/complaints will be placed on their schedule.

The role of the front office personnel should be discussed here. Many seasoned therapists have realized the power of a good receptionist as the first point-of-contact for patients attending the clinic. Considering the complexities of pain, it is recommended that therapists who are well versed in TNE train their front office staff, as well. In the ideal clinic, all front office staff would have developed a greater understanding of pain, allowing them to understand patients better, help patients, empathize with patients, develop an understanding of the challenges therapists face, and become an asset rather than a liability to the therapists providing TNE.

An additional consideration should be given to students attending therapy clinics for their clinical rotations. As recently discussed, it is best to have all staff and all visiting students develop some familiarity with TNE. Not only will this strategy help with the uniformity of treatment, should students provide some of the patient care, but it should also allow students exposure to the TNE approach. It has been shown that therapists struggle with pain (Louw, Louw et al., 2009) and therapy students have poor beliefs regarding chronic pain (Latimer, Maher et al., 2004). Employers implementing such an early exposure of TNE to students may find themselves in the early stages of developing future employees.

5.6: Tools and Props

If a patient following knee replacement surgery attends physical therapy, it is commonplace for the therapist to gather all necessary tools, such as a goniometer and a tape measure, prior to entering the treatment room to allow him or her to perform their job at an optimal level. If a patient with chronic pain secondary to central sensitization attends therapy, are there any tools that can be used to treat that patient, especially with a TNE approach? The evidence for TNE calls for pictures, metaphors and examples (Louw, Diener et al., 2011). In the previous chapter, we emphasized the need for developing a resource of metaphors and images to help with the conduct of TNE. We would recommend that clinicians create a three ring binder with large, colorful images to use for TNE. The binder may include images highlighted in chapter 4, including an ankle sprain, speeding bus, action potential, rusted nail, body nervous system, amazing X-rays, etc. Furthermore, simple black and white pictures that can be drawn upon can be prepared and readied in advance, such as a brain to highlight the neuromatrix or a clip art image of a lion allowing for the personalization of yellow flags. Therapists should also consider removing and/or replacing provocative images in their clinic, which may be contrary to the TNE message. Examples may be anatomical or pathoanatomical wall charts, old fear-inducing spine or joint models, or even removing the red "bulging" disc so commonly portrayed in all therapy spine models.

5.7: Measuring Progress

It is highly recommended that clinicians use validated outcome measures similar to the ones found in TNE studies (Louw, Diener et al., 2011). In a systematic review of TNE for chronic musculoskeletal pain, several outcome measures were highlighted. We do not recommend that all outcome measures described in the studies be used. It is important to realize that many clinics and institutions will have their own rules and regulations asking for the use of specific outcome measures. This section only aims to provide guidelines and insight into the clinical use of these outcome measures from a neuroscience perspective.

Pain scientists and therapists who truly understand chronic pain would argue that asking a patient for their pain rating does not provide any significant value. Despite this, pain ratings and pain scores have become ubiquitous in clinical practice. Asking for patients' pain ratings is often mandated by insurance carriers or healthcare policies. However, the word 'pain' is considered a provocative word and may be a significant source for firing up the pain neuromatrix (Moseley, 2007).

In fact, asking patients over and over about their pain may increase the pain ratings (Wilson, Williams et al., 2009). It is important to acknowledge that all pain ratings and pain scores are still only subjective measures and not a truly valid rating of a patient's perception of their pain.

Most clinicians will agree that the pain ratings given by patients with chronic pain have little to no clinical value. A significant number of studies on chronic pain have shown that pain fluctuates constantly and does not correlate to injury or the disease process. Therapists should therefore carefully monitor their use of the word 'pain' during evaluations and treatment sessions. Furthermore, therapists need to guard against substituting a patients "ache" with the word 'pain.' As an example, a patient may present with a primary complaint of a "deep burning ache" in their leg. By referring to the "deep burning ache," or just "ache," the word 'pain' can be avoided and may have therapeutic value (Maitland, 1986). Another way to avoid speaking the word 'pain' might be to present patients with a visual analogue scale and ask them to mark their 'rating of their complaint' rather than asking and emphasizing their 'pain' rating. The most commonly used scales for pain ratings in TNE are the Numeric Pain Rating Scale (NPRS) and Visual Analog Scale (VAS) (Moseley, 2002; Moseley, 2003; Ryan, Gray et al., 2010; Van Oosterwijck, Nijs et al., 2011).

A second, and arguably more important, measure is function. The focus of TNE is the reconceptualization of pain to allow patients to improve their function despite its presence. Function is important for all stakeholders: the patient, the clinician, insurance (third-party payers) and the physician. The Oswestry Disability Index, Roland Morris Disability Questionnaire, Neck Disability Index and DASH for upper extremity may be some choices. We recommended that for wide-spread, total-body pain, the functional tool closest to the area of main concern be chosen rather than a series of these outcome measures (Louw, Diener et al., 2011).

The Oswestry Disability Index (ODI) is a 10-item questionnaire that assesses different aspects of physical function. Each item is scored from 0 to 5, with higher values representing greater disability. The total score is multiplied by two and expressed as a percentage. The ODI has been shown to be a valid and reliable measure of disability related to LBP (Deyo, Battie et al., 1998; Fritz and Irrgang, 2001; Hakkinen, Kautiainen et al., 2007). A change of five points (10%) has been proposed as the minimally important change (MIC) (Ostelo, Deyo et al., 2008).

The 18-item Roland Morris Disability Questionnaire (RMDQ) is widely used to measure function related to spinal disorders (Moseley, 2002; Moseley, 2003; Moseley, Hodges et al., 2004; Grotle, Brox et al., 2005; Mannion, Denzler et al., 2007) and has been shown to be a reliable and valid method for measurement of self-perceived disability due to LBP (Roland and Morris, 1983; Roland and Morris, 1983; Moseley, Nicholas et al., 2004).

The Neck Disability Index (NDI) was developed in 1991 as a modification of the ODI and was the first instrument designed to assess self-rated disability in patients with neck pain (Vernon and Mior, 1991; Vernon, 2008). The NDI is scored from 0 (good function) to 50 (poor function), and the percentage of disability can be obtained when the score is multiplied by two. The NDI is a valid and reliable instrument sensitive to measure changes within a population of patients with neck pain (Vernon and Mior, 1991; Vernon, 2008).

In chapter 1, it was shown how fear avoidance is a powerful psychometric measure that is correlated to a high risk of developing chronic pain (Vlaeyen, Kole-Snijders et al., 1995; Moseley, 2004; Meeus, Nijs et al., 2010). Fear avoidance of Work and Physical Activity is well studied and can readily be applied to clinical practice (Fritz and George, 2002; Louw, Diener et al., 2011). The Fear Avoidance Beliefs Questionnaire (FABQ) is a 16-item questionnaire that was designed to quantify fear and avoidance beliefs in individuals with LBP. It has been adapted successfully to individuals with neck pain. The FABQ has two subscales: a four-item scale to measure fear avoidance beliefs about physical activity and a seven-item scale to measure fear-avoidance beliefs about work. Each item is scored from 0 to 6 with possible scores ranging between 0 and 24 and 0 and 42 for the physical activity and work subscales, respectively, with higher scores representing an increase in fear-avoidance beliefs. The FABQ has demonstrated acceptable levels of reliability and validity in previous LBP studies (Grotle, Vollestad et al., 2006; Poiraudeau, Rannou et al., 2006; Cleland, Fritz et al., 2008). Presence of avoidance behavior is associated with increased risk of prolonged disability and work loss. It is reported that FABQ-PA >14 and FABQ-W scores >34 are associated with a higher likelihood of not returning to work (Burton, Waddell et al., 1999; Fritz and George, 2002).

5.8: Combining TNE with Physical Therapy

There is a misconception that TNE might encourage therapists to become counselors and stop using their conventional physical treatments. There is little to no evidence to suggest that TNE is helpful on its own; there is greater evidence for its use in conjunction with other commonly used physical therapy interventions (Puentedura, Brooksby et al., 2009; Louw, Diener et al., 2011; Louw, Puentedura et al., 2011). Following the theme of this textbook, we highly recommend that TNE be supported and utilized within the model of movement and exercise.

Current best evidence for chronic pain, such as fibromyalgia, calls for a combination of cognitive therapy, such as TNE, as well as exercise (Busch, Barber et al., 2007). Several high-quality RCT's have indicated the use of TNE with manual therapy, including spinal mobilization and manipulation (Moseley, 2002), soft tissue treatment/massage (Moseley, 2002), neural tissue mobilization (Moseley, 2002), spinal stabilization exercises (Moseley, 2002; Moseley, 2003; Ryan, Gray et al., 2010), home exercises (Moseley, 2002), circuit training (Ryan, Gray et al., 2010), and aerobic exercise (Ryan, Gray et al., 2010). While some studies on TNE have conducted as education-only sessions (Moseley, 2003; Moseley, 2004; Moseley, Hodges et al., 2004; Meeus, Nijs et al., 2010; Van Oosterwijck, Nijs et al., 2011), it is recommended that TNE be incorporated with movement therapy.

5.9: Deep Learning

When a patient is confronted with the TNE message, he or she will have to make a decision, as in all healthcare education. Clinical experience tells us that patients will likely make one of three choices (Figure 5.1).

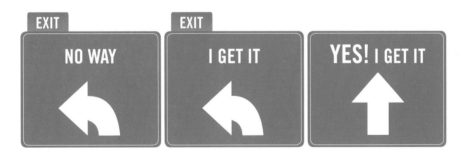

Figure 5.1: Our clinical experience tells us that when confronted with the TNE message, patients will likely make one of three choices.

NO WAY

It is important for therapists to realize that some patients may not be ready for this style of therapy or even the message. Each patient is on a quest to seek help for his or her condition and has a choice to accept your approach or not. This is not unique to TNE and applies to all kinds of therapy, including manual therapy, exercise and modalities. Unfortunately, TNE may evoke significant response in some patients, especially those not ready to receive the new information about pain.

Patients may become upset, challenge your intentions, and likely not come back to see you again. Most therapists would find this to be a devastating situation, but we would advise that they view it from the proper vantage point. Chronic pain is challenging. This approach has scientific evidence, follows the current best-evidence and is based on the latest neuroscience view of pain. There are many reasons why a patient may choose not to accept your TNE approach. These could include the following: the patient is not ready to accept the new pain message, the patient is still searching for passive treatment options, the patient still believes the answer is in their tissues, or the patient has numerous emotional issues that may need resolving prior to progressing accordingly.

Clinical experience indicates that approximately 5-10% of patients may fit into this category. They don't return to therapy. From a clinical perspective, therapists are advised not to force patients down the TNE pathway. If they miss a follow-up appointment or fail to return, they are likely communicating they do not want to pursue the TNE approach, and it may not be advisable to call the patient to reschedule.

I GET IT

Unfortunately, the majority of patients fit into this category. They receive the TNE message, seemingly understand the message and then proceed to just go through the motions. In this case, the patients undergo a superficial learning process. They will attend therapy but often miss appointments and never truly make progress. These patients are often passed from therapist to therapist or run out of insurance coverage for their visits.

There is no doubt that these patients cause significant clinical frustration for therapists. To ensure a more favorable response to TNE, therapists should try a series of strategies. First, identify patients you are currently treating who need TNE, and then schedule an appropriate time for such a TNE session. Teach the patient a new approach regarding their pain and reinforce it at each session as a means to have a patient undergo a deeper understanding of his or her pain.

YES! I GET IT

The ultimate goal of TNE is a deep learning process. During deep learning, a patient receives the message, internalizes the messages, applies it to his or her situation and positive changes occur (Crabtree, Royeen et al., 2001; Wittmann-Price and Godshall, 2009). The therapist sees positive changes in behavior, function and compliance with exercise (Louw, Puentedura et al., 2011).

5.10: How Much TNE?

Another common misconception of TNE is that a therapist needs to 'mentally prepare' for a long, exhausting session in which he or she may spend a long time to try and obtain the optimum deep learning experience. The aims of chapters 3, 4 and 5 were to make therapists aware that these sessions need not be exhausting. Education, as with any form of therapy, needs to be adequately paced. Additionally, not all patients will have the same number and depth of yellow flags in their presentation. As an example, a patient's only yellow flag may be fear, and they may only need a short, quick correction of thought to result in a superior outcome. A helpful strategy with which to view TNE is to visualize a barrier.

In some patients, the barrier to making a positive change may be small. For example, a patient may believe that a bulging disc is a significant reason for their pain and a reason to avoid movement, exercise and ADL's. The TNE session for such a patient may be a quick, 10-minute discussion of bulging discs. The patient's beliefs may be altered and their fear reduced. He or she will then be more willing to move, exercise, participate in therapy, and return to function. It could reasonably be argued that therapists already perform such sessions on a daily basis while helping a patient with a knee replacement or rotator cuff repair understand more about their condition, set goals, ease fears and develop a plan of care. The change in language is a key component of TNE, this textbook and clinical practice. We encourage therapists to continue this daily task but with a new pain vocabulary as the educational model.

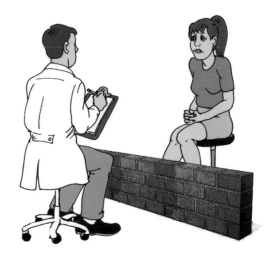

In some patients the barriers are bigger. These patients may have several inappropriate beliefs and more complex yellow flags; therefore, they will need more education. This will likely take a few sessions to address issues such as widespread pain, high levels of fear, job issues, failed treatment, etc. In a simplistic model, these patients will have several of the signs and symptoms associated with central sensitization and several yellow flags (Watson and Kendall, 2000). In such a scenario, the patient may conceivably be seen for eight visits and TNE sessions would be constantly imbedded into the movement-based approaches of exercise and manual therapy (Moseley, 2002; Louw, Puentedura et al., 2011). Given the larger barrier, TNE is a bigger part of the therapy sessions.

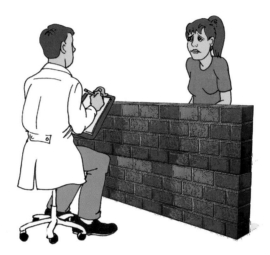

A third, more complex clinical issue involves an even larger and wider barrier. These patients may have all the above, plus many other issues. Most of their psychometric measures will be "off the charts." There may be significant barriers to improvement, which may include abuse or history of abuse, a deep sense of being wronged and even true psychological issues (Hauser, Kosseva et al., 2011). These patients will likely have significant psychological factors, such as depression, which is strongly associated with chronic pain (Goldenberg, 1999; Pae, Luyten et al., 2008).

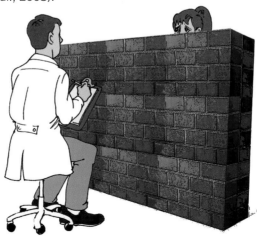

A simplistic therapeutic approach may be for the therapist to see these patients as not being appropriate candidates for therapy and refer them for psychological counseling. Ultimately, they will need a multi-disciplinary approach, including movement-based therapy. We believe TNE should be attempted for these patients (Louw, Diener et al., 2012). These sessions will likely be of longer durations and the overall prognosis will be diminished compared to the previous two clinical barrier scenarios.

5.11: Who Needs TNE?

Perhaps the most difficult, and important, aspect of TNE is the determination of the correct patient for such an approach. This is not unique to TNE and applies to all therapeutic interventions. Current research into the sub-classification of low back pain, for example, encourages therapists to classify patients into specific sub-groups that are more likely to benefit from certain therapeutic interventions (Fritz, Cleland et al., 2007; Fritz, Lindsay et al., 2007). It could be argued that all patients, regardless of their presenting symptoms, will need some form of TNE. Patient education is a critical component of any therapeutic encounter, so why not provide the latest pain neuroscience education from the get-go. As an example, a patient following knee replacement or an ankle sprain will need information about their condition and how to promote their healing and rehabilitation. The clinician could provide all of the key messages of TNE and 'biologize' the message using appropriate metaphors and carefully considering use of threatening words.

Specific indications for TNE include patients with central sensitization (Nijs, Van Houdenhove et al., 2010; Nijs, Paul van Wilgen et al., 2011), chronic pain (Louw, Diener et al., 2011), patients who have had multiple treatment "failures," patients referred to therapy specifically for TNE (e.g., marketing to a physician), patients with high levels of fear, and patients displaying various pain catastrophizing characteristics. Apart from the aforementioned list, therapists are also encouraged to listen attentively to a patient's history and symptoms to identify any specific comments that may need addressing through a TNE approach. For example, during the course of a treatment a patient states she is a little worried as she has an upcoming nerve conduction test to rule out carpal tunnel syndrome (CTS). Given the complexity of CTS, an attentive therapist may choose to flag this statement, explore the patient's beliefs regarding CTS and deliver a neuroscience view of CTS, alleviating stress and anxiety in the patient.

5.12: How Do We Get Physicians On-Board?

The development and evidence for TNE provides an avenue for marketing. TNE research has not only been published in therapy-related journals but also medical journals, which are viewed more favorably by referral sources (Louw, Diener et al., 2011). Chronic pain is a major issue. Therapists armed with TNE evidence, along with the will and compassion to help patients with chronic pain, are likely to receive a sympathetic ear from referral sources. Strategies include finding and keeping TNE articles on file to be able to assist in marketing TNE. Therapists are encouraged to develop various flyers and brochures to help educate referral sources about your use of TNE in clinical practice. Marketing TNE should be directed to physicians, nurse practitioners, physician assistants, the general public, colleagues, support groups and patients.

Chapter 5 References

Burton, A. K., G. Waddell, et al. (1999). Information and advice to patients with back pain can have a positive effect. A randomized controlled trial of a novel educational booklet in primary care. *Spine, 24*(23): 2484-2491.

Busch, A. J., K. A. Barber, et al. (2007). Exercise for treating fibromyalgia syndrome. *Cochrane Database Syst Rev,* (4): CD003786.

Christensen, F. B., I. Laurberg, et al. (2003). Importance of the back-cafe concept to rehabilitation after lumbar spinal fusion: a randomized clinical study with a 2-year follow-up. *Spine, 28*(23): 2561-2569.

Cleland, J. A., J. M. Fritz, et al. (2008). Psychometric properties of the Fear-Avoidance Beliefs Questionnaire and Tampa Scale of Kinesiophobia in patients with neck pain. *Am J Phys Med Rehabil, 87*(2): 109-117.

Crabtree, J. L., C. B. Royeen, et al. (2001). The effects of learning through discussion in a course in occupational therapy: a search for deep learning. *J Allied Health, 30*(4): 243-247.

Deyo, R. A., M. Battie, et al. (1998). Outcome measures for low back pain research. A proposal for standardized use. *Spine (Phila Pa 1976), 23*(18): 2003-2013.

Fritz, J. M., J. A. Cleland, et al. (2007). Subgrouping patients with low back pain: evolution of a classification approach to physical therapy. *J Orthop Sports Phys Ther, 37*(6): 290-302.

Fritz, J. M. and S. Z. George (2002). Identifying psychosocial variables in patients with acute work-related low back pain: the importance of fear-avoidance beliefs. *Phys Ther, 82*(10): 973-983.

Fritz, J. M. and J. J. Irrgang (2001). A comparison of a modified Oswestry Low Back Pain Disability Questionnaire and the Quebec Back Pain Disability Scale. *Phys Ther, 81*(2): 776-788.

Fritz, J. M., W. Lindsay, et al. (2007). Is there a subgroup of patients with low back pain likely to benefit from mechanical traction? Results of a randomized clinical trial and subgrouping analysis. *Spine, 32*(26): E793-800.

Goldenberg, D. L. (1999). Fibromyalgia syndrome a decade later: what have we learned? *Archives of Internal Medicine, 159*(8): 777-785.

Grotle, M., J. I. Brox, et al. (2005). Clinical course and prognostic factors in acute low back pain: patients consulting primary care for the first time. *Spine, 30*(8): 976-982.

Grotle, M., N. K. Vollestad, et al. (2006). Clinical course and impact of fear-avoidance beliefs in low back pain: prospective cohort study of acute and chronic low back pain: II. *Spine, 31*(9): 1038-1046.

Hakkinen, A., H. Kautiainen, et al. (2007). Changes in the total Oswestry Index and its ten items in females and males pre- and post-surgery for lumbar disc herniation: a 1-year follow-up. *Eur Spine J, 16*(3): 347-352.

Hauser, W., M. Kosseva, et al. (2011). Emotional, physical, and sexual abuse in fibromyalgia syndrome: a systematic review with meta-analysis. *Arthritis Care & Research, 63*(6): 808-820.

Henrotin, Y. E., C. Cedraschi, et al. (2006). Information and low back pain management: a systematic review. *Spine, 31*(11): E326-334.

Houben, R. M., R. W. Ostelo, et al. (2005). Health care providers' orientations towards common low back pain predict perceived harmfulness of physical activities and recommendations regarding return to normal activity. *Eur J Pain, 9*(2): 173-183.

Latimer, J., C. Maher, et al. (2004). The attitudes and beliefs of physiotherapy students to chronic back pain. *Clin J Pain, 20*(1): 45-50.

Louw, A. (2013). *Your Fibromyalgia Workbook: A Neuroscience Approach.* Minneapolis, OPTP.

Louw, A., I. Diener, et al. (2011). The effect of neuroscience education on pain, disability, anxiety, and stress in chronic musculoskeletal pain. *Archives of Physical Medicine and Rehabilitation, 92*(12): 2041-2056.

Louw, A., I. Diener, et al. (2012). Preoperative education addressing postoperative pain in total joint arthroplasty: Review of content and educational delivery methods. *Physiotherapy Theory and Practice.*

Louw, A., Q. Louw, et al. (2009). Preoperative Education for Lumbar Surgery for Radiculopathy. *South African Journal of Physiotherapy, 65*(2): 3-8.

Louw, A., E. L. Puentedura, et al. (2011). Use of an abbreviated neuroscience education approach in the treatment of chronic low back pain: A case report. *Physiotherapy Theory and Practice.*

Louw, A., E. L. Puentedura, et al. (2012). Use of an abbreviated neuroscience education approach in the treatment of chronic low back pain: A case report. *Physiotherapy Theory and Practice, 28*(1): 50-62.

Maitland, G. D. (1986). *Vertebral Manipulation.* London, Butterworths.

Mannion, A. F., R. Denzler, et al. (2007). A randomised controlled trial of post-operative rehabilitation after surgical decompression of the lumbar spine. *Eur Spine J, 16*(8): 1101-1117.

Meeus, M., J. Nijs, et al. (2010). Pain Physiology Education Improves Pain Beliefs in Patients With Chronic Fatigue Syndrome Compared With Pacing and Self-Management Education: A Double-Blind Randomized Controlled Trial. *Arch Phys Med Rehabil, 91*(8): 1153-1159.

Mintken, P. E., C. DeRosa, et al. (2008). AAOMPT clinical guidelines: A model for standardizing manipulation terminology in physical therapy practice. *The Journal of Orthopaedic and Sports Physical Therapy, 38*(3): A1-6.

Moseley, G. L. (2003). Joining forces - combining cognition-targeted motor control training with group or individual pain physiology education: a successful treatment for chronic low back pain. *J Man Manip Therap, 11*(2): 88-94.

Moseley, G. L. (2003). Unravelling the barriers to reconceptualisation of the problem in chronic pain: the actual and perceived ability of patients and health professionals to understand the neurophysiology. *J Pain, 4*(4): 184-189.

Moseley, G. L. (2004). Evidence for a direct relationship between cognitive and physical change during an education intervention in people with chronic low back pain. *Eur J Pain, 8*(1): 39-45.

Moseley, G. L. (2005). Widespread brain activity during an abdominal task markedly reduced after pain physiology education: fMRI evaluation of a single patient with chronic low back pain. *Aust J Physiother, 51*(1): 49-52.

Moseley, G. L. (2007). Reconceptualising pain according to modern pain sciences. *Physical Therapy Reviews, 12*: 169-178.

Moseley, G. L., M. K. Nicholas, et al. (2004). A randomized controlled trial of intensive neurophysiology education in chronic low back pain. *Clin J Pain, 20*(5): 324-330.

Moseley, L. (2002). Combined physiotherapy and education is efficacious for chronic low back pain. *Aust J Physiother, 48*(4): 297-302.

Nijs, J., C. Paul van Wilgen, et al. (2011). How to explain central sensitization to patients with 'unexplained' chronic musculoskeletal pain: practice guidelines. *Man Ther, 16*(5): 413-418.

Nijs, J., B. Van Houdenhove, et al. (2010). Recognition of central sensitization in patients with musculoskeletal pain: Application of pain neurophysiology in manual therapy practice. *Man Ther, 15*(2): 135-141.

Ostelo, R. W., R. A. Deyo, et al. (2008). Interpreting change scores for pain and functional status in low back pain: towards international consensus regarding minimal important change. *Spine (Phila Pa 1976), 33*(1): 90-94.

Pae, C. U., P. Luyten, et al. (2008). The relationship between fibromyalgia and major depressive disorder: a comprehensive review. *Current Medical Research and Opinion, 24*(8): 2359-2371.

Poiraudeau, S., F. Rannou, et al. (2006). Fear-avoidance beliefs about back pain in patients with subacute low back pain. *Pain, 124*(3): 305-311.

Puentedura, E. J., C. L. Brooksby, et al. (2009). Rehabilitation following lumbosacral percutaneous nucleoplasty: a case report. *J Orthop Sports Phys Ther, 40*(4): 214-224.

Roland, M. and R. Morris (1983). A study of the natural history of back pain. Part I: development of a reliable and sensitive measure of disability in low-back pain. *Spine (Phila Pa 1976), 8*(2): 141-144.

Roland, M. and R. Morris (1983). A study of the natural history of low-back pain. Part II: development of guidelines for trials of treatment in primary care. *Spine (Phila Pa 1976), 8*(2): 145-150.

Ryan, C. G., H. G. Gray, et al. (2010). Pain biology education and exercise classes compared to pain biology education alone for individuals with chronic low back pain: a pilot randomised controlled trial. *Man Ther, 15*(4): 382-387.

Van Oosterwijck, J., J. Nijs, et al. (2011). Pain neurophysiology education improves cognitions, pain thresholds, and movement performance in people with chronic whiplash: A pilot study. *J Rehabil Res Dev, 48*(1): EPub ahead of print

Vernon, H. (2008). The Neck Disability Index: state-of-the-art, 1991-2008. *Journal of Manipulative and Physiological Therapeutics, 31*(7): 491-502.

Vernon, H. and S. Mior (1991). The Neck Disability Index: a study of reliability and validity. *Journal of Manipulative and Physiological Therapeutics, 14*(7): 409-415.

Vlaeyen, J. W., A. M. Kole-Snijders, et al. (1995). Fear of movement/(re)injury in chronic low back pain and its relation to behavioral performance. *Pain, 62*(3): 363-372.

Watson, P. and N. Kendall (2000). Assessing psychosocial yellow flags. *Topical Issues in Pain 2*. L. S. Gifford. Falmouth, CNS Press.

Wilson, D., M. Williams, et al. (2009). Language and the pain experience. *Physiotherapy Research International: The Journal for Researchers and Clinicians in Physical Therapy, 14*(1): 56-65.

Wittmann-Price, R. A. and M. Godshall (2009). Strategies to promote deep learning in clinical nursing courses. *Nurse Educ, 34*(5): 214-216.

Chapter 6

The Bigger Picture of Pain

6.1: Introduction

In Chapters 3 and 4, we outlined the various biological systems that are engaged to protect during a pain experience in response to threat (Figure 6.1) (Sapolsky, 1994). These systems include immune, sympathetic, parasympathetic, endocrine, linguistic, motor and more. These systems are activated in response to a threat, which we can metaphorically describe as a lion entering the room (Louw, 2013; Louw, 2013).

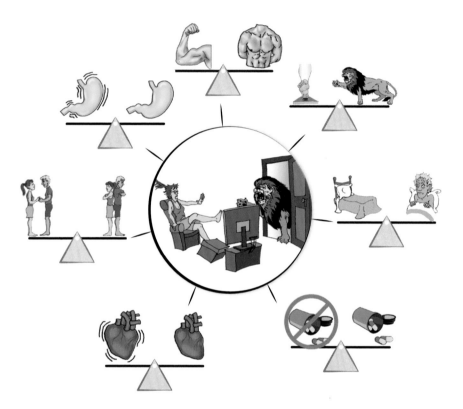

Figure 6.1: The various biological systems engaged to protect during a pain experience in response to threat.

The activation and regulation of the various bodily systems are complex and driven primarily by changes in catecholamines, such as adrenaline and cortisol. The stress response alters the catecholamines, resulting in huge, body-wide systems altering the physical and mental health of the patient. With prolonged alteration in these catecholamines, there are various long lasting, potentially irreversible changes that may occur in patients with chronic pain (Figure 6.2) (Harden, Duc et al., 1994; Madden, 2003; Riva, Mork et al., 2012).

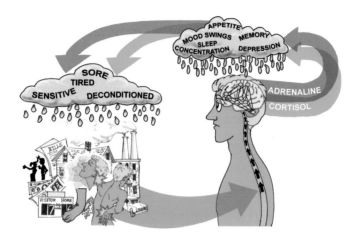

Figure 6.2: With prolonged alteration of catecholamines, long lasting and potentially irreversible changes may occur in patients with chronic pain.

It is imperative that therapists realize TNE is but one treatment strategy that may help patients with chronic pain. There is high-level evidence for aerobic exercise to help people with chronic pain, such as fibromyalgia (Busch, Barber et al., 2007). In each chapter of this textbook, including this one, we strongly urge therapists to utilize TNE while performing all the other physical modalities of exercise and manual therapy (Louw, Diener et al., 2011).

In this chapter, we will discuss how movement-based therapy can help patients in chronic pain from a neuroscience perspective. Most of the treatments utilized in therapy are rooted in biomechanical models, and it is imperative that therapists be consistent in their message. For example, a patient may receive a well designed and executed TNE session, but when the therapist applies a physical treatment such as manual therapy or exercise, he or she might reach for the anatomical model to explain the use of the physical treatment. This would add to the patient's confusion and likely undo any gains achieved through the TNE.

Additionally, this chapter will provide therapists with additional tools, such as dietary guidance, sleep hygiene, meditation, goal setting, pacing of exercise and activity, and more. A common complaint therapists may have is that they lack knowledge of "what to do with patients like this." By the end of this chapter, there will be an exhaustive list of treatment options for the patient with chronic pain.

In the section that follows, we will systematically explore each output system. The columns will indicate the immediate response of the system during an acute stress response, e.g., lion jumping in the room. The second column will describe the changes to the system if the stressor remains, e.g., lion following you around for weeks, months or years. In the final column treatment options are described, specifically directed at the signs and symptoms associated with the long term changes in each system.

6.2: Sympathetic Nervous System (SNS)

With an immediate stress response, the SNS is activated to respond to the threat. The SNS acts primarily via adrenaline (epinephrine), which is a fast acting neurotransmitter (Yanagida, 1995; Baron and Janig, 2004). Normally, it is thought to be fully active for only a few minutes at the most. Adrenaline causes pupils to dilate, heart rate to increase and blood to be diverted to areas in immediate need. Cortisol, a more potent and longer lasting catecholamine, has a similar effect to adrenaline and is likely to be more involved in the prolonged stress response (Sapolsky, 1998).

Over time, patients may experience adrenal fatigue. Adrenal fatigue is poorly defined and is disputed in medical literature (Nippoldt, 2010). The term adrenal fatigue is often used to describe nonspecific symptoms such as tiredness, difficulty sleeping and changes in appetite. Adrenal fatigue is thought to describe the inability of the adrenal glands to produce adequate quantities of cortisol (Baschetti, 2001; Tanriverdi, Karaca et al., 2007). With altered catecholamines, nerve sensitivity will increase, likely due to ion channel sensitivity to adrenaline (Devor, 2005).

Long-term patients may experience symptoms of a more sensitive gastrointestinal (GI) system as blood is diverted to other body areas (Sarzi-Puttini, Atzeni et al., 2006; Bradley, 2008; Schweinhardt, Sauro et al., 2008). Adrenaline is also thought to be a key contributor to the development and maintenance of trigger points (Bennett and Goldenberg, 2011).

It also proposed that increased adrenaline, heart rate and blood pressure results in more turbulent blood flow, potentially contributing to increased damage to the walls of blood vessels and, ultimately, atherosclerosis (Sapolsky, 1994).

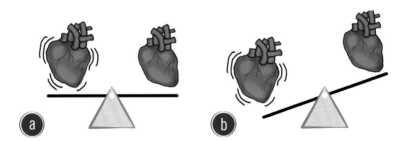

Figure 6.3: A system in balance (a) versus a system under constant stress and the various effects of a prolonged stress response (b).

Table 6.1: Effects of acute and prolonged stress on activity in the Sympathetic Nervous System

Acute Response to Threat	Long Term Changes	Potential Treatment Options
• Dilated pupils • Increased heart rate • Blood diverted to areas in need of extra blood and oxygen • Hypervigilance • Awake	• Adrenal fatigue • Increased nerve sensitization • Sleep disturbance (deep phases) • Changes in GI system • Increased development of trigger points • Fatigue • Irritability • Increased risk for atherosclerosis • Increased pain	• TNE to decrease the stressor • Skillful delivery of medication • Aerobic exercise • Relaxation • Meditation • Diaphragmatic breathing

6.3: Muscle/Motor System

In the acute stress response, blood is diverted via catecholamine activation to areas in need of immediate protection or action, i.e., larger muscle groups. In the acute phase, larger leg muscles, such as the gluteal muscles, gastrocnemius and soleus as well as quadriceps, may be needed to run away (flight response to stress). Larger muscles in the upper body may be activated, such as the deltoids, biceps and triceps, to defend (Sapolsky, 1994).

In the acute phase, smaller, less important muscles often pay the price. Blood, energy and oxygen is diverted away from postural muscles (Wakefield, Holtermann et al., 2011). Over time, lack of activity of these postural muscles may lead to postural disorders developing (Edmondston, Chan et al., 2007). Overactive muscles shorten and become more prone to trigger points (Fernandez-de-Las-Penas, Simons et al., 2007), and lengthened muscles weaken. Postural muscles also become ischemic as blood and oxygen is diverted from the muscle, which may additionally contribute to the pain (Larsson, Cai et al., 1995).

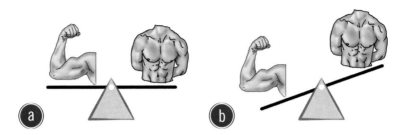

Figure 6.4: A motor system in balance with synergistic action of mobilizing and stabilizing muscles (a) versus a motor system under constant stress where mobilizing muscles are overactive in comparison to stabilizing/postural muscles (b).

When faced with a threat, stabilizing muscles, such as transversus abdominis and lumbar multifidus, experience delays in contraction (Moseley, Nicholas et al., 2004; Moseley and Hodges, 2005; Moseley and Hodges, 2006). With an impending threat, e.g., lion, the immediate need for joint protection via spinal stabilization is likely to be questioned by the brain and central nervous system. The stabilizing system is likely to disengage at the time in favor of a flight response (avoidance of threat). Numerous studies have shown that pain changes motor control related to spinal stabilization (Hodges and Richardson, 1998; Hodges and Richardson, 1999; Hodges, 2000). Furthermore, therapists need to remember that the motor cortex will be engaged in the pain neuromatrix, and this will likely impact motor control, as well (Tsao and Hodges, 2007; Puentedura and Louw, 2012). Similar research has demonstrated that pain affects the deep cervical spine flexors, which are designed to provide stabilization and protection in the cervical spine (Jull, Kristjansson et al., 2004; Jull, Falla et al., 2009).

Another interesting finding is that muscles rich in proprioceptive innervation are also affected in persistent pain states. With persistent pain states, such as fibromyalgia, it is well established that balance and coordination are affected over time (Jones, Horak et al., 2009).

Table 6.2: Effects of acute and prolonged stress on activity on the Muscle/Motor System

Acute Response to Threat	Long Term Changes	Potential Treatment Options
• Larger muscles activate in the legs to run away, i.e., glutes, hamstring and quadriceps • Larger upper extremity muscles activate to protect, i.e., hit, push, etc. • Smaller postural muscles deactivate (posture is not important right now) • Stabilizing muscles deactivate (stabilization is not important right now), for example, transversus abdominis, multifidus and deep neck flexors • Although likely a larger proprioceptive issue, it should be noted that smaller muscles containing a high number of proprioceptive fibers likely deactivate, influencing balance and proprioception	• Muscle imbalances • Fatigue • Trigger points • Balance and proprioception issues • Loss of joint protection	• Spinal stabilization • Reduce the threat, i.e., TNE • Aerobic exercise • Postural correction • Stretches • Relaxation • Balance retraining • Trigger point therapy • Diet • Hydration • Biofeedback

6.4: Endocrine System

It is now well established that pain is a neuro-endocrine-immune response. The main culprit responsible for the endocrine changes is the catecholamine cortisol. Cortisol is more formally known as hydrocortisone and is a glucocorticoid steroid hormone produced by the adrenal gland. Cortisol is produced in response to stress and low levels of blood glucocorticosteroids (Sapolsky, 1998).

The primary function of cortisol is to increase blood sugar, suppress the immune system and aid in fat, protein and carbohydrate metabolism. The release of cortisol from the adrenal gland is controlled by the hypothalamus. The secretion of corticotropin-releasing hormone (CRH) by the hypothalamus triggers anterior pituitary secretion of adrenocorticotropic hormone (ACTH). ACTH is carried by the cells to the vascular cortex where it triggers blood secretion. Cortisol also prevents the release of substances in the body that cause inflammation. This is why cortisol is used to treat conditions resulting from overactivity of the B-cell mediated antibody response such as inflammatory and rheumatoid diseases, and allergies. Low-potency hydrocortisone is used to treat skin problems such as rashes, eczema and others (Pae, Luyten et al., 2008; Van Houdenhove, Van Den Eede et al., 2009; Riva, Mork et al., 2012). Cortisol also has a daily pattern; levels peak in the early and late mornings, after which they decrease and bottom out between midnight and 4 am or 3-5 hours after sleep initiation.

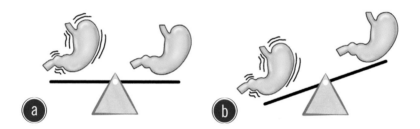

Figure 6.5: An endocrine system in balance (a) versus one under constant stress where cortisol levels are higher (b).

Cortisol is affected by changes in ACTH, depression, psychological stress, and physiological stressors such as illness, surgery, fear, injury and pain. Over time, cortisol dysregulation is associated with proteolysis, resulting in muscle wasting as well as reduction in bone formation, e.g., stress dwarfism in kids under stress such as in war zones. Furthermore, cortisol works along with adrenaline to create short-term memories. Long-term exposure to cortisol damages hippocampus cells, limiting learning and altering memory. Systemically, cortisol changes lead to increased blood pressure, increases in the vascular system's sensitivity to adrenaline, shut down of the reproductive system leading to low libido and temporary infertility, weight gain, appetite changes and obesity (Sapolsky, 1994). Over time, the endocrine system changes affect the immune system significantly (see later).

Table 6.3: Effects of acute and prolonged stress on activity in the Endocrine System

Acute Response to Threat	Long Term Changes	Potential Treatment Options

• Very similar to adrenaline
• Shunt blood
• Mobilize energy
• Increase vigilance
	• Changes in tissues:
	  ○ Fatigue
	  ○ Sensitivity
	  ○ "Sore, tired, sluggish"
	  ○ Deconditioned
	  ○ Potential failure
	
	• Brain
	  ○ Memory changes
	  ○ Weight gain
	  ○ Mood swings
	  ○ Problems with focus and concentration
	  ○ Sleep disturbance
	  ○ Changes in appetite
		• Decrease the threat, i.e., TNE
		• Aerobic exercise
		• Relaxation
		• Breathing exercise
		• Biofeedback
		• Diet

6.5: Pain System

Pain is an output by the brain based on the perception of threat (Moseley, 2003). The main "system" is the brain and central nervous system. With an immediate stress response due to a threat, e.g., a lion in the room, pain may not be produced by the brain because of the bigger threat to survival, in this case the lion. As an example, if a person were to run from the room to escape the lion and they happen to step on a nail or thumbtack, it would not likely produce pain. Pain felt from the nail or thumbtack injury while trying to escape a bigger threat (lion) would not be helpful for overall survival. Once the immediate threat has dissipated (lion chase concluded), pain may be produced by the brain to make you aware of the nail or thumbtack in the foot, which will no doubt require attention.

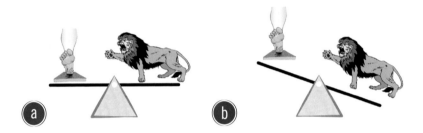

Figure 6.6: With a system in balance, pain from a nail in the foot or an attack from a lion would be weighed (a) and the brain would likely conclude that the threat of a lion attack is of greater concern than a nail; therefore, pain would not be produced (b).

This concept is highlighted by unfortunate individuals who arrive at hospital emergency departments impaled by sharp objects and with significant tissue damage, yet they experience little to no pain (Dimsdale and Dantzer, 2007). Over time though, pain will be experienced and likely increased. With persistent threat, failed treatments, different explanations for pain, etc., the "pain system," primarily the sensitivity of the nervous system, will be increased and patients will develop an extra-sensitive nervous system (Nijs, Van Houdenhove et al., 2010; Louw, 2012; Louw, Butler et al., 2013).

The clinical picture is dominated by central sensitization (Meeus and Nijs, 2007; Latremoliere and Woolf, 2009), decreased pressure pain thresholds (Fernandez-de-las-Penas, de la Llave-Rincon et al., 2009), sensitivity to movement and decreased activity and function. Terminology that applies here includes hyperalgesia and allodynia. Allodynia is pain after stimulation that is not normally painful and hyperalgesia refers to an increased response to a stimulus that is normally painful (Wall and Melzack, 2005).

Table 6.4: Effects of acute and prolonged stress on activity in the Pain System

Acute Response to Threat	Long Term Changes	Potential Treatment Options
• Down regulated	• Overactive • Hypersensitive • Hyperalgesia • Allodynia	• Reduce threat, i.e., TNE • Engage the endogenous pain mechanisms, i.e., TNE • Skillful delivery of medication • Modalities as needed • Aerobic exercise • Aquatic therapy

6.6: Immune System

As stated before, the latest view of pain includes pain as a neuro-endocrine-immune response. The immune system is very complex and, from a therapy point of view, represents a new frontier. It is now well established that the immune system plays a significant role in persistent pain states, widespread pain, body part recognition and inflammation (Miller, Cohen et al., 2002; Thacker, Clark et al., 2007; Togo, Natelson et al., 2009). The immune system is slow and changes occur over time. In an acute stress state, spending time and energy on a sore throat will not be needed, and the workings of the immune system are likely to be put on hold. This may lead to a heightened vulnerability in patients as their immunity to pathogens is suppressed.

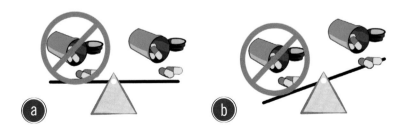

Figure 6.7: With a system in balance (a) the immune system is able to handle any threats, whereas when a system is under stress and out of balance (b), efficient activity of the immune system may be compromised.

Over time, however, immune molecules are altered by the workings of the catecholamines, especially cortisol (Adler, Kinsley et al., 1999; Staud, 2004; Bonifazi, Suman et al., 2006; Weissbecker, Floyd et al., 2006; Wingenfeld, Wagner et al., 2007; Bradley, 2008; Carvalho, Correa et al., 2008; Izquierdo-Alvarez, Bocos-Terraz et al., 2008; Stisi, Venditti et al., 2008). Altered cortisol causes some immune molecules, such as interleukin-1 (IL-1), interleukin 6 (IL-6) and tumor necrosis factor alpha (TNF-α), to proliferate over time and may contribute to increased pain states. It is now well established that these immune molecules are implicated in increased neuropathic pain via ion channel activation (Devor, 2005; Maizels and McCarberg, 2005; Arnold, 2006; Fujii, Ozaki et al., 2008; Martinez-Lavin and Solano, 2009) as well as neurogenic inflammation (Marinus, Moseley et al., 2011). During infections, trauma or injury, cytokines such as interleukin 6 (IL-6) increase 1000-fold, thus allowing more cytokine-specific ion channels to open up, potentially resulting in increased sensitivity. This is the process that is seen to occur in the flu.

Adding to the complexity of pain, it is also now well established that the immune system is likely to change the blood-brain and blood-spinal cord barriers (Beggs, Liu et al., 2010; Echeverry, Shi et al., 2011). This change is thought to be one of the mechanisms involved in the spreading of pain, receptor field changes, problems with laterality construction and disinhibition of the somatosensory homunculus. With poorer representation of the body part in the brain, pain will likely be increased to help defend. With persistent threat, therapists may see patients develop immune deficiency over time; they will get the flu or infections more often and take longer to recover. Memory changes, a sensitive nervous system, spreading pain, problems with body part recognition and pain are all thought to be tied to changes in the immune system response associated with persistent threat (pain).

Table 6.5: Effects of acute and prolonged stress on activity in the Immune System

Acute Response to Threat	Long Term Changes	Potential Treatment Options
• Initially nothing • Start slowing down gradually	• Immune deficiency • More prone to infection, sore throats, flu, etc. • Prolonged swelling and inflammation of tissues • Hypersensitive nerves • Tender to palpation • Memory changes • Problems with left/right discrimination • Disowning body parts • Spreading pain • Old injury sites and surgery sites increase sensitivity	• Understand more about the biology of what is happening, i.e., TNE • Medication • Goal setting • Coping strategies • Humor • Diet • Aerobic exercise • Social interaction

6.7: Reproductive System

Most people would agree that if they were faced with an imminent threat to their survival (a lion entering the room), their last thought would be about engaging in sexual reproduction. In the immediate stress response, sexual function and sexual desire is suppressed or put on hold. This is partly due to hormones but may also be due to the pain neuromatrix utilizing the brain's areas associated with emotions and arousal. Prolonged stress will lead to lower sex drive and infertility. This biological mechanism of sexual down-regulation can also be affected by weight gain, lower self-esteem and even abuse, which has been shown to be prevalent in chronic pain patients (Weissbecker, Floyd et al., 2006). Furthermore, a sensitive nervous system may also cause painful intercourse, which may contribute to the pain experience and further reduce interest in sexual activity.

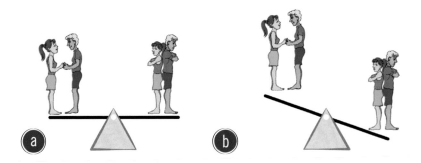

Figure 6.8: With a reproductive system in balance (a) desire and arousal will be dependent upon environmental effects (partner response, location, etc.), whereas with a system under stress and out of balance (b), desire and arousal is suppressed.

Table 6.6: Effects of acute and prolonged stress on activity in the Reproductive System

Acute Response to Threat	Long Term Changes	Potential Treatment Options
• Inhibited sexual interest and function	• Low libido • Self-confidence issues • Hyperalgesia • Infertility • Pain • Depression	• Education • Aerobic exercise • Woman's health specialist • Counseling • Medication • Biofeedback • Relaxation • Meditation

6.8: Language

When confronted by sudden stressful situations, people often respond linguistically in an uncharacteristic, and perhaps disinhibited, manner. Should a lion jump into the room, there's likely to be a very colorful linguistic response. This is typically loud and may involve swearing (Stephens, Atkins et al., 2009; Stephens and Umland, 2011). Over time, continued stress and pain may cause a linguistic change. Patients with persistent pain become less expressive, softer spoken and withdrawn. Even if patients tend to "talk a lot," clinicians will recognize that it is primarily focused on the pain they are experiencing. Patients may also describe the process of struggling to find words. Language is also likely impacted by social withdrawal, which is part of the fear avoidance model and associated with persistent pain (Vlaeyen and Linton, 2000).

Table 6.7: Effects of acute and prolonged stress on Language

Acute Response to Threat	Long Term Changes	Potential Treatment Options
• Short • Sharp • Abrasive • Expressive • Loud	• Softer • Less expressive • Difficulty finding words	• Skillful subjective examination and questioning • Safe, healing and welcoming clinical environment • Individualized care • Counseling • Therapeutic neuroscience education

6.9: Mood

In the acute stress response, moods are typically anxious, fearful, nervous and stressed. Hypervigilance is part of the overall mood, dealing with the impending threat. Over time, pain can take a significant toll on mood (Hamilton, Affleck et al., 2008; Schweinhardt, Sauro et al., 2008). All of the previously discussed biological changes occur and can lead to changes in mood. Depression sets in and is well described in patients with chronic pain (Sarzi-Puttini, Atzeni et al., 2006; Bradley, 2008; Izquierdo-Alvarez, Bocos-Terraz et al., 2008; Schweinhardt, Sauro et al., 2008; Louw, Puentedura et al., 2012). With the changes in cortisol and the inability to regulate cortisol, mood swings occur. Patients may also develop apathy, irritability, anger and frustration.

Table 6.8: Effects of acute and prolonged stress on Mood

Acute Response to Threat	Long Term Changes	Potential Treatment Options
• Stressed • Nervous • Anxious	• Depression • Mood swings • Apathy • Irritability • Anger • Frustration	• Safe, healing and welcoming clinical environment • Educate patient, i.e., TNE • Aerobic exercise • Humor • Diet • Relaxation • Meditation • Social interaction

6.10: Respiration

Most therapists should have little problem figuring out the respiratory responses to acute and prolonged stress. In the acute phase, breathing is fast, shallow and uses accessory muscles. This response coincides with the increased heart rate and adrenaline. Over time, the altered respiration pattern may lead to muscle imbalances, decreased blood flow, decreased oxygenation of tissues, and even pain. This accessory breathing pattern may also, over time, contribute to fatigue. It is hypothesized that prolonged accessory apical breathing may lead to potential health repercussions, e.g., development of pneumonia.

Table 6.9: Effects of acute and prolonged stress on Respiration

Acute Response to Threat	Long Term Changes	Potential Treatment Options
• Fast • Shallow • Accessory muscles	• Muscle imbalances • Decreased blood flow and oxygenation of tissue ○ Potential increased nerve sensitivity • Fatigue	• Diaphragmatic breathing • Biofeedback • Relaxation • Aerobic exercise

6.11: Sleep

When faced with immediate danger, such as a roaring African lion, it is not time for sleep. With the adrenal system activated, a hypervigilant state is present (Yanagida, 1995; Baron and Janig, 2004). Pupils dilate, hair stands up on the back of the neck and hearing increases to an acute level. Over time, cortisol causes similar changes in the adrenal system and causes significant interference with sleep. Patients with chronic pain have significant problems with sleep, especially falling asleep, accessing the deeper restorative phases of sleep or staying asleep (Sarzi-Puttini, Atzeni et al., 2006; Shah, Feinberg et al., 2006; Theadom, Cropley et al., 2007; Bigatti, Hernandez et al., 2008; Emad, Ragab et al., 2008; Hamilton, Affleck et al., 2008).

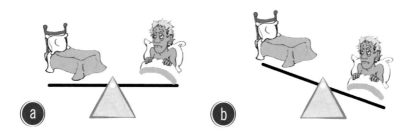

Figure 6.9: With a sleep system in balance (a) sleepiness and wakefulness are appropriately cycled, whereas with a system under stress and out of balance (b), wakefulness will disrupt sleep patterns.

Overall, the sleep disturbance has a significant effect on fatigue (Sarzi-Puttini, Atzeni et al., 2006; Theadom, Cropley et al., 2007; Hamilton, Affleck et al., 2008). Furthermore, sleep deprivation is associated with memory changes, which is prevalent in patients with chronic pain (Luerding, Weigand et al., 2008). A system often associated with sleep issues is the parasympathetic nervous system (PNS). The PNS may be altered, causing changes in sleep, the nourishing of cells and the healing of tissues.

Table 6.10: Effects of acute and prolonged stress on Sleep

Acute Response to Threat	Long Term Changes	Potential Treatment Options
• No sleep • Vigilance • Adrenaline	• Difficulty falling asleep • Fatigue • No deep phases of sleep • Sensitivity • Irritability • Decreased memory	• Education • Medication • Diet • Sleep hygiene • Relaxation • Meditation • Breathing • Biofeedback • Journaling • Aerobic exercise

Therapists continue to struggle when treating patients with chronic pain (Wolff, Michel et al., 1991; Latimer, Maher et al., 2004; Louw, Louw et al., 2009). A common complaint from therapists is that they have "no idea what to do" with such patients. A quick review of the treatment options listed in the columns in Tables 6.1 to 6.10 should give them some viable options. What we would like to stress is that there are many strategies therapists can include as a part of their treatment sessions, as well as the TNE.

A therapist providing patient education (TNE) will also need to develop and utilize an aerobic exercise program for his or her patient, including education on its importance and instruction in a home exercise program. Along with exercise, there should be discussion about a sleep hygiene program, diaphragmatic breathing, relaxation, stretching and more. It is quickly apparent that there is much therapists can do to treat such patients. A quick review of treatment options would include discussion of skillful delivery of medication, TNE, aerobic exercise, spinal stabilization, posture correction strategies, relaxation, meditation, diet, sleep hygiene, journaling, coping strategies, social interaction, humor, manual therapy, modalities, aquatic therapy, developing a safe and welcoming healing environment, goal setting, pacing and graded exposure, and more.

For the rest of this chapter, we provide some guidelines for the clinical application of these treatments. These guidelines are by no means comprehensive, but they are based on the neuroscience theme of the textbook, allowing for a more rounded biopsychosocial approach to treating patients in pain.

6.12: Guidelines for Treating Patients with Chronic Pain

6.12a: Skillful Delivery of Medication

Even with the advent of the doctorate in physical therapy (DPT) and the inclusion of pharmacology into therapy curriculums, we would strongly advise that all pharmacological questions be directed to the patient's treating physician. A therapist should, however, develop an understanding of medications as they pertain to pain management so that they may help patients understand how a medicine may influence their pain experience. It is well established that low dose anti-depressants and membrane stabilizing medication may help patients in chronic pain (Arnold, Crofford et al., 2007; Goldenberg, 2007; Hauser, Bernardy et al., 2009). Low dose anti-depressants, often referred to as selective serotonin reuptake inhibitors (SSRIs), likely help modulate pain by enhancing the endogenous mechanisms of the brain (Hauser, Bernardy et al., 2009). It is believed that membrane-stabilizing medications deactivate ion channels, thus modulating the action potential of the axons, resulting in a nerve that's less prone to fire. Clinically, patients who are too sensitive to move, exercise or be touched in therapy may have the ability to engage in much-needed movement-based therapy due to medication lowering the sensitivity of their nervous system. Ideally, patients can be slowly tapered off the medication over time. It is important to realize that most of the membrane stabilizing medications take several weeks to have a clinical effect on pain and sensitivity. Additionally, there seems to be a patient-specific characteristic or individuality to the current membrane stabilizing drugs. Patients may report that they have taken a certain membrane stabilizing drug and it did not help them, yet when switched to similar medication, they get much-needed relief.

6.12b: Therapeutic Neuroscience Education

The theme of this textbook is TNE, which has been already been described in detail. One of the main mechanisms behind TNE is the ability to help patients reconceptualize their pain experience (Moseley, 2007). In essence, by understanding more about their pain, especially the biology and physiology of their pain experience, the threat can be lessened. We have represented these threats metaphorically as an African lion and the resultant system responses.

If a small African lion cub walked into a room (Figure 6.10), the systems need not engage. If adrenaline and cortisol do not activate, because the threat is perceived to be small, it is likely that almost none of the stress system responses cataloged in the previous sections will be needed. Thus, TNE can have a significant biological effect on patients and should likely be the cornerstone of this approach.

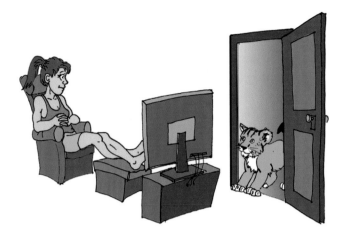

Figure 6.10: If a small lion cub were to enter the room, it might not necessarily engage the stress response systems.

6.12c: Aerobic Exercise

The overall health benefits of aerobic exercise cannot be overstated. For example, in the classic experiment the Dallas Bed Rest Study, researchers recruited six college students to spend their summer in bed. After just three weeks in bed, the subjects experienced deterioration in cardiovascular fitness that was equivalent to 20 years of aging. Thirty years later, five of the six subjects were retested. Only two had continued to exercise with any regularity, and all had gained weight and body fat. Even so, the declines from 30 years of aging were less than those they had suffered during the original three weeks of bed rest.

Immediately after being retested, the five men were put on an aerobic exercise program, which included regular walking, jogging and cycling. In just six months, the declines they had suffered over the previous 30 years were completely reversed (McGavock, Hastings et al., 2009).

In general terms, aerobic exercise (Figure 6.11) has also shown evidence in helping with the following:

- **Cognitions** (Uysal, Tugyan et al., 2005; Pontifex and Hillman, 2008; van Uffelen, Chin et al., 2008; Smith, Blumenthal et al., 2010)

- **Quality of life** (Stringer, Berezovskaya et al., 1998; Chatzitheodorou, Kabitsis et al., 2007; Dittrich, Gunther et al., 2008; Gondoh, Sensui et al., 2009; Reid, Baron et al., 2010)

- **Cardiovascular fitness** (Kramer and McDonald, 2006; O'Brien, Nixon et al., 2010)

- **Muscle tone** (O'Brien, Nixon et al., 2010)

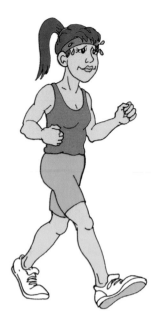

- **Oxygenation of the brain** (Caglar, Sabuncuoglu et al., 2005; Bollo, Williams et al., 2010)

- **Inhibition of gray matter loss** (Gondoh, Sensui et al., 2009)

- **Increase in overall brain size** (Colcombe, Erickson et al., 2006; Clinic, 2007).

For specific diagnoses, aerobic exercise has shown efficacy in treating patients with the following:
- **Muscle disease** (Voet, van der Kooi et al., 2010)

- **HIV** (Stringer, Berezovskaya et al., 1998; O'Brien, Nixon et al., 2010)

- **Stroke** (Quaney, Boyd et al., 2009)

- **Rheumatoid arthritis** (RA) (Hurkmans, van der Giesen et al., 2009)

Figure 6.11: Aerobic exercise has demonstrated significant health benefits.

- **Panic disorders** (Wedekind, Sprute et al., 2008)

- **Osteoarthritis** (Roos, 2002; Hart, Haaland et al., 2008)

- **Migraines** (Dittrich, Gunther et al., 2008)

- **Heart disease** (Deley, Kervio et al., 2005; Zhang, Liu et al., 2007)

- **Post-traumatic stress disorders** (PTSD) (Newman and Motta, 2007)

- **Low back pain** (Sculco, Paup et al., 2001; Tritilanunt and Wajanavisit, 2001; Hoffman, Shepanski et al., 2005; Ferreira, Ferreira et al., 2007)

- **Fibromyalgia** (gold evidence Cochrane) (Wigers, Stiles et al., 1996; Jentoft, Kvalvik et al., 2001; Dobkin, Da Costa et al., 2006; Busch, Barber et al., 2007)

- **Pregnancy** (Kramer and McDonald, 2006)

- **Diabetes** (Rossi, Santoro et al., 2005)

- **Brain injury** (Jackson, Turner-Stokes et al., 2001)

- **Cystic fibrosis** (Boas, Danduran et al., 2000)

- **Chronic fatigue syndrome** (Fulcher and White, 1997).

The list is lengthy and impressive.

In terms of neuroscience education for pain, aerobic exercise should be seen as a very powerful tool in helping the patient in chronic pain. There is overwhelming evidence for the importance of aerobic exercise in patients with chronic pain (Gowans, deHueck et al., 2001; Sim and Adams, 2002; Goldenberg, Burckhardt et al., 2004; Bonifazi, Suman et al., 2006; Busch, Barber et al., 2007; Rooks, Gautam et al., 2007; Brosseau, Wells et al., 2008; Carville, Arendt-Nielsen et al., 2008). Aerobic exercise in and of itself has been shown to help decrease pain, causing an immediate post-exercise hypoalgesia (Koltyn, Garvin et al., 1996; Hoffman, Shepanski et al., 2004; Bruce, Fries et al., 2005; Hoffman, Shepanski et al., 2005; Chatzitheodorou, Kabitsis et al., 2007; Hoffman and Hoffman, 2007; Hurkmans, van der Giesen et al., 2009; Sharma, Ryals et al., 2010). There is also ample evidence that aerobic exercise has the following effects:

- **Improves sleep** (Catai, Chacon-Mikahil et al., 2002; Yamamoto, Mohri et al., 2007; Ucok, Aycicek et al., 2009; Reid, Baron et al., 2010)

- **Improves motor function** (Quaney, Boyd et al., 2009)

- **Improves memory** (Miles and Hardman, 1998; Uysal, Tugyan et al., 2005; Pontifex, Hillman et al., 2009)

- **Improves cortisol changes** (Wedekind, Sprute et al., 2008)

- **Aids the immune system** (Stringer, Berezovskaya et al., 1998; Woods, Ceddia et al., 1999; Boas, Danduran et al., 2000; Bauer and Weisser, 2002; Castellano and White, 2008; Haaland, Sabljic et al., 2008)

- **Decreases chronic inflammation** (Haaland, Sabljic et al., 2008)

- **Decreases anxiety** (Newman and Motta, 2007)

- **Decreases depression symptoms** (Dimeo, Bauer et al., 2001; Oman and Oman, 2003; Blumenthal, Babyak et al., 2007; Newman and Motta, 2007)

- **Improves mood** (Petruzzello and Tate, 1997; Sculco, Paup et al., 2001; Hoffman and Hoffman, 2007)

- **Decreases nerve sensitivity** (Nathan, Wilcox et al., 2001)

- **Is just as effective as anti-depressants in patients with chronic pain** (Blumenthal, Babyak et al., 2007).

Therapists must have the necessary skills to effectively highlight the importance and benefit of an aerobic exercise program to their patient. Patients in chronic pain are often reluctant to engage in exercise because they experience pain with activity and movements, and they may believe the pain signals harm to their tissues. TNE aims to help patients reconceptualize their pain (Moseley, 2007). Once the TNE has helped a patient reconceptualize their pain, the patient needs to be introduced to the benefit of aerobic exercise through a neuroscience approach. Benefits would include changes in adrenaline, decreased activation of the ion channels, decreased firing of the nervous system, decreased upregulation of the central nervous system, improved respiration, improved sleep, decreased pain, improved immunity, regulation of cortisol, improved oxygenation of the brain, improved mood, improved cognitions, improved memory, improved appetite, lifting of depression, oxygenation and energizing of tissues, decreased sensitivity of tissues, and improved blood flow throughout the body.

Once a patient has been educated via TNE to reconceptualize their pain and persuaded as to the neurophysiological benefits of aerobic exercise, therapists may consider various strategies to help patients remain compliant with their home exercise program (HEP). Strategies include the following:

- **Keeping an exercise log book** (Cox, Burke et al., 2003; Mailloux, Finno et al., 2006; Moseley, 2006; Hurling, Catt et al., 2007; Wu, Keyes et al., 2010)

- **Providing no more than five exercises for HEP** (Duncan and Pozehl, 2002; Medina-Mirapeix, Escolar-Reina et al., 2009)

- **Educating the patient more about the importance of exercise** (Friedrich, Gittler et al., 1998; Friedrich, Gittler et al., 2005; Mori, Sogg et al., 2006; Mayoux-Benhamou, Giraudet-Le Quintrec et al., 2008; Medina-Mirapeix, Escolar-Reina et al., 2009)

- **Making the exercises personal to the patient rather than a generic approach** (Scales and Miller, 2003; Asenlof, Denison et al., 2005)

- **Treating pain before and even during the exercise program** (Engstrom and Oberg, 2005; Dobkin, Sita et al., 2006; Medina-Mirapeix, Escolar-Reina et al., 2009)

- **Keeping instructions simple** (Lysack, Dama et al., 2005; Ainsworth and Hagino, 2006)

- **Constantly motivating patients** (Scales and Miller, 2003; Ainsworth and Hagino, 2006)

- **Using low-cost equipment** (Ainsworth and Hagino, 2006).

In addition to such strategies, therapists may want to consider the use of electronic aids to help patients in the current and ever-evolving technical world, such as the Internet, smart phones and their applications, etc. In a recent study, a fully automated Internet and mobile phone-based motivation and action support system was shown to significantly increase and maintain the level of physical activity in healthy adults (Hurling, Catt et al., 2007). The test group received tailored solutions for perceived barriers, a weekly schedule to plan their exercise sessions with mobile phone and email reminders, a message board to share their experiences with others, and feedback on their level of physical activity. We would strongly urge therapists to begin looking at the use of modern technology to help remind patients about their exercise program.

While we are on the subject of modern technology enhancing patient care, therapists might also consider the delivery of TNE via the use of these new technological devices. As an example, in a recent case study (Louw et al., 2013 – submitted for publication), a patient with chronic pain following thoracic outlet surgery received a single one-on-one clinic session with a therapist who examined the patient and delivered a TNE session. After the initial and only on-site consultation, the patient was monitored, educated, advised and progressed with respect to exercise, activity, movement and goals via e-mail (Figure 6.12).

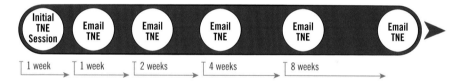

Figure 6.12: Timeframe of a single case study involving therapeutic neuroscience education (TNE) delivered in a hybrid on-site and distance format via email.

In this case, the patient not only reported significant recovery but also had the financial benefit of limiting expensive travel and time. We propose that approaches such as this may be of significant benefit for patients in remote areas, and future research should aim to investigate such avenues. With the expansion of technology, tele-health needs to be expanded and adequately researched for its efficacy and cost-savings advantages, including the delivery of TNE (Tousignant, Boissy et al.; Thomas, Burton et al., 2004).

Out of all the strategies we might utilize clinically, having patients write out (pen and paper) a schedule for their exercise, specifying day, date, time and activity, has allowed patients to be a lot more compliant (Heiden, Testa et al., 2009). This approach was recently replicated in a student-exercise study (Schwartz, 2010).

Students were randomized into three groups to measure compliance. One group was instructed to exercise at least once for twenty minutes during the following week with no further parameters provided. A second group was given the same challenge, but this group was given a detailed education session about the importance of exercise in reducing the risk of heart disease, as further motivation. A third group was asked to commit to exercising at a specific time, on a specific day, at a designated location and write that commitment using pen and paper. Results from this study showed that after a week, only 29% of the students in the first group reported having completed their exercise tasks. Compliance rose modestly for the second group (to 39%) by the provision of educational motivation. The third group reported greatest compliance (91%), and the researchers concluded that exercise, especially for personal health reasons, is a habit (Schwartz, 2010). By having the students commit to the task and build it into their daily schedule, it became a routine and much easier to follow. Most people will realize that a major reason they might struggle to exercise is through falling out of the habit or routine. Therapists should endeavor to create or build a routine for their patients.

Two important considerations in aerobic exercise are dosage and frequency. To explore this we should revisit the definition of aerobic exercise. Aerobic exercise is working out at an intensity of 60-70% of one's age-predicted maximum heart rate (HR). Commonly, age predicted max HR is calculated as 220 minus a person's age. So, as an example, a 40-year-old patient would have a max HR of 180 (220 minus 40). In this example, 60% of max HR would be 108 (180 X 0.6) and 70% of max HR would be 126 (180 X 0.7), and this would mean that our 40-year-old patient should be exercising at a target HR of 108–126 beats per minute.

With reference to pain, it has been shown that aerobic exercise at >50% VO_2 max and for a duration >10 min is required to elicit exercise analgesia (Hoffman, Shepanski et al., 2004). Without discussing the complexities of individualized max HR and VO_2 max, it is suggested that most patients in chronic pain should aim to raise their exercise HR to 100–110 beats per minute. Clinically, therapists should realize this is probably not that much elevated from the resting heart rate of most patients in chronic pain. A brisk walk may be all that is needed. Patients are often fearful that aerobic exercise will mean running a marathon or enduring boot camp-style vigorous exercises. This perception may cause undue stress and fear, which may in turn increase pain. Therapists should seek to calm any fears and anxiety associated with aerobic exercise by reviewing the above information with their patient.

A good example of this approach is a study on patients with chronic fatigue syndrome (Fulcher and White, 1997). Patients with chronic fatigue syndrome started with 5-15 minutes of walking, five days per week, and tolerated it well. By adding 1-2 minutes per day, they worked their way up to 30 minutes. They had the choice to substitute walking with bicycling or swimming. After the 12-week study, more than half the patients reported feeling substantially better. After one year, 63% of the participants were still doing very well. In a second group of patients, who were given stretches and relaxation exercises, only 25% reported improvement at the same follow up point.

Once again, the benefits of aerobic exercise cannot be overstated, even for chronic pain. This section should not be taken lightly since the therapist will face a huge challenge ahead of them. It has been shown in patients with chronic heart failure that only 22% adhere to their HEP; further data shows that in cardiac rehabilitation in patients who have had a heart attack, only one in seven follow through with their exercise program and make long lasting changes (Capomolla, Ceresa et al., 2002).

All of this information is good news. The evidence for exercise is compelling, but....the patient is in pain! The biggest issue therapists will face is the patient's pain. They know that exercise is good for them; they know it may even help, but you (the therapist) do not understand...they hurt, and the more they exercise, the more they hurt! It cannot be stressed enough that exercise should only be discussed once a patient has developed a better understanding of their pain. The key message of TNE is that tissues and injuries heal over time. Once they have healed, tissues can be sore, sensitive and deconditioned; a significant proportion of the continued pain is more likely due to an oversensitive nervous system. The 'alarm system' is too sensitive in the patient with chronic pain. It only takes a few pulls on the resistance band for the alarm to go off. The important message to have the patient understand is that their alarm is not signaling further injury but 'sensitivity.' It may be helpful to review or draw the extra-sensitive nerves for a patient as they embark on exercise (Figure 6.13).

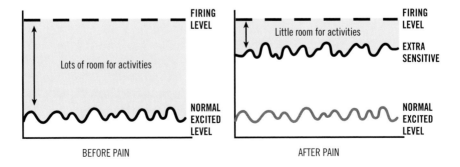

Figure 6.13: Explaining that the nervous system may be 'extra sensitive' and that is why activity increases pain.

Patients can also be taught mantras or self-talk. This is frequently done by athletes. For example, a marathon runner trying to qualify for the Olympic team will prepare himself not only physically, but mentally. In this case, an experienced marathon runner will know the real race only starts 20 miles into the race. He may mentally prepare through self-talk or mantras for that time of the race when the going will get tough. Patients in pain are really no different. Patients should learn – "sore but safe" or "hurt does not equal harm."

Conversely, there are other mantras that are more likely to be detrimental to the patient in chronic pain. Two in particular are worthy of discussion – "no pain; no gain" (Figure 6.14) and "if it hurts, don't do it" (Figure 6.15).

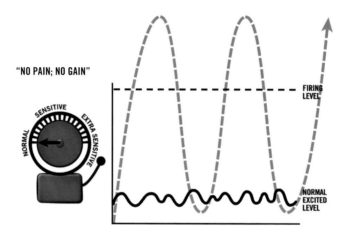

Figure 6.14: The detrimental consequences of following a 'no pain; no gain' mantra when a patient has chronic pain.

In the "no pain; no gain" approach, patients may push themselves hard, disregard the pain barrier and push right through it. Pain protects, so the patient will crash. He or she may valiantly try again, and the same will happen. This is the classic 'boom-bust' cycle, which will overwhelm the patient, and they will learn that it does not help to push hard into pain. With failure, resentment, depression and even fear, pain is likely to be increased and will be produced earlier over time to protect.

In an acute injury, e.g., an athlete rehabilitating from an ankle sprain, this model of "no pain; no gain" may pose no problems, but it will likely not work in the patient with chronic pain. It is, however, worth noting that an athlete who fights their way through "no pain; no gain" likely understands their pain. They know what it means and do not fear it. Once again, knowledge is important in reducing fear. Pain that is understood does not induce fear and anxiety.

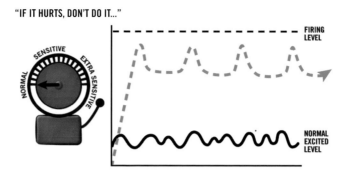

"IF IT HURTS, DON'T DO IT..."

Figure 6.15: The detrimental consequences of following a 'if it hurts, don't do it' mantra when a patient has chronic pain.

The second mantra, "if it hurts, don't do it," is probably much more common in patients with chronic pain. This approach is riddled with fear, anxiety and uncertainty. It could also be argued that an approach such as this wakens the alarm system by making patients focus on the exact moment he or she experiences pain. Given the sensitivity of the nervous system, a patient's ability to execute meaningful progressive tasks and exercise will be diminished considerably, and no progress will be made. In fact, given that fear and anxiety will increase nerve sensitivity, the tolerances will decrease over time, limiting exercise and movement more and more. This is the classic fear avoidance model.

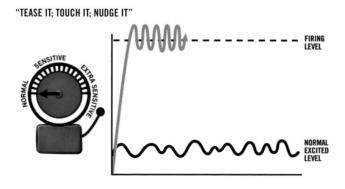

"TEASE IT; TOUCH IT; NUDGE IT"

Figure 6.16: The concept of exercising and performing activities to the point of onset of discomfort or "tease it; touch it; nudge it," where 'it' is pain.

Because both of the previous approaches present significant limitations, therapists may be left questioning what they can or should do. An alternative approach of "tease it; touch it; nudge it" (Figure 6.16) appears to lead to better outcomes over time for this patient population. In such an approach, patients are instructed to exercise or do a task slightly into some discomfort but not to crash through it into pain or to stop short.

Armed with improved knowledge about the neurobiology of pain, mantras and coaching from the therapist, the patient will succeed. Over time, the pain threshold will increase as they reap the benefits of exercising, allowing them to push a little further with the exercise. Over time, the numbers, distance and time will increase: five minutes of walking becomes six, followed by seven, etc. (Figure 6.17).

"TEASE IT; TOUCH IT; NUDGE IT"

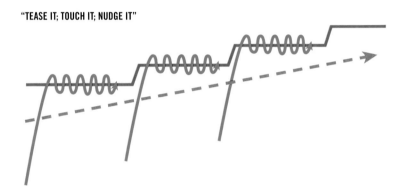

Figure 6.17: Over time, the patient will be able to perform more repetitions and longer sets over a longer time period as the pain threshold increases, allowing them to do more without experiencing their pain.

6.12d: Strengthening

In contrast to all the available research on aerobic exercise and pain, less is known about strengthening. Additionally, there does not appear to be any compelling evidence that patients in chronic pain will have become significantly weakened. Bed rest, limited movement and generally decreased functioning may take a toll, but most of these patients will have become deconditioned rather than exhibiting true muscle weakness. The available evidence for strengthening in patients with chronic pain suggests the use of lighter weight and resistance exercise along with higher repetitions (Valkeinen, Hakkinen et al., 2005; Brosseau, Wells et al., 2008). Clinically, it may be worth thinking of lighter-weight, higher-repetition exercises as toning exercises and another way to bring about increased heart rate, blood flow and oxygenation of tissues.

It should also be recognized how educating a patient that they are in need of strengthening exercises may give them the implication of weakness, which in turn may produce fear and anxiety. Resistance exercises should therefore be considered conditioning exercises. As with aerobic exercise, conditioning exercises should be preempted with TNE and a reminder to patients of the extra sensitivity of their nervous system. They should understand that receiving signals from the body part being exercised is normal and likely not signaling true tissue damage. Finally, conditioning exercises should not focus on pain. Patients should be encouraged to focus on a certain number of repetitions, duration or distance. Not only will this help to de-focus pain, but it should also reinforce the message that pain is not important in this case.

6.12e: Spinal Stabilization

The amount of research on spinal stabilization for low back pain over the past two decades has been truly impressive (Richardson, Jull et al., 1999; Richardson, Hodges et al., 2004). Much of that research has focused on muscle properties, fine-wire needle electromyography findings in healthy and painful volunteers, muscle contractile properties, pain inhibition, effect of fear and catastrophization on motor control, imaging studies, physical tests associated with motor control, and more (Hides, Richardson et al., 1995; Hides, Richardson et al., 1996; Hides, Richardson et al., 1996; Hodges and Richardson, 1997; Hodges, Cresswell et al., 1999; Hodges, 2001; Hodges, Cresswell et al., 2001; Hodges, Moseley et al., 2003; Moseley, Nicholas et al., 2004; Moseley and Hodges, 2005; Hides, Belavy et al., 2007). More recently, a research team from the same university developed similar research related to the cervical spine focusing on deep cervical spine flexors for cervical spine stabilization (Jull, Sterling et al., 2008). This research once again focused on muscle and contractile properties in symptomatic individuals and, subsequently, in patient groups with neck pain, headache and traumatic injuries to the cervical spine (Jull, Barrett et al., 1999; Falla, Bilenkij et al., 2004; Falla, Jull et al., 2004; Falla, Jull et al., 2004; Jull, Kristjansson et al., 2004; Falla, Jull et al., 2006; Falla, Jull et al., 2006; Falla, Jull et al., 2007; Falla, O'Leary et al., 2007). The purpose of this section discussing spinal stabilization is not to review spinal stabilization theory but to discuss the clinical application of spinal stabilization in patients with chronic pain.

Spinal stabilization has been proposed as a treatment for patients with chronic LBP (Hodges 2003, Cairns, Foster et al., 2006; Goldby, Moore et al., 2006; Critchley, Ratcliffe et al., 2007). Despite the popularity of spinal stabilization, controversy has ensued. The controversy has surrounded an approach whereby therapists teach patients a very specific approach that focuses on specific muscles, e.g., transversus abdominis, using a definite sequence of retraining those muscles, and equipment such as the biofeedback units and diagnostic ultrasound (Fritz, Whitman et al., 2005; Koumantakis, Watson et al., 2005; Cairns, Foster et al., 2006). This is often referred to as 'specific' spinal stabilization. This approach is summarized by Hodges as "firing the right muscles at the right time, in the right sequence for the right amount of time and then disengaging at the appropriate time" (Richardson, Hodges et al., 2004). This approach is attributed to researchers from Queensland university, including Hodges, Jull, Richardson and Hides (Richardson, Jull et al., 1999; Richardson, Hodges et al., 2004).

In contrast to the 'specific approach,' it has also been postulated that stabilization can be performed as a more generalized approach, i.e., one that's not overly concerned about specific muscles, sequences of contraction, or careful monitoring and quantification of contractions. This more generalized approach has been promoted mainly by Stuart McGill (Vera-Garcia, Brown et al., 2006; Fenwick, Brown et al., 2009; Sanchez-Zuriaga, Vera-Garcia et al., 2009). From the clinical perspective, therapists are likely to be using one approach or the other.

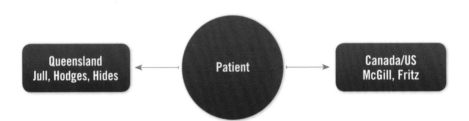

Figure 6.18: Spinal stabilization for low back pain can be approached from two differing points of view: a 'specific' motor control approach, promoted by researchers from Queensland, versus a more 'general' strengthening approach, advocated by researchers from Canada (McGill) and the US (Fritz).

The major contention surrounding the differing spinal stabilization approaches is the paucity of evidence for either approach. Current evidence, focusing on systematic reviews and high-quality randomized controlled trials, has failed to show that spinal stabilization exercises are superior to other forms of exercise and therapy for patients with LBP (Mannion, Caporaso et al., Koumantakis, Watson et al., 2005; Niemisto, Rissanen et al., 2005; Nilsson-Wikmar, Holm et al., 2005; Cairns, Foster et al., 2006; Critchley, Ratcliffe et al., 2007).

Once again, it is not our aim to describe spinal stabilization in detail but to offer useful strategies for patients with chronic LBP. While it may be appropriate to focus on a 'specific' motor control approach with some patients, we believe there is a stronger argument for a more 'generalized' approach for patients with chronic LBP. This is based on the realization that patients with persistent pain will struggle to perform small, well-coordinated tasks such as those required during the 'specific' spinal stabilization approach. Various factors may contribute to this struggle, including the motor cortex being utilized in the pain neuromatrix (Puentedura and Louw, 2012), decreased importance in fine motor control when facing threat (Sapolsky, 1994), altered cortical representation of the low back, i.e., smudging (Flor, 2000; Moseley, 2008), psychological issues affecting motor control (Moseley and Hodges, 2006), and problems with pelvic position sense (Luomajoki and Moseley, 2011). The 'generalized' approach we advocate for such patients would mean teaching patients a simple bracing exercise and then shifting focus quickly to more functional movements and tasks.

When considering spinal stabilization concepts from a TNE perspective, care should once again be given to the language used when educating patients about their need for stabilization. Patients may assume stabilization means "instability" or weakness, which may induce fear. Additionally, if a therapist decides to opt for the 'specific' spinal stabilization approach, with its stronger focus and emphasis on specific muscles and sequences of motor control retraining, the patient may become frustrated, as they will be unable to perform a simple abdominal drawing-in maneuver.

6.12f: Posture

If we recall the cascade of events that are likely to occur in the stress response, such as when a lion enters the room, we will understand how postural changes can occur, especially over a long period. Patients will likely report pain associated with postural demands, but this may also in part be due to blood flow changes, i.e., ischemia (Wakefield, Holtermann et al., 2011). It is important that therapists understand that even if posture is perceived to be poor, it may not correlate to pain and pathology (Lewis, Green et al., 2005; Lewis, Wright et al., 2005; Edmondston, Chan et al., 2007). A critical point to be made with respect to posture is that as long as there is the perception of threat, e.g., a lion in the room, there will be little chance for posture to be restored. Given the neuroscience premise of postural changes, therapists are clinically challenged to teach patients self-correcting exercises, develop reminder strategies and focus on aerobic exercise to help oxygenate the sensitive postural muscles (Larsson, Cai et al., 1995).

6.12g: Relaxation and Meditation

Relaxation styles, approaches and schools of thought are varied. Therapists may explore various strategies with their patients, but they should make it as uncomplicated as possible. Patients should be taught progressive relaxation (Hassett and Gevirtz, 2009). Patients may be asked to tighten muscles followed by relaxation: "feel it melting away." Relaxation exercises may be especially beneficial in the period before going to sleep, i.e., as part of the sleep hygiene program. Patients should also be taught small, easy relaxation activities to incorporate during busy daily tasks. This may include stopping activity after a reminder from a clock, timer, electronic media or simple reminder note. During these breaks, patients could take deep, cleansing breaths. Tied into relaxation and breathing, therapists with some training in meditation techniques may also wish to incorporate meditation into the relaxation regimen (Kaplan, Goldenberg et al., 1993).

6.12h: Diet

The issue of foods and their effect on pain can be a relative minefield. In general, therapists might consider two clinical approaches. First, they may wish to study the field of dietary approaches and pain from the various resources available (Barnard, 1998). A second approach may be to refer to a dietician and arrange an appropriate consultation with the patient. We would recommend that, regardless of the strategy chosen, every effort should be made to avoid adding any further financial concern to patients with chronic pain. We should not be in the business of selling or recommending special foods, supplements or diets to our patients. Many patients with chronic pain complaints are likely to spend a small fortune on various treatments, such as pillows, magnets, orthotics and more. We see no need to add further stressors to enhance the pain experience. Finally, the core components of TNE are education and empowerment for the patient, which is teaching them to help themselves. If it is deemed appropriate for a particular patient, a dietician can be brought onboard to help them make good food choices, learn to read dietary labels, etc.

6.12i: Sleep Hygiene

Sleep disturbance is well documented in patients with chronic pain (Sarzi-Puttini, Atzeni et al., 2006; Shah, Feinberg et al., 2006; Theadom, Cropley et al., 2007; Bigatti, Hernandez et al., 2008; Emad, Ragab et al., 2008; Hamilton, Affleck et al., 2008). Of all the treatment strategies, restoring a healthy sleep pattern may be the most beneficial and provide long-lasting benefits (Schaefer, Chandran et al., 2011; Mork and Nilsen, 2012; Wolfe, 2012). The National Sleep Foundation recommends adults sleep between seven and nine hours a day. In a study where subjects were placed in rooms with no windows to the outside so that they would be unaware if it was night or day, subjects slept an average of eight hours a day. Americans report an average of six and a half hours of sleep per day, which may even be overestimated. In a Chicago study, 699 middle-aged adults reported that they slept 7.5 hours per day, but wrist monitors, worn to detect the true amount of sleep they got, reported an average of only 6.1 hours per day (Lauderdale, Knutson et al., 2008).

Many strategies have been proposed to assist patients to sleep better. From the clinical perspective, it is recommended that therapists develop a check-list for their patient to systematically follow a set program. By having the patient add one additional strategy each night, the patient will steadily incorporate the strategies and develop a healthier sleeping pattern (Schwartz, 2010). Such strategies include the following:

- **Shut the lights and television off**–Lights and television stimulate the nervous system, and keeping them on till late night makes it more difficult to sleep. Ideally, have patients shut off all non-essential lights and turn the television off one hour prior to bedtime. Patients should use this time for breathing, relaxation, reading and gentle stretches to prepare their body for sleep.

- **No naps during the day**–Stating this to a patient may upset them. However, sleep cycles have been studied extensively, and if a person sleeps in the day for more than a 20-minute nap, it will have a negative effect on night sleep, which they need (Schwartz, 2010).

- **No caffeine after morning or early afternoon**–Caffeine is a stimulant and thus keeps you awake (Currie, Wilson et al., 1995). In an ideal world, patients with persistent pain should attempt to wean themselves completely off caffeine. Apart from the stimulating effect, it is also linked to muscle tenderness and trigger points (Fernandez-De-Las-Penaz, Arendt-Nielsen et al., 2010). It has been shown that the caffeine from one soft drink in the late morning will still be circulating in the system late in the evening (Schwartz, 2010). Patients who drink caffeinated beverages should try to limit them to the morning and, maybe, early afternoon, to give them the best chance to sleep.

- **Park your ideas**–When someone has a lot of 'stuff' on their mind, for instance, remembering to take the trash out, remembering the parent-teacher meeting next Monday and remembering to pay the water bill tomorrow, the brain is kept busy. Relaxing in such a scenario will be challenging. Patients may consider keeping a little note pad and pen next to their bed. When they go to bed, they should be encouraged to write all their thoughts down. It can be seen as a way to give the brain permission to "let go" since the messages are 'parked,' not lost, and will be ready for the morning.

- **Darken and cool your room** – Melatonin is a hormone that is part of the human sleep cycle and aids sleeping (Klerman, Goldenberg et al., 2001). Melatonin works at its best in cooler temperatures and when a room is dark. Patients should close the curtains, pull down the shades, shut the lights off, close the doors and cool the room, or use a fan.

- **No kids or animals in bed** – Sleep is vital in the recovery process, and having kids or animals in bed will make it more difficult to get to sleep, and stay asleep, due to movement and extra body heat.

- **No alcohol** – Alcohol is a double-edged sword. On one hand, it may be a relaxant and reduce stress and anxiety. On the other hand, it is a diuretic and will interfere with sleep when increased bathroom breaks occur. Moderation is likely the key as well as avoiding alcohol late at night and before bed.

- **Limit water intake in the evening** – Hydration is important, and patients should keep with the recommendations set out to stay properly hydrated. Once again, patients should ensure they hydrate during the day and early evening but avoid large volumes of water right before bed. Too much water intake in the late evenings will most likely lead to several bathroom breaks during the night, when sleep is needed the most.

- **Stay in bed** – Patients should force themselves to sleep and not wake in the morning. If they have trouble going to bed or wake up early, they should force themselves to sleep. In the evening, if they set a time such as 9PM to go to bed and they find themselves struggling, they should lie still and close their eyes, even if they're still wide awake. The same applies for waking in the mornings. If they wake and it's still early, they should stay in bed and keep their eyes closed. After doing this for a few days, these "closed-eye" sessions will transfer into sleep (Schwartz, 2010).

- **Exercise** – It should be no surprise that exercise enhances sleep. There are many reasons for this, and some include flushing catecholamines such as adrenaline and cortisol out of the blood. Both chemicals increase alertness and thus hinder sleep.

The aforementioned list is a start. Therapists are once again encouraged to develop a personalized list for their patients and have patients use it as a checklist. The following is a clinic example:

Below, you will find a series of strategies to help you with your sleep. Changing sleep patterns may take a few days/weeks. Keep at it. Research has shown that if/when you make these changes, they will kick in quickly and translate to increased sleep, helping you feel refreshed, have more energy, have less pain and a change in mood. As you complete a task, check it off.

☐ Set a time to go to bed, and no…1AM is not an option.

☐ Lights, TV and computer off. One hour prior to bed time, quiet the house down.

☐ No large volumes of water prior to going to bed, to avoid going to the bathroom a lot.

☐ Limit alcoholic beverages to early evening; it makes you go to the bathroom as well.

☐ Keep bedroom dark and cool.

☐ No kids or animals in bed.

☐ Park your ideas – put a notepad and pen next to your bed and write all last-minute thoughts down (pay bills, call Sally, etc.) – so the brain can let it go and sleep.

☐ In the hour prior to sleep, relax, breathe, stretch, meditate and read.

☐ No checking e-mails prior to bed, as it will keep your brain going.

☐ Turn lights off when going to bed. If you cannot sleep, close your eyes and relax until you finally fall asleep. Studies have shown this quiet time quickly translates to sleep, and there's another extra hour every night.

☐ Have a set wake-up time. As with going to bed, if you wake up early, stay in bed and relax with your eyes closed. This, too, will translate to sleep.

☐ Keep caffeine to a minimum, especially in late afternoons and evening.

☐ No naps. Yes – this may make you tear up the paper, but naps mess up evening sleep patterns. If you want a nap, quick cat naps of no more than 20 minutes will refresh without messing up the night sleep rhythm.

☐ Exercise such as aerobic exercise (walking) helps reduce stress chemicals in the body and thus will help you sleep better.

☐ Medicine should be taken per your doctor's advice.

☐ Other.

6.12j: Journaling

Chronic pain is complex and cognitive treatment calls for reflection. Deep learning requires a patient to receive the message aimed at cognitive change, internalize it and apply it to their problem, i.e., pain (Sandberg and Barnard, 1997). Journaling is commonly used in psychology and is yet another strategy to help patients in pain focus on positive change, reflect on events and even slow down. Journaling could fit easily into the sleep hygiene program, specifically during the hour before bed as part of the process of turning lights off, television off, stretches, relaxation and meditation, as well as reading. Patients who are not interested in extensive journaling could reflect on a few positive thoughts from the day, or even a single thought, and enter it into the daily logbook they keep regarding their exercise program (Moseley, 2006).

6.12k: Coping Skills

The ultimate goal of treatment is independence. Patients should be taught ways to "help themselves." This is a core strategy in recovery. Coping strategies are vital tools in helping a patient develop mastery over a problem and his or her life, and reduce fear and anxiety (Gifford, 1998). It has even been shown that coping strategies, such as a means to take control of a situation like a "flare up," has a positive effect on the immune system (Rabin, 1999). Clinically, therapists are encouraged to teach patients to engage in these coping tasks when they experience "a bad day." Furthermore, therapists may even place a reminder/sticker on the inside of a patient's home exercise program (HEP) folder to remind them. Strategies include the following:

- **Problem solve**–Patients need to see the cause/relationship aspects of why they experience more pain on a particular day or time. For example, they may have overdone a certain task, such as sitting too long in front of a computer or doing excessive loads of laundry, and this can be rectified in the future. Keeping true to the TNE message, specifically chapter 1, the overload can also be some emotional issue that may have caused a bad day. By recognizing an event and how it impacted pain, they can develop a deeper understanding of their pain.

- **Reduce nociception**–Any possible measure to reduce nociception should be used, specifically the ones patients have found beneficial in the past. This may include application of ice, heat or a TENS unit.

- **Active approaches**–Patients should be encouraged to pursue active approaches to help their pain, particularly exercises like aerobic activities, such as a brisk walk, or specific stretches. Patients may even be asked to perform only a very special set of exercises on a bad day, e.g., ones marked with a red dot or walk for five minutes only.

- **Get away**—Often a particular environment will impact pain considerably. Patients should be taught to escape the immediate "here and now" with some strategies. This may include getting up from a chair in a cubicle and going to the drinking fountain once every hour and, as they walk, take in deep breaths and begin to relax. Patients with private offices may close the door, lie on the floor and do a few breathing and relaxation exercises. A housewife may step outside the house, walk down the sidewalk for a few minutes, turn around and return. Clocks, timers, applications or simple sticky notes can be used to remind patients to periodically "get away."

- **No on or off switch**—Patients should be discouraged from "doing nothing." The tendency is for a patient experiencing a bad day to shut down, go home (or to the couch) and do nothing; this tendency should be discouraged. Patients may indeed re-schedule or re-prioritize tasks on a "bad day," but they should be encouraged to perform at least *some* of their scheduled tasks.

The end result of a coping strategy such as this is self-care. A patient finds ways he or she can help themself and becomes less dependent on the healthcare provider.

6.12l: Social Interaction

Social interaction is very important. It is well established that patients with chronic pain withdraw from life as they experience disuse, depression and disability (Vlaeyen, Kole-Snijders et al., 1995). Patients in pain limit their time out in the community, they avoid family gatherings, do not go to the mall or movies, and often see their time out of the house as a time to gather supplies while living in a self-appointed confinement. It is interesting to note that social interaction plays a significant role in keeping the immune system healthy (Rabin, 1999), and patients should be encouraged to get out of their comfort zone and experience life. Clinically, therapists might encourage patients to develop a written plan to attend a movie, attend a family gathering, meet someone at the mall for lunch, etc.

6.12m: Humor

Patients in pain don't laugh (Falkenberg, Jarmuzek et al., 2011). Patients with chronic pain laugh even less (Bokarius, Ha et al., 2011; Bozikas, Kosmidis et al., 2011). Apart from effects of pain, it is estimated that people, in general, laugh a lot less than they used to. When did you last experience a good old belly laugh? As with social interaction, it has been shown that humor correlates to a healthier immune system (Rabin, 1999), and therapists may use humor as a strategy to help with pain and lift depression (Falkenberg, Buchkremer et al., 2011). Therapists may consider joke books in the waiting room, cartoon-of-the-day, joke telling, and even more importantly, not take themselves too seriously in the clinic.

6.12n: Manual Therapy

The application of manual therapy for chronic pain can also be a double-edged sword. Skillful delivery of manual therapy techniques has a significant potential to alter nociception and, ultimately, a pain experience (Fernandez-Carnero, Fernandez-de-las-Penas et al., 2008; Beneciuk, Bishop et al., 2009; La Touche, Paris-Alemany et al., 2012). A significant concern, however, is the model in which manual therapy tends to be presented to the patient. Manual therapy is often based on a single faulty structure phenomenon, i.e., a local joint. In the past, manual therapy dogma has implored therapists to find the single faulty structure, possibly reproduce the patient's pain, and then set about "fixing" that pain (Maitland, 1986; Grieve, 1991). Pain is more complex. Tissue problems and pain are poorly correlated. The patient's pain may well be elicited by a manual technique at a single level, but could that pain be experienced due to a sensitive nervous system, such as central sensitization, and fueled by high fear levels? Another concern with a manual therapy approach to chronic pain is the creation of dependence. Manual therapy is a passive approach, making the patient dependent on the therapist to manipulate/move the joint and "fix" the problem. This is a direct contrast to the ultimate goal of independence and self-help. Once again, this "find it and fix it" model perpetuates the notion of a joint or a muscle as a single fault for the pain, fueling a biomedical approach (Nijs, Roussel et al., 2012).

Therapists should carefully consider the use of manual therapy in their patients with chronic pain states. Manual therapy, put into the right framework, can be very helpful. For example, if manual therapy is used to help gain some movement and increase blood flow, and is not proposed as 'fixing a structural issue,' it may be a better model for a patient in chronic pain. Patients can be educated that the manual technique is being used to jumpstart some movement and help recovery, but the more active approach will help long-term. Manual therapy needs a paradigm shift. For too long, therapists have viewed manual techniques through biomedical glasses. What follows next is an example of such a shift, in this case, The Maitland Concept. Geoff Maitland, an icon and pioneer in manual therapy, is likely part of the fabric of all modern manual therapists. No matter what approach a therapist may profess to use, there will likely be many aspects of The Maitland Concept in use, for example, clinical reasoning, graded mobilization, etc. The following editorial (www.ispinstitute.com) describes the contribution of this valuable manual therapy approach, but from a neuroscience perspective.

A Neuroscience View of the Maitland Concept

This editorial is likely to cause outrage from two different groups. On the one hand, the pain scientists may take issue with our comments in this editorial and, on the other, manual therapists may be upset and think we are trying to tinker with a fundamental element of manual therapy. Neither of these is our intention. We are preparing a series of pain lectures for serious manual therapists who have a strong Maitland influence. Sure, the lectures will feature all the good parts of the neuromatrix: pain as an output, multiple systems, and neuroplastic events surrounding a pain experience. The more we work on the lectures and reflect about trying to "keep everyone happy," the more we find ourselves wondering if what we do now is so much better than before. Yes, we may use fancy words, such as neuroscience, periaqueductal gray area and hyperalgesia, but we believe we may find a few neuroscience gems if we carefully view Geoff Maitland's approach:

- **Approach to the patient**—The Maitland Concept is an approach to the patient. The patient is the cornerstone of the equation, not the treatment technique. This central theme is very important in pain, especially considering that pain experiences are individual and personal. Focus on a patient, including his and her goals, knowledge, aspirations and expectations, helps treatment to be directed to the individual. In a simple procedural approach, such as injection therapy, it's about the technique. Over the years, we have observed hundreds of therapists in their practice, be it students, novice therapists or experienced, skilled masters. Manual techniques can be taught and learned, but how a therapist interacts with and views the patient is vital. For example, right now there's a huge interest in spinal manipulation by physical therapists. Week after week, we see young, go-getter therapists learning the skills to perform these techniques well from the mechanical viewpoint. However, we're not sure how their patients actually view or experience these techniques. If we were to watch a video from years gone by of Geoff Maitland treating a patient, we would not presume to challenge his hand skills. But there's more…it's how he does what he does. It's all about…the patient!

- **Severity and irritability** – We have heard plenty of criticism of severity and irritability recognition over the years. Many therapists who regularly see patients with chronic pain believe that a large proportion of the severity and irritability we have detected for years in a typical Maitland evaluation is likely due to irritability of symptoms due to nervous system sensitization, rather than irritability in tissues. The premise is that careful examination may reveal a patient presenting with tissues injured in such a manner that it causes severe pain, and processes such as inflammation of damaged tissue are aggravated (flared) by aggressive examination and treatment. If we set aside the incorrect notion of 'tissues causing pain' and the poorly understood biological processes in the original intent of the screening for severity and irritability, Maitland at least taught therapists to carefully examine patients and follow rule number one in medicine – do no harm. It is also interesting that Maitland did allow for examination and treatment of patients with high severity and irritability but through use of lighter techniques. So, there was no 'fight through the pain,' nor 'stop short of pain.' Instead, there was gentle, graded exposure to movement and hands-on treatment in a safe, accepting healing environment.

- **Focusing on signs and symptoms** – If therapists were to buy Maitland's textbook for an update on the latest pathologies related to spinal disorders they would be in for a surprise. Maitland never really discussed or focused on specific pathological issues, but rather signs and symptoms. Watching Geoff Maitland examining a patient with right-sided neck pain with limited rotation to the right and extension, you'll notice the patient is never provided a biological explanation of their pain. Treatment simply focused on clearing the signs and symptoms. Sure, current research suggests that patients need to be educated, but if we consider how negative biomedical information (herniation, bulges, tear, rip, torn) has induced fear and anxiety, it could be argued that de-emphasizing these anatomical issues may have been an important part in treatment. Day after day, you might see therapists displaying their knowledge: "look at me, I am so smart and let me tell you everything you need to know (and more) about your bulging disc." De-emphasizing tissue injury is a critical part of therapeutic neuroscience education.

- **Gentle oscillations**—Think back to the years Geoff Maitland developed his concept of manual therapy. He worked with and was influenced by Cyriax, Grieve and Kaltenborn. Have you ever seen a video of Cyriax performing a manipulation? Sure, Cyriax was highly skilled, but he was in an era of aggressive, strong manual therapy. Maitland introduced a gentle series of oscillatory techniques believed to help people recover from pain and disability. This approach has so many interesting pain implications. The first has to do with the pain gate theory. Yes, Melzack has exhorted us to move beyond the pain gate, but gentle oscillating large amplitude motions can be seen as a modulation effect on nociceptive input to the central nervous system. Secondly, gentle mobilizations that are always under the patient's control are safe and allow for movement and therapy in a less fearful environment. Lastly, and by no means least, could gentle repetitive oscillations on a spinal level, often at various angles, help restore body maps in the brain? A patient experiences pain at L4. Gentle oscillations at 30-60 seconds, angled cephalad or caudad may, in fact, help solidify that level (L4) in the brain, thus altering its representation. Ever notice how a patient moves better after a few PA mobilizations as part of the examination, even after receiving no "treatment"?

- **Test and re-test**—A cornerstone of the Maitland Concept is the test, re-test or within-session changes approach. Test a patient's ability to flex his or her shoulder: it elevates to 90 degrees flexion. Lie down, treat and then re-test. Now the arm rises to 100 degrees. In pain science, we know the importance of vision. In the now famous rubber hand illusion, we can trick the brain to feel sensation in a rubber hand. Apart from various complex neuroplastic events in the brain, vision is VERY powerful and often dominates. Think of mirror therapy. Surely a brain is smart enough to "know" it's not my hand or foot, but vision wins. How powerful for a brain to see the same arm five minutes later being raised a lot higher. Could this change the perception of threat? By the way, for this to work, you had better know your stuff and make sure it gets better!!

- **Clinical reasoning**—Likely the biggest contribution of the Maitland Concept is clinical reasoning: teaching us to think critically. It's interesting that every pain class we teach starts with this – how you think, critical thinking, thinking about your thinking. The more complex pain becomes, the more important thinking becomes: making fewer errors in reasoning and judgment. The more complex pain gets, the more lateral thinking may be required: analytical assessment, constant assessment, etc. Since pain is so complex and individualized, recipes are less likely to work for chronic pain compared to something like grade I acute ankle sprains; surely clinical reasoning is needed more than ever before. Clinical reasoning includes patient education and changing the patient's reasoning about their condition, care and prognosis.

- **Hands-on and manipulation**—Yes, we know…current best-evidence for chronic pain asks us to reconsider hands-on treatment, since chronic pain is less about a specific joint and more about bigger, larger systems and issues such as endocrine, immune, brain and more. It must, however, be stated that various hands-on treatments, particularly manipulation, have shown activation of the descending inhibitory mechanisms to help modulate acute pain. Modulating acute pain may just be one of the most potent ways to treat chronic pain… prevent it! Hands-on, human touch and interaction are vital components of treatment in patients with a pain experience. Maitland, as much as he may have been criticized for "not showing exercises," focused on treatment that was seemingly very beneficial for the acute and sub-acute patients. Did we mention hands-on is important? We love this quote: "The more impressive the procedure, the more powerful the placebo effect."

- **Placebo**—Placebo is not 'nothing,' as in a sham or fake treatment, but is instead enhancing the endogenous mechanisms in the brain to modulate pain. Entrenched in this is the power of expectation. We recently published a clinical prediction rule for cervical spine manipulation and found patient expectations was one of the predictors of success. It is proposed that people coming to therapy who are expecting to be treated carry endogenous healing inside of them; they expect to get better. Imagine what patients must have "carried within them" driving to see….Geoff Maitland!

- **Language**—Yes, Aussies have a very unique language, but this is not about that. We are driven by insurance companies and regulatory groups to ask for pain ratings. We know asking people their pain rating results in increased pain and heightened sensitivity. In the Maitland Approach, if a patient reported their hip pain as a deep, bruising ache, the therapist was asked to always refer to that complaint as 'your deep, bruising ache.' We have become accustomed to call everything 'pain.' We know the word 'pain' is a powerful activator or propellant of the pain neuromatrix. Could "deep, bruising ache" cause a less sensitive response than 'pain'? We think so.

- **Slump test**—Geoff Maitland, in a video interview, described to Mark Jones how he worked out some of the mechanics of the slump test. Neck flexion increased leg pain. Surely, there must be more. Yes, the "neural tension" of those days was crude, viewed from our current vantage point, but it shows bigger thinking, looking somewhere else and…clinical reasoning.

After reading this simple editorial about The Maitland Concept, we hope you are just as amazed as we are, looking back at our profession's infancy and pioneers like Geoff Maitland, at our explosion of knowledge and how we have grown as therapists, and now scientists, to stand upon the building blocks of our indoctrination and see the bigger, broader picture – to see how it really is.

6.12o: Modalities

In this short discussion of modalities, we hope to highlight similar issues to those for manual therapy, discussed earlier. Skillful delivery of modalities such as electrical stimulation, TENS, etc., should be seen as valuable tools to help reduce nociception and may significantly impact a patient's pain experience (Iversen, Chhabriya et al., 2011). The proposed mechanism of action for electrical modalities involves the pain gate. Even though Ron Melzack, one of the authors of the pain gate more than 50 years ago, is now asking therapists to move beyond the pain gate and take on the brain, the pain gate can still be seen as another mechanism to alter a patient's pain experience (Melzack, 1996; Wall, 1996; Melzack, 1999). However, with your new neuroscience understanding of pain, it may be interesting to consider how a modality such as TENS and electrical stimulation influences a pain experience. Sure, the pain gate may apply here, but consider this: why would a patient's pain be affected by an electrical stimulation device that is not plugged in to a power source, but the patient believes it is plugged in? (Bayer, Baer et al., 1991). Once again, as with the previous discussion of manual therapy, therapists need to consider the paradigm in which they utilize these modalities. Beliefs alter pain; just as altering nociception may alter pain. Modalities should therefore also be used for patients with chronic pain to potentially alter pain, allow for normalized movement and function, and allow exercise and thus progression over time.

The biggest drawback for modalities is the tendency to become dependent upon its use. Modalities are inherently passive, and patients get a message of having to 'go to therapy, lie on a table and receive the treatment.' This goes against the current evidence for a more active, self-help approach. Therapists may consider modalities whereby a patient can be taught and become self-reliant, e.g., TENS, to help them with their pain (Gifford, 1998; Khadilkar, Milne et al., 2005). As with pharmacological approaches, patients may develop a tolerance and, over time, find less relief from such modalities. Therapists are advised to teach patients to not use the devices all the time and use it specific to a task and not pain. Focusing on "when it hurts" is contrary to the TNE message. Patients should rather focus on using a TENS during a specific task with which they usually struggle, e.g., standing to cook a meal.

6.12p: Aquatic Therapy

There is evidence for the use of aquatic therapy in patients with chronic pain such as fibromyalgia (Evcik, Yigit et al., 2008; Louw, Puentedura et al., 2011). Unfortunately, aquatic therapy has seemingly become a dumping ground for patients with chronic pain and therapists are encouraged to view aquatic therapy from a different perspective. The warmth of the water as well as the buoyancy will help patients move more than they may be able to on land. This freedom to move allows for increased blood flow and oxygen and, from a larger neuroscience perspective, allows healthy stimulation and mapping of body parts in the somatosensory and motor homunculi. Once again, the main concern will be dependence. Patients may become reluctant to "leave the water" and believe they cannot function outside the water. Therapists should listen to their patients for evidence of poor cognitions, which will need addressing with TNE. Patients may say, "I will never be able to do without pool therapy." In such a scenario, therapists should lay out the plan of care and explain to the patient that the aquatic environment should be but a first step, to allow them to get moving. Over time, they will be transitioning to more and more land-based therapy and exercises. This process can be compared to using a walker after a knee replacement. In the beginning it is important; it helps you get going, and over time, you transition to more independent activities.

Specific to the treatment followed during the aquatic therapy session, therapists are encouraged to follow the exercise principles already discussed, including focusing on cardiovascular exercise, toning exercise versus strength, and general stabilization. As with the land-based exercises, therapists should be careful about the way they explain the approach, i.e., not doing 'strengthening' exercises in the pool, which implies weakness. Finally, aquatic therapy should be performed under direct supervision by a clinician and this would, once again, be an ideal time to filter TNE to the patient, session-by-session.

6.12q: Welcoming, Safe Healing Environment

All of the treatment options discussed so far relate to this concept. We truly believe therapists will often underestimate the ability to create a welcoming and safe healing environment. Similarly, research projects are sterile and try to account for all outside factors, yet this phenomenon will creep into the study findings, as well. Patients with chronic pain are often treated poorly, as if they have some kind of plague. Creating a welcoming clinical environment of warmth is a great start. Considering that the definition of pain is a product by the brain based on perception of threat, it should make sense that such a healing environment can alter a pain experience. How does this look clinically? It starts at the front desk. As discussed in chapter 5, front office staff should have pain science knowledge and thus start the process of educating and encouraging in the waiting room. Therapists should listen to the patients and allow time for questions and answers. Another critical component is to keep a patient with a specific therapist. Too often, patients will be passed on from therapist to therapist, therapist to therapist assistant and, sometimes, therapist to technician. All of this impacts the patient's recovery significantly. In fact, we would challenge therapists to keep the patients all to themselves. 'Own your patient.'

6.12r: Goal Setting, Pacing and Graded Exposure

One of the biggest issues that patients with chronic pain struggle with is setting appropriate goals. Patients often fall into one of two categories. One, a patient may not have any goals. Two, and more common, patients may have goals but they are poorly defined, non-specific or so far out of reach that they may not see a need to try to achieve them. There are many components to goal setting and various descriptions of pacing, graded exposure, etc. (de Jong, Vlaeyen et al., 2005; de Jong, Vangronsveld et al., 2008; George and Zeppieri, 2009; Meeus, Nijs et al., 2010; Goudsmit, Nijs et al., 2012). In its simplest form, any task can be broken into smaller parts. Therapists do it all the time. For example, a patient following knee replacement will go through weeks of therapy with the ultimate goals of walking, riding a bike, going up stairs, etc. Naturally, none of these activities can be performed one day after surgery. How do we set goals and help patients take small steps to accomplishing their therapy goals? (Gladwell, 2006) Here is an example:

- Ask your patient to write down some goals at home and bring them in. At first, don't be specific. Have them bring them in and then start molding them until they are measurable, broken down to small pieces and within reach.

- These first goals tend to be vague. See the example below that a recent patient e-mailed to the therapist:

Goals
1. Improve quality of life
2. Improve heart rate during cardio
3. Be happier and more positive
4. Reduce anxiety
5. Improve marriage
6. Have more energy
7. Know how it feels to be pain-free for a week

- As you can see, the goals at this early stage are very vague.

- These written goals may help with TNE. They can give you more information needed to address educational issues. Point 4 (reduce anxiety) is such an example. This can very easily be turned into a question: "what are you anxious about?" Maybe it's increased pain with therapy, which then allows for a small refresher education session about what pain actually means: 'sensitivity' versus 'injury.'

- We do recommend functional goals, i.e., tasks that can readily be measured and have meaning towards recovery.

- We also, however, require "deep desires." These may help patients give it another try. One clinically meaningful way we seek these would be as follows: "*Suzy, if I could reach behind your back and magically switch off your pain . . . get rid of all it, what would you do again?*" Patients often say things like take up dancing, play a round of golf, take a road trip or run a 5K race. The interesting thing is that there is likely no reason they cannot do any of these, given education, time and rehabilitation. This usually comes as a shock, for instance: "*There is nothing in your examination that shows me you are not able to do…. Sure, maybe not tomorrow, but it can be done.*" Maybe Suzy was a runner and her "dream goal is to run a half-marathon." No reason she cannot run a half-marathon, just not next week. As she becomes healthier, stronger and able to push a little more, there is no reason why she could not do the local 5K race by a certain date. Sure, it will be slow, but she would have done it. After that, a few more and then a 10K, etc.

- Once goals are set, they need to be broken down into smaller, more manageable pieces that will keep the patient motivated and on task, and not cause undue increased pain. Here is a good example of a patient with fibromyalgia we treated recently (Louw, Puentedura et al., 2011):

  o She brought her list. One main goal was to "clean her house."

  o Can you see how vague it is?

  o So, we asked her to make a list of tasks that constitute "clean the house."

  o After she brought the list (vacuuming, dusting, sweeping, mopping, etc.), we asked her if she could only do one task, which one would it be. She chose vacuuming. Can you see we're now down to a specific task?

  o Then, how many rooms need vacuuming? She answered five.

  o We asked her next – if you could only vacuum one room, which one would it be? Living room. Then? Entry way and so forth. Soon the rooms were labeled A, B, C, D and E.

  o Then (the important part), we asked her – if she was to go home, take the vacuum out of the closet and vacuum a room today, how much of a room could she do, put the vacuum away and still be OK...not wiped out on the couch? She answered a half of one room. Now, we changed the room labels to have her vacuum half a room at a time and gave her a vacuuming schedule:

Day	Room	Day	Room
1	A1	6	C2
2	A2	7	D1
3	B1	8	D2
4	B2	9	E1
5	C1	10	E2

○ Now we have a plan. In 10 days from now, this patient may actually have vacuumed her whole house! What a win.

○ In regards to pacing and graded exposure, therapists may consider the following. Meals don't have to be cooked in one session. Dinner can gradually be prepared from AM to PM with rest periods between cutting vegetables for relaxation, stretches and exercise. All laundry does not have to be done in one day. One load per day is more than enough to keep a household going. Later, an AM load and a PM load can be done compared to "doing all of it in one shot." All the floors do not need to be swept at the same time. Answering five e-mails at a time is progress instead of sitting in front of a computer for hours. Weeding a garden can be broken up with neatly placed stakes. Walking exercise can be done in two or three small walks a day.

• Set time-specific goals. Patients who know they need to be ready for a task by a certain date will be more motivated. The goal may be to cook a complete meal. It may start in the AM or the day before to prepare some ingredients. As the patient gets better, stronger and accomplishes more, set a date (calendar) and have him/her invite someone for dinner. Another example may be walking. Walking is steadily increasing, so look for a community event, e.g., a charity walk on a certain date.

• Discuss barriers. Often, patients struggling with pain don't see how they can do it. Have them share the barriers, e.g., 'I'm too busy,' 'I have too much pain,' etc. Use your TNE to educate and convince them; break the tasks down even further.

6.13: Conclusion

Therapists should take a few minutes and view the extensive list and discussions of treatments. As we started this chapter, we commented that therapists often express frustration because they don't know what to do with patients with chronic pain. This chapter aimed to show therapists the vast number of strategies that can be used for such patients. All of these suggested treatments should be "bathed" in neuroscience and ultimately in TNE. We do not make this statement lightly. It has been reported that the late Dr. Patrick Wall, one of the original authors of the pain gate theory, believed therapists to be the ideal profession to take on chronic pain. Why therapists? Therapists are in a unique position because they possess most of the qualities needed to treat chronic pain: knowledge of biology, knowledge and use of movement and exercise, cheaper treatment provides within the healthcare community, the sheer number of therapists available to help chronic pain, etc. There is so much we can offer these patients.

Chapter 6 References

(2009). Exercise may slow or reverse brain decline. Aerobic exercise benefits executive-control brain function, and may enable the brain to continue to grow and develop. *Duke Med Health News, 15*(3): 3.

Adler, G. K., B. T. Kinsley, S. Hurwitz, C. J. Mossey and D. L. Goldenberg (1999). Reduced hypothalamic-pituitary and sympathoadrenal responses to hypoglycemia in women with fibromyalgia syndrome. *Am J Med, 106*(5): 534-543.

Ainsworth, K. D. and C. C. Hagino (2006). A survey of Ontario chiropractors: their views on maximizing patient compliance to prescribed home exercise. *J Can Chiropr Assoc, 50*(2): 140-155.

Arnold, L. M. (2006). Biology and therapy of fibromyalgia. New therapies in fibromyalgia. *Arthritis Res Ther, 8*(4): 212.

Arnold, L. M., L. J. Crofford, S. A. Martin, J. P. Young and U. Sharma (2007). The effect of anxiety and depression on improvements in pain in a randomized, controlled trial of pregabalin for treatment of fibromyalgia. *Pain Medicine, 8*(8): 633-638.

Asenlof, P., E. Denison and P. Lindberg (2005). Individually tailored treatment targeting motor behavior, cognition, and disability: 2 experimental single-case studies of patients with recurrent and persistent musculoskeletal pain in primary health care. *Phys Ther, 85*(10): 1061-1077.

Barnard, N. (1998). *Foods That Fight Pain.* New York, Three Rivers Press.

Baron, R. and W. Janig (2004). The role of the sympathetic nervous system in pain processing. *The Pain System in Normal and Pathological States: A Primer for Clinicians.* L. Villanueva, A. Dickenson and H. Ollat. Seattle, IASP Press.

Baschetti, R. (2001). Chronic fatigue syndrome, decreased exercise capacity, and adrenal insufficiency. *Archives of Internal Medicine, 161*(12): 1558-1559.

Bauer, T. and B. Weisser (2002). [Effect of aerobic endurance exercise on immune function in elderly athletes]. *Praxis (Bern 1994), 91*(5): 153-158.

Bayer, T. L., P. E. Baer and C. Early (1991). Situational and psychophysiological factors in psychologically induced pain. *Pain, 44*(1): 45-50.

Beggs, S., X. J. Liu, C. Kwan and M. W. Salter (2010). Peripheral nerve injury and TRPV1-expressing primary afferent C-fibers cause opening of the blood-brain barrier. *Molecular Pain, 6*: 74.

Beneciuk, J. M., M. D. Bishop and S. Z. George (2009). Effects of upper extremity neural mobilization on thermal pain sensitivity: a sham-controlled study in asymptomatic participants. *The Journal of Orthopaedic and Sports Physical Therapy, 39*(6): 428-438.

Bennett, R. M. and D. L. Goldenberg (2011). Fibromyalgia, myofascial pain, tender points and trigger points: splitting or lumping? *Arthritis Research & Therapy, 13*(3): 117.

Bigatti, S. M., A. M. Hernandez, T. A. Cronan and K. L. Rand (2008). Sleep disturbances in fibromyalgia syndrome: relationship to pain and depression. *Arthritis Rheum, 59*(7): 961-967.

Blumenthal, J. A., M. A. Babyak, P. M. Doraiswamy, L. Watkins, B. M. Hoffman, K. A. Barbour, S. Herman, W. E. Craighead, A. L. Brosse, R. Waugh, A. Hinderliter and A. Sherwood (2007). Exercise and pharmacotherapy in the treatment of major depressive disorder. *Psychosom Med, 69*(7): 587-596.

Boas, S. R., M. J. Danduran, S. A. McColley, K. Beaman and M. R. O'Gorman (2000). Immune modulation following aerobic exercise in children with cystic fibrosis. *Int J Sports Med, 21*(4): 294-301.

Bokarius, A., K. Ha, R. Poland, V. Bokarius, M. H. Rapaport and W. W. Ishak (2011). Attitude toward humor in patients experiencing depressive symptoms. *Innovations in Clinical Neuroscience, 8*(9): 20-23.

Bollo, R. J., S. C. Williams, C. S. Peskin and U. Samadani (2010). When the air hits your brain: cerebral autoregulation of brain oxygenation during aerobic exercise allows transient hyperoxygenation: case report. *Neurosurgery, 67*(2): E507-509.

Bonifazi, M., A. L. Suman, C. Cambiaggi, A. Felici, G. Grasso, L. Lodi, M. Mencarelli, M. Muscettola and G. Carli (2006). Changes in salivary cortisol and corticosteroid receptor-alpha mRNA expression following a 3-week multidisciplinary treatment program in patients with fibromyalgia. *Psychoneuroendocrinology, 31*(9): 1076-1086.

Bozikas, V. P., M. H. Kosmidis, M. Giannakou, A. Adamopoulou, X. Gonda, K. Fokas and G. Garyfallos (2011). Humor appreciation of captionless cartoons in obsessive-compulsive disorder. *Annals of General Psychiatry, 10*(1): 31.

Bradley, L. A. (2008). Pathophysiologic mechanisms of fibromyalgia and its related disorders. *J Clin Psychiatry, 69 Suppl 2*: 6-13.

Brosseau, L., G. A. Wells, P. Tugwell, M. Egan, K. G. Wilson, C. J. Dubouloz, L. Casimiro, V. A. Robinson, J. McGowan, A. Busch, S. Poitras, H. Moldofsky, M. Harth, H. M. Finestone, W. Nielson, A. Haines-Wangda, M. Russell-Doreleyers, K. Lambert, A. D. Marshall and L. Veilleux (2008). Ottawa Panel evidence-based clinical practice guidelines for aerobic fitness exercises in the management of fibromyalgia: part 1. *Phys Ther, 88*(7): 857-871.

Brosseau, L., G. A. Wells, P. Tugwell, M. Egan, K. G. Wilson, C. J. Dubouloz, L. Casimiro, V. A. Robinson, J. McGowan, A. Busch, S. Poitras, H. Moldofsky, M. Harth, H. M. Finestone, W. Nielson, A. Haines-Wangda, M. Russell-Doreleyers, K. Lambert, A. D. Marshall and L. Veilleux (2008). Ottawa Panel evidence-based clinical practice guidelines for strengthening exercises in the management of fibromyalgia: part 2. *Phys Ther, 88*(7): 873-886.

Bruce, B., J. F. Fries and D. P. Lubeck (2005). Aerobic exercise and its impact on musculoskeletal pain in older adults: a 14 year prospective, longitudinal study. *Arthritis Res Ther, 7*(6): R1263-1270.

Busch, A. J., K. A. Barber, T. J. Overend, P. M. Peloso and C. L. Schachter (2007). Exercise for treating fibromyalgia syndrome. *Cochrane Database Syst Rev*(4): CD003786.

Caglar, E., H. Sabuncuoglu, T. Keskin, S. Isikli, S. Keskil and F. Korkusuz (2005). In vivo human brain biochemistry after aerobic exercise: preliminary report on functional magnetic resonance spectroscopy. *Surg Neurol, 64 Suppl 2*: S53-56; discussion S56-57.

Cairns, M. C., N. E. Foster and C. Wright (2006). Randomized controlled trial of specific spinal stabilization exercises and conventional physiotherapy for recurrent low back pain. *Spine, 31*(19): E670-681.

Capomolla, S., M. Ceresa, A. Civardi, A. Lupo, A. Ventura, M. Scabini, P. Leonelli, G. Salvaneschi, A. Petocchi, G. Pinna, M. Ferrari, O. Febo, A. Caporotondi, G. Guazzotti, M. T. La Rovere, M. Gnemmi, R. Maestri and F. Cobelli (2002). [Home exercise therapy in chronic congestive heart failure: observational study of factors affecting adherence to the program]. *Ital Heart J Suppl, 3*(11): 1098-1105.

Carvalho, L. S., H. Correa, G. C. Silva, F. S. Campos, F. R. Baiao, L. S. Ribeiro, A. M. Faria and D. d'Avila Reis (2008). May genetic factors in fibromyalgia help to identify patients with differentially altered frequencies of immune cells? *Clin Exp Immunol, 154*(3): 346-352.

Carville, S. F., S. Arendt-Nielsen, H. Bliddal, F. Blotman, J. C. Branco, D. Buskila, J. A. Da Silva, B. Danneskiold-Samsoe, F. Dincer, C. Henriksson, K. G. Henriksson, E. Kosek, K. Longley, G. M. McCarthy, S. Perrot, M. Puszczewicz, P. Sarzi-Puttini, A. Silman, M. Spath and E. H. Choy (2008). EULAR evidence-based recommendations for the management of fibromyalgia syndrome. *Ann Rheum Dis, 67*(4): 536-541.

Castellano, V. and L. J. White (2008). Serum brain-derived neurotrophic factor response to aerobic exercise in multiple sclerosis. *J Neurol Sci, 269*(1-2): 85-91.

Catai, A. M., M. P. Chacon-Mikahil, F. S. Martinelli, V. A. Forti, E. Silva, R. Golfetti, L. E. Martins, J. S. Szrajer, J. S. Wanderley, E. C. Lima-Filho, L. A. Milan, J. A. Marin-Neto, B. C. Maciel and L. Gallo-Junior (2002). Effects of aerobic exercise training on heart rate variability during wakefulness and sleep and cardiorespiratory responses of young and middle-aged healthy men. *Braz J Med Biol Res, 35*(6): 741-752.

Chatzitheodorou, D., C. Kabitsis, P. Malliou and V. Mougios (2007). A pilot study of the effects of high-intensity aerobic exercise versus passive interventions on pain, disability, psychological strain, and serum cortisol concentrations in people with chronic low back pain. *Phys Ther, 87*(3): 304-312.

Clinic, M. (2007). Aerobic exercise increases size of aging brain. *Mayo Clin Health Lett, 25*(5): 4.

Colcombe, S. J., K. I. Erickson, P. E. Scalf, J. S. Kim, R. Prakash, E. McAuley, S. Elavsky, D. X. Marquez, L. Hu and A. F. Kramer (2006). Aerobic exercise training increases brain volume in aging humans. *J Gerontol A Biol Sci Med Sci, 61*(11): 1166-1170.

Cox, K. L., V. Burke, T. J. Gorely, L. J. Beilin and I. B. Puddey (2003). Controlled comparison of retention and adherence in home- vs center-initiated exercise interventions in women ages 40-65 years: The S.W.E.A.T. Study (Sedentary Women Exercise Adherence Trial). *Prev Med, 36*(1): 17-29.

Critchley, D. J., J. Ratcliffe, S. Noonan, R. H. Jones and M. V. Hurley (2007). Effectiveness and cost-effectiveness of three types of physiotherapy used to reduce chronic low back pain disability: a pragmatic randomized trial with economic evaluation. *Spine, 32*(14): 1474-1481.

Critchley, D. J., J. Ratcliffe, S. Noonan, R. H. Jones and M. V. Hurley (2007). Effectiveness and cost-effectiveness of three types of physiotherapy used to reduce chronic low back pain disability: a pragmatic randomized trial with economic evaluation. *Spine (Phila Pa 1976), 32*(14): 1474-1481.

Currie, S. R., K. G. Wilson and S. T. Gauthier (1995). Caffeine and chronic low back pain. *Clin J Pain, 11*(3): 214-219.

de Jong, J. R., K. Vangronsveld, M. L. Peters, M. E. Goossens, P. Onghena, I. Bulte and J. W. Vlaeyen (2008). Reduction of pain-related fear and disability in post-traumatic neck pain: a replicated single-case experimental study of exposure in vivo. *J Pain, 9*(12): 1123-1134.

de Jong, J. R., J. W. Vlaeyen, P. Onghena, C. Cuypers, M. den Hollander and J. Ruijgrok (2005). Reduction of pain-related fear in complex regional pain syndrome type I: the application of graded exposure in vivo. *Pain, 116*(3): 264-275.

Deley, G., G. Kervio, B. Verges, A. Hannequin, M. F. Petitdant, S. Salmi-Belmihoub, B. Grassi and J. M. Casillas (2005). Comparison of low-frequency electrical myostimulation and conventional aerobic exercise training in patients with chronic heart failure. *Eur J Cardiovasc Prev Rehabil, 12*(3): 226-233.

Devor, M. (2005). Response of nerves to injury in relation to neuropathic pain. *Melzack and Wall's Textbook of Pain.* S. McMahon and M. Koltzenburg. Edinburgh, Elsevier.

Dimeo, F., M. Bauer, I. Varahram, G. Proest and U. Halter (2001). Benefits from aerobic exercise in patients with major depression: a pilot study. *Br J Sports Med, 35*(2): 114-117.

Dimsdale, J. E. and R. Dantzer (2007). A biological substrate for somatoform disorders: importance of pathophysiology. *Psychosomatic Medicine, 69*(9): 850-854.

Dittrich, S. M., V. Gunther, G. Franz, M. Burtscher, B. Holzner and M. Kopp (2008). Aerobic exercise with relaxation: influence on pain and psychological well-being in female migraine patients. *Clin J Sport Med, 18*(4): 363-365.

Dobkin, P. L., D. Da Costa, M. Abrahamowicz, M. Dritsa, R. Du Berger, M. A. Fitzcharles and I. Lowensteyn (2006). Adherence during an individualized home based 12-week exercise program in women with fibromyalgia. *J Rheumatol, 33*(2): 333-341.

Dobkin, P. L., A. Sita and M. J. Sewitch (2006). Predictors of adherence to treatment in women with fibromyalgia. *Clin J Pain, 22*(3): 286-294.

Duncan, K. A. and B. Pozehl (2002). Staying on course: the effects of an adherence facilitation intervention on home exercise participation. *Prog Cardiovasc Nurs, 17*(2): 59-65, 71.

Echeverry, S., X. Q. Shi, S. Rivest and J. Zhang (2011). Peripheral nerve injury alters blood-spinal cord barrier functional and molecular integrity through a selective inflammatory pathway. *The Journal of Neuroscience: The Official Journal of the Society for Neuroscience, 31*(30): 10819-10828.

Edmondston, S. J., H. Y. Chan, G. C. Ngai, M. L. Warren, J. M. Williams, S. Glennon and K. Netto (2007). Postural neck pain: an investigation of habitual sitting posture, perception of 'good' posture and cervicothoracic kinaesthesia. *Man Ther, 12*(4): 363-371.

Emad, Y., Y. Ragab, F. Zeinhom, G. El-Khouly, A. Abou-Zeid and J. J. Rasker (2008). Hippocampus dysfunction may explain symptoms of fibromyalgia syndrome. A study with single-voxel magnetic resonance spectroscopy. *J Rheumatol, 35*(7): 1371-1377.

Engstrom, L. O. and B. Oberg (2005). Patient adherence in an individualized rehabilitation programme: a clinical follow-up. *Scand J Public Health, 33*(1): 11-18.

Evcik, D., I. Yigit, H. Pusak and V. Kavuncu (2008). Effectiveness of aquatic therapy in the treatment of fibromyalgia syndrome: a randomized controlled open study. *Rheumatol Int, 28*(9): 885-890.

Falkenberg, I., G. Buchkremer, M. Bartels and B. Wild (2011). Implementation of a manual-based training of humor abilities in patients with depression: a pilot study. *Psychiatry Research, 186*(2-3): 454-457.

Falkenberg, I., J. Jarmuzek, M. Bartels and B. Wild (2011). Do depressed patients lose their sense of humor? *Psychopathology, 44*(2): 98-105.

Falla, D., G. Bilenkij and G. Jull (2004). Patients with chronic neck pain demonstrate altered patterns of muscle activation during performance of a functional upper limb task. *Spine, 29*(13): 1436-1440.

Falla, D., G. Jull, P. Hodges and B. Vicenzino (2006). An endurance-strength training regime is effective in reducing myoelectric manifestations of cervical flexor muscle fatigue in females with chronic neck pain. *Clin Neurophysiol, 117*(4): 828-837.

Falla, D., G. Jull and P. W. Hodges (2004). Feedforward activity of the cervical flexor muscles during voluntary arm movements is delayed in chronic neck pain. *Exp Brain Res, 157*(1): 43-48.

Falla, D., G. Jull, S. O'Leary and P. Dall'Alba (2006). Further evaluation of an EMG technique for assessment of the deep cervical flexor muscles. *J Electromyogr Kinesiol, 16*(6): 621-628.

Falla, D., G. Jull, A. Rainoldi and R. Merletti (2004). Neck flexor muscle fatigue is side specific in patients with unilateral neck pain. *Eur J Pain, 8*(1): 71-77.

Falla, D., G. Jull, T. Russell, B. Vicenzino and P. Hodges (2007). Effect of neck exercise on sitting posture in patients with chronic neck pain. *Phys Ther, 87*(4): 408-417.

Falla, D., S. O'Leary, A. Fagan and G. Jull (2007). Recruitment of the deep cervical flexor muscles during a postural-correction exercise performed in sitting. *Man Ther, 12*(2): 139-143.

Fenwick, C. M., S. H. Brown and S. M. McGill (2009). Comparison of different rowing exercises: trunk muscle activation and lumbar spine motion, load, and stiffness. *Journal of Strength and Conditioning Research/National Strength & Conditioning Association, 23*(5): 1408-1417.

Fernandez-Carnero, J., C. Fernandez-de-las-Penas and J. A. Cleland (2008). Immediate hypoalgesic and motor effects after a single cervical spine manipulation in subjects with lateral epicondylalgia. *J Manipulative Physiol Ther, 31*(9): 675-681.

Fernandez-de-las-Penas, C., A. I. de la Llave-Rincon, J. Fernandez-Carnero, M. L. Cuadrado, L. Arendt-Nielsen and J. A. Pareja (2009). Bilateral widespread mechanical pain sensitivity in carpal tunnel syndrome: evidence of central processing in unilateral neuropathy. *Brain, 132*(Pt 6): 1472-1479.

Fernandez-de-Las-Penas, C., D. Simons, M. L. Cuadrado and J. Pareja (2007). The role of myofascial trigger points in musculoskeletal pain syndromes of the head and neck. *Curr Pain Headache Rep, 11*(5): 365-372.

Fernandez-De-Las-Penaz, C., L. Arendt-Nielsen and R. Gerwin (2010). *Tension-Type and Cervicogenci Headache: Pathology, Diagnosis, and Management.* Sudbury, Jones and Bartlett.

Ferreira, M. L., P. H. Ferreira, J. Latimer, R. D. Herbert, P. W. Hodges, M. D. Jennings, C. G. Maher and K. M. Refshauge (2007). Comparison of general exercise, motor control exercise and spinal manipulative therapy for chronic low back pain: A randomized trial. *Pain, 131*(1-2): 31-37.

Flor, H. (2000). The functional organization of the brain in chronic pain. *Prog Brain Res, 129*: 313-322.

Friedrich, M., G. Gittler, M. Arendasy and K. M. Friedrich (2005). Long-term effect of a combined exercise and motivational program on the level of disability of patients with chronic low back pain. *Spine (Phila Pa 1976), 30*(9): 995-1000.

Friedrich, M., G. Gittler, Y. Halberstadt, T. Cermak and I. Heiller (1998). Combined exercise and motivation program: effect on the compliance and level of disability of patients with chronic low back pain: a randomized controlled trial. *Arch Phys Med Rehabil, 79*(5): 475-487.

Fritz, J. M., J. M. Whitman and J. D. Childs (2005). Lumbar spine segmental mobility assessment: an examination of validity for determining intervention strategies in patients with low back pain. *Arch Phys Med Rehabil, 86*(9): 1745-1752.

Fujii, Y., N. Ozaki, T. Taguchi, K. Mizumura, K. Furukawa and Y. Sugiura (2008). TRP channels and ASICs mediate mechanical hyperalgesia in models of inflammatory muscle pain and delayed onset muscle soreness. *Pain, 140*(2): 292-304.

Fulcher, K. Y. and P. D. White (1997). Randomised controlled trial of graded exercise in patients with the chronic fatigue syndrome. *BMJ, 314*(7095): 1647-1652.

George, S. Z. and G. Zeppieri (2009). Physical therapy utilization of graded exposure for patients with low back pain. *J Orthop Sports Phys Ther, 39*(7): 496-505.

Gifford, L. S. (1998). Tissue and input related mechanisms. Topical Issues in Pain. L. S. Gifford. Falmouth, NOI Press.

Gifford, L. S., Ed. (1998). *Topical Issues in Pain.* Falmouth, NOI Press.

Gladwell, P. (2006). A practical guide to goalsetting. *Topical Issues in Pain 5.* L. S. Gifford. Falmouth, CNS Press.

Goldby, L. J., A. P. Moore, J. Doust and M. E. Trew (2006). A randomized controlled trial investigating the efficiency of musculoskeletal physiotherapy on chronic low back disorder. *Spine, 31*(10): 1083-1093.

Goldenberg, D. L. (2007). Pharmacological treatment of fibromyalgia and other chronic musculoskeletal pain. Best practice & research. *Clinical Rheumatology, 21*(3): 499-511.

Goldenberg, D. L., C. Burckhardt and L. Crofford (2004). Management of fibromyalgia syndrome. *JAMA, 292*(19): 2388-2395.

Gondoh, Y., H. Sensui, S. Kinomura, H. Fukuda, T. Fujimoto, M. Masud, T. Nagamatsu, H. Tamaki and H. Takekura (2009). Effects of aerobic exercise training on brain structure and psychological well-being in young adults. *J Sports Med Phys Fitness, 49*(2): 129-135.

Goudsmit, E. M., J. Nijs, L. A. Jason and K. E. Wallman (2012). Pacing as a strategy to improve energy management in myalgic encephalomyelitis/chronic fatigue syndrome: a consensus document. *Disability and Rehabilitation, 34*(13): 1140-1147.

Gowans, S. E., A. deHueck, S. Voss, A. Silaj, S. E. Abbey and W. J. Reynolds (2001). Effect of a randomized, controlled trial of exercise on mood and physical function in individuals with fibromyalgia. *Arthritis Rheum, 45*(6): 519-529.

Grieve, G. (1991). *Mobilisation of the Spine.* London, Churchill Livingstone.

Haaland, D. A., T. F. Sabljic, D. A. Baribeau, I. M. Mukovozov and L. E. Hart (2008). Is regular exercise a friend or foe of the aging immune system? A systematic review. *Clin J Sport Med, 18*(6): 539-548.

Hamilton, N. A., G. Affleck, H. Tennen, C. Karlson, D. Luxton, K. J. Preacher and J. L. Templin (2008). Fibromyalgia: the role of sleep in affect and in negative event reactivity and recovery. *Health Psychol, 27*(4): 490-497.

Harden, R. N., T. A. Duc, T. R. Williams, D. Coley, J. C. Cate and R. H. Gracely (1994). Norepinephrine and epinephrine levels in affected versus unaffected limbs in sympathetically maintained pain. *Clin J Pain, 10*(4): 324-330.

Hart, L. E., D. A. Haaland, D. A. Baribeau, I. M. Mukovozov and T. F. Sabljic (2008). The relationship between exercise and osteoarthritis in the elderly. *Clin J Sport Med, 18*(6): 508-521.

Hassett, A. L. and R. N. Gevirtz (2009). Nonpharmacologic treatment for fibromyalgia: patient education, cognitive-behavioral therapy, relaxation techniques, and complementary and alternative medicine. *Rheumatic Disease Clinics of North America, 35*(2): 393-407.

Hauser, W., K. Bernardy, N. Uceyler and C. Sommer (2009). Treatment of fibromyalgia syndrome with antidepressants: a meta-analysis. *JAMA: The Journal of the American Medical Association, 301*(2): 198-209.

Heiden, E., M. Testa and D. Musolf (2009). *Faster, Better, Stronger,* HarperCollins.

Hides, J. A., D. L. Belavy, W. Stanton, S. J. Wilson, J. Rittweger, D. Felsenberg and C. A. Richardson (2007). Magnetic resonance imaging assessment of trunk muscles during prolonged bed rest. *Spine, 32*(15): 1687-1692.

Hides, J. A., C. A. Richardson and G. Jull (1996). Multifidus muscle recovery is not automatic after resolution of acute first-episode low back pain. *Spine, 21*: 2763-2769.

Hides, J. A., C. A. Richardson and G. A. Jull (1995). Magnetic resonance imaging and ultrasonography of the lumbar multifidus muscle. Comparison of two different modalities. *Spine, 20*(1): 54-58.

Hides, J. A., C. A. Richardson and G. A. Jull (1996). Multifidus muscle recovery is not automatic after resolution of acute, first-episode low back pain. *Spine, 21*(23): 2763-2769.

Hodges, P., A. Cresswell and A. Thorstensson (1999). Preparatory trunk motion accompanies rapid upper limb movement. *Exp Brain Res, 124*(1): 69-79.

Hodges, P. W. (2000). The role of the motor system in spinal pain: implications for rehabilitation of the athlete following lower back pain. *J Sci Med Sport, 3*(3): 243-253.

Hodges, P. W. (2001). Changes in motor planning of feedforward postural responses of the trunk muscles in low back pain. *Exp Brain Res, 141*(2): 261-266.

Hodges, P. W. (2003). Core stability exercise in chronic low back pain. *Orthop Clin North Am, 34*(2): 245-254.

Hodges, P. W., A. G. Cresswell and A. Thorstensson (2001). Perturbed upper limb movements cause short-latency postural responses in trunk muscles. *Exp Brain Res, 138*(2): 243-250.

Hodges, P. W., G. L. Moseley, A. Gabrielsson and S. C. Gandevia (2003). Experimental muscle pain changes feedforward postural responses of the trunk muscles. *Experimental Brain Research. Experimentelle Hirnforschung. Experimentation cerebrale, 151*(2): 262-271.

Hodges, P. W. and C. A. Richardson (1997). Relationship between limb movement speed and associated contraction of the trunk muscles. *Ergonomics, 40*(11): 1220-1230.

Hodges, P. W. and C. A. Richardson (1998). Delayed postural contraction of transversus abdominis in low back pain associated with movement of the lower limb. *J Spinal Disord, 11*(1): 46-56.

Hodges, P. W. and C. A. Richardson (1999). Altered trunk muscle recruitment in people with low back pain with upper limb movement at different speeds. *Arch Phys Med Rehabil, 80*(9): 1005-1012.

Hoffman, M. D. and D. R. Hoffman (2007). Does aerobic exercise improve pain perception and mood? A review of the evidence related to healthy and chronic pain subjects. *Curr Pain Headache Rep, 11*(2): 93-97.

Hoffman, M. D., M. A. Shepanski, S. P. Mackenzie and P. S. Clifford (2005). Experimentally induced pain perception is acutely reduced by aerobic exercise in people with chronic low back pain. *J Rehabil Res Dev, 42*(2): 183-190.

Hoffman, M. D., M. A. Shepanski, S. B. Ruble, Z. Valic, J. B. Buckwalter and P. S. Clifford (2004). Intensity and duration threshold for aerobic exercise-induced analgesia to pressure pain. *Arch Phys Med Rehabil, 85*(7): 1183-1187.

Hurkmans, E., F. J. van der Giesen, T. P. Vliet Vlieland, J. Schoones and E. C. Van den Ende (2009). Dynamic exercise programs (aerobic capacity and/or muscle strength training) in patients with rheumatoid arthritis. *Cochrane Database Syst Rev*(4): CD006853.

Hurling, R., M. Catt, M. D. Boni, B. W. Fairley, T. Hurst, P. Murray, A. Richardson and J. S. Sodhi (2007). Using internet and mobile phone technology to deliver an automated physical activity program: randomized controlled trial. *J Med Internet Res, 9*(2): e7.

Iversen, M. D., R. K. Chhabriya and N. Shadick (2011). Predictors of the use of physical therapy services among patients with rheumatoid arthritis. *Physical Therapy, 91*(1): 65-76.

Izquierdo-Alvarez, S., J. P. Bocos-Terraz, J. L. Bancalero-Flores, L. Pavon-Romero, E. Serrano-Ostariz and C. A. de Miquel (2008). Is there an association between fibromyalgia and below-normal levels of urinary cortisol? *BMC Res Notes, 1*: 134.

Jackson, D., L. Turner-Stokes, J. Culpan, A. Bateman, O. Scott, J. Powell and R. Greenwood (2001). Can brain-injured patients participate in an aerobic exercise programme during early inpatient rehabilitation? *Clin Rehabil, 15*(5): 535-544.

Jentoft, E. S., A. G. Kvalvik and A. M. Mengshoel (2001). Effects of pool-based and land-based aerobic exercise on women with fibromyalgia/chronic widespread muscle pain. *Arthritis Rheum, 45*(1): 42-47.

Jones, K. D., F. B. Horak, K. Winters-Stone, J. M. Irvine and R. M. Bennett (2009). Fibromyalgia is associated with impaired balance and falls. *J Clin Rheumatol, 15*(1): 16-21.

Jull, G., C. Barrett, R. Magee and P. Ho (1999). Further clinical clarification of the muscle dysfunction in cervical headache. *Cephalalgia, 19*(3): 179-185.

Jull, G., E. Kristjansson and P. Dall'Alba (2004). Impairment in the cervical flexors: a comparison of whiplash and insidious onset neck pain patients. *Man Ther, 9*(2): 89-94.

Jull, G., M. Sterling, D. Falla, S. P. O'Leary and J. Treleaven (2008). *Whiplash, Headache, and Neck Pain: Research-Based Directions for Physical Therapies.* Philadelphia, Churchill Livingston.

Jull, G. A., D. Falla, B. Vicenzino and P. W. Hodges (2009). The effect of therapeutic exercise on activation of the deep cervical flexor muscles in people with chronic neck pain. *Man Ther, 14*(6): 696-701.

Kaplan, K. H., D. L. Goldenberg and M. Galvin-Nadeau (1993). The impact of a meditation-based stress reduction program on fibromyalgia. *General Hospital Psychiatry, 15*(5): 284-289.

Khadilkar, A., S. Milne, L. Brosseau, G. Wells, P. Tugwell, V. Robinson, B. Shea and M. Saginur (2005). Transcutaneous electrical nerve stimulation for the treatment of chronic low back pain: a systematic review. *Spine, 30*(23): 2657-2666.

Klerman, E. B., D. L. Goldenberg, E. N. Brown, A. M. Maliszewski and G. K. Adler (2001). Circadian rhythms of women with fibromyalgia. *The Journal of Clinical Endocrinology and Metabolism, 86*(3): 1034-1039.

Koltyn, K. F., A. W. Garvin, R. L. Gardiner and T. F. Nelson (1996). Perception of pain following aerobic exercise. *Med Sci Sports Exerc, 28*(11): 1418-1421.

Koumantakis, G. A., P. J. Watson and J. A. Oldham (2005). Trunk muscle stabilization training plus general exercise versus general exercise only: randomized controlled trial of patients with recurrent low back pain. *Physical Therapy, 85*(3): 209-225.

Kramer, M. S. and S. W. McDonald (2006). Aerobic exercise for women during pregnancy. *Cochrane Database Syst Rev, 3*: CD000180.

La Touche, R., A. Paris-Alemany, J. S. Mannheimer, S. Angulo-Diaz-Parreno, M. D. Bishop, A. Lopez-Valverde-Centeno, H. von Piekartz and J. Fernandez-Carnero (2012). Does Mobilization of the Upper Cervical Spine Affect Pain Sensitivity and Autonomic Nervous System Function in Patients With Cervico-craniofacial Pain?: A Randomized-controlled Trial. *The Clinical Journal of Pain.*

Larsson, S. E., H. Cai, Q. Zhang, R. Larsson and P. A. Oberg (1995). Microcirculation in the upper trapezius muscle during sustained shoulder load in healthy women--an endurance study using percutaneous laser-Doppler flowmetry and surface electromyography. *Eur J Appl Physiol Occup Physiol, 70*(5): 451-456.

Latimer, J., C. Maher and K. Refshauge (2004). The attitudes and beliefs of physiotherapy students to chronic back pain. *Clin J Pain, 20*(1): 45-50.

Latremoliere, A. and C. J. Woolf (2009). Central sensitization: a generator of pain hypersensitivity by central neural plasticity. *The Journal of Pain: Official Journal of the American Pain Society, 10*(9): 895-926.

Lauderdale, D. S., K. L. Knutson, L. L. Yan, K. Liu and P. J. Rathouz (2008). Self-reported and measured sleep duration: how similar are they? *Epidemiology 19*(6): 838-845.

Lewis, J. S., A. Green and C. Wright (2005). Subacromial impingement syndrome: the role of posture and muscle imbalance. *Journal of Shoulder and Elbow Surgery / American Shoulder and Elbow Surgeons ... [et al.], 14*(4): 385-392.

Lewis, J. S., C. Wright and A. Green (2005). Subacromial impingement syndrome: the effect of changing posture on shoulder range of movement. *The Journal of Orthopaedic and Sports Physical Therapy, 35*(2): 72-87.

Louw, A. (2012). *Your Nerves Are Having Back Surgery.* Minneapolis, OPTP.

Louw, A. (2013). *Why Do I Hurt? A Neuroscience Approach to Pain.* Minneapolis, OPTP.

Louw, A. (2013). *Your Fibromyalgia Workbook: A Neuroscience Approach.* Minneapolis, OPTP.

Louw, A., D. S. Butler, I. Diener and E. J. Puentedura (2013). Development of a Preoperative Neuroscience Educational Program for Patients with Lumbar Radiculopathy. *American Journal of Physical Medicine & Rehabilitation / Association of Academic Physiatrists.*

Louw, A., I. Diener, D. S. Butler and E. J. Puentedura (2011). The effect of neuroscience education on pain, disability, anxiety, and stress in chronic musculoskeletal pain. *Archives of Physical Medicine and Rehabilitation, 92*(12): 2041-2056.

Louw, A., Q. Louw and L. C. C. Crous (2009). Preoperative Education for Lumbar Surgery for Radiculopathy. *South African Journal of Physiotherapy 65*(2): 3-8.

Louw, A., E. L. Puentedura and P. Mintken (2011). Use of an abbreviated neuroscience education approach in the treatment of chronic low back pain: A case report. *Physiotherapy Theory and Practice.*

Louw, A., E. L. Puentedura and P. Mintken (2012). Use of an abbreviated neuroscience education approach in the treatment of chronic low back pain: a case report. *Physiotherapy Theory and Practice 28*(1): 50-62.

Luerding, R., T. Weigand, U. Bogdahn and T. Schmidt-Wilcke (2008). Working memory performance is correlated with local brain morphology in the medial frontal and anterior cingulate cortex in fibromyalgia patients: structural correlates of pain-cognition interaction. *Brain, 131*(Pt 12): 3222-3231.

Luomajoki, H. and G. L. Moseley (2011). Tactile acuity and lumbopelvic motor control in patients with back pain and healthy controls. *British Journal of Sports Medicine 45*(5): 437-440.

Lysack, C., M. Dama, S. Neufeld and E. Andreassi (2005). A compliance and satisfaction with home exercise: a comparison of computer-assisted video instruction and routine rehabilitation practice. *J Allied Health, 34*(2): 76-82.

Madden, K. S. (2003). Catecholamines, sympathetic innervation and immunity. *Brain Behav Immun, 17*(S1): 5-10.

Mailloux, J., M. Finno and J. Rainville (2006). Long-term exercise adherence in the elderly with chronic low back pain. *Am J Phys Med Rehabil, 85*(2): 120-126.

Maitland, G. D. (1986). *Vertebral Manipulation.* London, Butterworths.

Maizels, M. and B. McCarberg (2005). Antidepressants and antiepileptic drugs for chronic non-cancer pain. *Am Fam Physician, 71*(3): 483-490.

Mannion, A. F., F. Caporaso, N. Pulkovski and H. Sprott Spine stabilisation exercises in the treatment of chronic low back pain: a good clinical outcome is not associated with improved abdominal muscle function. *Eur Spine J, 21*(7): 1301-1310.

Marinus, J., G. L. Moseley, F. Birklein, R. Baron, C. Maihofner, W. S. Kingery and J. J. van Hilten (2011). Clinical features and pathophysiology of complex regional pain syndrome. *Lancet Neurology, 10*(7): 637-648.

Martinez-Lavin, M. and C. Solano (2009). Dorsal root ganglia, sodium channels, and fibromyalgia sympathetic pain. *Med Hypotheses, 72*(1): 64-66.

Mayoux-Benhamou, A., J. S. Giraudet-Le Quintrec, P. Ravaud, K. Champion, E. Dernis, D. Zerkak, C. Roy, A. Kahan, M. Revel and M. Dougados (2008). Influence of patient education on exercise compliance in rheumatoid arthritis: a prospective 12-month randomized controlled trial. *J Rheumatol, 35*(2): 216-223.

McGavock, J. M., J. L. Hastings, P. G. Snell, D. K. McGuire, E. L. Pacini, B. D. Levine and J. H. Mitchell (2009). A forty-year follow-up of the Dallas Bed Rest and Training study: the effect of age on the cardiovascular response to exercise in men. *The Journals of Gerontology. Series A, Biological Sciences and Medical Sciences, 64*(2): 293-299.

Medina-Mirapeix, F., P. Escolar-Reina, J. J. Gascon-Canovas, J. Montilla-Herrador, F. J. Jimeno-Serrano and S. M. Collins (2009). Predictive factors of adherence to frequency and duration components in home exercise programs for neck and low back pain: an observational study. *BMC Musculoskelet Disord, 10*: 155.

Meeus, M. and J. Nijs (2007). Central sensitization: a biopsychosocial explanation for chronic widespread pain in patients with fibromyalgia and chronic fatigue syndrome. *Clinical Rheumatology, 26*(4): 465-473.

Meeus, M., J. Nijs, J. Van Oosterwijck, V. Van Alsenoy and S. Truijen (2010). Pain Physiology Education Improves Pain Beliefs in Patients With Chronic Fatigue Syndrome Compared With Pacing and Self-Management Education: A Double-Blind Randomized Controlled Trial. *Arch Phys Med Rehabil, 91*(8): 1153-1159.

Melzack, R. (1996). Gate control theory: on the evolution of pain. *Pain Forum, 5*: 128-138.

Melzack, R. (1999). From the gate to the neuromatrix. *Pain Suppl, 6*: S121-126.

Miles, C. and E. Hardman (1998). State-dependent memory produced by aerobic exercise. *Ergonomics 41*(1): 20-28.

Miller, G. E., S. Cohen and A. K. Ritchey (2002). Chronic psychological stress and the regulation of pro-inflammatory cytokines: a glucocorticoid-resistance model. *Health Psychol, 21*(6): 531-541.

Mori, D. L., S. Sogg, P. Guarino, J. Skinner, D. Williams, A. Barkhuizen, C. Engel, D. Clauw, S. Donta and P. Peduzzi (2006). Predictors of exercise compliance in individuals with Gulf War veterans illnesses: Department of Veterans Affairs Cooperative Study 470. *Mil Med 171*(9): 917-923.

Mork, P. J. and T. I. Nilsen (2012). Sleep problems and risk of fibromyalgia: longitudinal data on an adult female population in Norway. *Arthritis and Rheumatism, 64*(1): 281-284.

Moseley, G. L. (2003). A pain neuromatrix approach to patients with chronic pain. *Man Ther, 8*(3): 130-140.

Moseley, G. L. (2006). Do training diaries affect and reflect adherence to home programs? *Arthritis Rheum, 55*(4): 662-664.

Moseley, G. L. (2007). Reconceptualising pain according to modern pain sciences. *Physical Therapy Reviews, 12*: 169-178.

Moseley, G. L. (2008). I can't find it! Distorted body image and tactile dysfunction in patients with chronic back pain. *Pain, 140*(1): 239-243.

Moseley, G. L. and P. W. Hodges (2005). Are the changes in postural control associated with low back pain caused by pain interference? *The Clinical Journal of Pain, 21*(4): 323-329.

Moseley, G. L. and P. W. Hodges (2005). Are the changes in postural control associated with low back pain caused by pain interference? *Clin J Pain, 21*(4): 323-329.

Moseley, G. L. and P. W. Hodges (2006). Reduced variability of postural strategy prevents normalization of motor changes induced by back pain: a risk factor for chronic trouble? *Behav Neurosci, 120*(2): 474-476.

Moseley, G. L., M. K. Nicholas and P. W. Hodges (2004). Does anticipation of back pain predispose to back trouble? *Brain : a Journal of Neurology, 127*(Pt 10): 2339-2347.

Moseley, G. L., M. K. Nicholas and P. W. Hodges (2004). Does anticipation of back pain predispose to back trouble? *Brain, 127*(Pt 10): 2339-2347.

Nathan, P. A., A. Wilcox, P. S. Emerick and et al. (2001). Effects of an aerobic exercise program on median nerve conduction and symptoms associated with carpal tunnel syndrome. *Journal of Occupational and Environmental Medicine, 43*(10): 840-843.

Newman, C. L. and R. W. Motta (2007). The effects of aerobic exercise on childhood PTSD, anxiety, and depression. *Int J Emerg Ment Health, 9*(2): 133-158.

Niemisto, L., P. Rissanen, S. Sarna, T. Lahtinen-Suopanki, K. A. Lindgren and H. Hurri (2005). Cost-effectiveness of combined manipulation, stabilizing exercises, and physician consultation compared to physician consultation alone for chronic low back pain: a prospective randomized trial with 2-year follow-up. *Spine, 30*(10): 1109-1115.

Nijs, J., N. Roussel, C. Paul van Wilgen, A. Koke and R. Smeets (2012). Thinking beyond muscles and joints: Therapists' and patients' attitudes and beliefs regarding chronic musculoskeletal pain are key to applying effective treatment. *Man Ther.*

Nijs, J., B. Van Houdenhove and R. A. Oostendorp (2010). Recognition of central sensitization in patients with musculoskeletal pain: Application of pain neurophysiology in manual therapy practice. *Man Ther, 15*(2): 135-141.

Nilsson-Wikmar, L., K. Holm, R. Oijerstedt and K. Harms-Ringdahl (2005). Effect of three different physical therapy treatments on pain and activity in pregnant women with pelvic girdle pain: a randomized clinical trial with 3, 6, and 12 months follow-up postpartum. *Spine, 30*(8): 850-856.

Nippoldt, T. (2010). Mayo Clinic office visit. Adrenal fatigue. An interview with Todd Nippoldt, M.D. *Mayo Clinic Women's HealthSource, 14*(3): 6.

O'Brien, K., S. Nixon, A. M. Tynan and R. Glazier (2010). Aerobic exercise interventions for adults living with HIV/AIDS. *Cochrane Database Syst Rev, 8*: CD001796.

Oman, R. F. and K. K. Oman (2003). A case-control study of psychosocial and aerobic exercise factors in women with symptoms of depression. *J Psychol, 137*(4): 338-350.

Pae, C. U., P. Luyten, D. M. Marks, C. Han, S. H. Park, A. A. Patkar, P. S. Masand and B. Van Houdenhove (2008). The relationship between fibromyalgia and major depressive disorder: a comprehensive review. *Current Medical Research and Opinion, 24*(8): 2359-2371.

Petruzzello, S. J. and A. K. Tate (1997). Brain activation, affect, and aerobic exercise: an examination of both state-independent and state-dependent relationships. *Psychophysiology, 34*(5): 527-533.

Pontifex, M. B. and C. H. Hillman (2008). Neuroelectric measurement of cognition during aerobic exercise. *Methods, 45*(4): 271-278.

Pontifex, M. B., C. H. Hillman, B. Fernhall, K. M. Thompson and T. A. Valentini (2009). The effect of acute aerobic and resistance exercise on working memory. *Med Sci Sports Exerc, 41*(4): 927-934.

Puentedura, E. J. and A. Louw (2012). A neuroscience approach to managing athletes with low back pain. *Physical Therapy in Sport: Official Journal of the Association of Chartered Physiotherapists in Sports Medicine, 13*(3): 123-133.

Quaney, B. M., L. A. Boyd, J. M. McDowd, L. H. Zahner, J. He, M. S. Mayo and R. F. Macko (2009). Aerobic exercise improves cognition and motor function poststroke. *Neurorehabil Neural Repair, 23*(9): 879-885.

Rabin, B. S. (1999). *Stress, Immune Function and Health.* New York, Wiley-Liss.

Reid, K. J., K. G. Baron, B. Lu, E. Naylor, L. Wolfe and P. C. Zee (2010). Aerobic exercise improves self-reported sleep and quality of life in older adults with insomnia. *Sleep Med.*

Richardson, C., P. Hodges and J. Hides (2004). *Therapeutic Exercise For Lumbopelvic Stabilization.* London, Churchill Livingstone.

Richardson, C., G. A. Jull, P. Hodges and J. Hides (1999). *Therapeutic Exercise For Spinal Segmental Stabilization in Low Back Pain.* London, Churchill Livingstone.

Riva, R., P. J. Mork, R. H. Westgaard and U. Lundberg (2012). Comparison of the cortisol awakening response in women with shoulder and neck pain and women with fibromyalgia. *Psychoneuroendocrinology, 37*(2): 299-306.

Riva, R., P. J. Mork, R. H. Westgaard, T. Okkenhaug Johansen and U. Lundberg (2012). Catecholamines and heart rate in female fibromyalgia patients. *Journal of Psychosomatic Research, 72*(1): 51-57.

Rooks, D. S., S. Gautam, M. Romeling, M. L. Cross, D. Stratigakis, B. Evans, D. L. Goldenberg, M. D. Iversen and J. N. Katz (2007). Group exercise, education, and combination self-management in women with fibromyalgia: a randomized trial. *Arch Intern Med, 167*(20): 2192-2200.

Roos, E. (2002). [Physical activity can influence the course of early arthritis. Both strength training and aerobic exercise provide pain relief and functional improvement]. *Lakartidningen, 99*(45): 4484-4489.

Rossi, M., G. Santoro, R. Ricco, F. Pentimone and A. Carpi (2005). Effect of chronic aerobic exercise on cutaneous microcirculatory flow response to insulin iontophoresis and to ischemia in elderly males. *Int J Sports Med, 26*(7): 558-562.

Sanchez-Zuriaga, D., F. J. Vera-Garcia, J. M. Moreside and S. M. McGill (2009). Trunk muscle activation patterns and spine kinematics when using an oscillating blade: influence of different postures and blade orientations. *Archives of Physical Medicine and Rehabilitation, 90*(6): 1055-1060.

Sandberg, J. and Y. Barnard (1997). Deep learning is difficult. *Instruc Sci, 25*(1): 15-36.

Sapolsky, R. (1994). *Why Zebras Don't Get Ulcers.* New York, W.H. Freeman and Company

Sapolsky, R. M. (1994). *Why Zebras Don't Get Ulcers.* New York, Freeman.

Sapolsky, R. M. (1998). *Why zebras don't get ulcers: an updated guide to stress, stress-related diseases, and coping.* New York, W.H. Freeman and Co.

Sarzi-Puttini, P., F. Atzeni, A. Diana, A. Doria and R. Furlan (2006). Increased neural sympathetic activation in fibromyalgia syndrome. *Ann N Y Acad Sci, 1069*: 109-117.

Scales, R. and J. H. Miller (2003). Motivational techniques for improving compliance with an exercise program: skills for primary care clinicians. *Curr Sports Med Rep, 2*(3): 166-172.

Schaefer, C., A. Chandran, M. Hufstader, R. Baik, M. McNett, D. Goldenberg, R. Gerwin and G. Zlateva (2011). The comparative burden of mild, moderate and severe fibromyalgia: results from a cross-sectional survey in the United States. *Health and Quality of Life Outcomes, 9*: 71.

Schwartz, T. (2010). *The Way We're Working Isn't working.* New York, NY, Free Press.

Schweinhardt, P., K. M. Sauro and M. C. Bushnell (2008). Fibromyalgia: a disorder of the brain? *Neuroscientist, 14*(5): 415-421.

Sculco, A. D., D. C. Paup, B. Fernhall and M. J. Sculco (2001). Effects of aerobic exercise on low back pain patients in treatment. *Spine J, 1*(2): 95-101.

Shah, M. A., S. Feinberg and E. Krishnan (2006). Sleep-disordered breathing among women with fibromyalgia syndrome. *J Clin Rheumatol, 12*(6): 277-281.

Sharma, N. K., J. M. Ryals, B. J. Gajewski and D. E. Wright (2010). Aerobic exercise alters analgesia and neurotrophin-3 synthesis in an animal model of chronic widespread pain. *Phys Ther, 90*(5): 714-725.

Sim, J. and N. Adams (2002). Systematic review of randomized controlled trials of nonpharmacological interventions for fibromyalgia. *Clin J Pain, 18*(5): 324-336.

Smith, P. J., J. A. Blumenthal, B. M. Hoffman, H. Cooper, T. A. Strauman, K. Welsh-Bohmer, J. N. Browndyke and A. Sherwood (2010). Aerobic exercise and neurocognitive performance: a meta-analytic review of randomized controlled trials. *Psychosom Med, 72*(3): 239-252.

Staud, R. (2004). Fibromyalgia pain: do we know the source? *Curr Opin Rheumatol, 16*(2): 157-163.

Stephens, R., J. Atkins and A. Kingston (2009). Swearing as a response to pain. *Neuroreport, 20*(12): 1056-1060.

Stephens, R. and C. Umland (2011). Swearing as a response to pain-effect of daily swearing frequency. *The Journal of Pain: Official Journal of the American Pain Society, 12*(12): 1274-1281.

Stisi, S., C. Venditti and I. Sarracco (2008). [Distress influence in fibromyalgia.]. *Reumatismo, 60*(4): 274-281.

Stringer, W. W., M. Berezovskaya, W. A. O'Brien, C. K. Beck and R. Casaburi (1998). The effect of exercise training on aerobic fitness, immune indices, and quality of life in HIV+ patients. *Med Sci Sports Exerc, 30*(1): 11-16.

Tanriverdi, F., Z. Karaca, K. Unluhizarci and F. Kelestimur (2007). The hypothalamo-pituitary-adrenal axis in chronic fatigue syndrome and fibromyalgia syndrome. *Stress, 10*(1): 13-25.

Thacker, M. A., A. K. Clark, F. Marchand and S. B. McMahon (2007). Pathophysiology of peripheral neuropathic pain: immune cells and molecules. *Anesthesia and Analgesia, 105*(3): 838-847.

Theadom, A., M. Cropley and K. L. Humphrey (2007). Exploring the role of sleep and coping in quality of life in fibromyalgia. *J Psychosom Res, 62*(2): 145-151.

Thomas, K., D. Burton, L. Withrow and B. Adkisson (2004). Impact of a preoperative education program via interactive telehealth network for rural patients having total joint replacement. *Orthop Nurs, 23*(1): 39-44.

Togo, F., B. H. Natelson, G. K. Adler, J. E. Ottenweller, D. L. Goldenberg, Z. R. Struzik and Y. Yamamoto (2009). Plasma cytokine fluctuations over time in healthy controls and patients with fibromyalgia. *Experimental Biology and Medicine, 234*(2): 232-240.

Tousignant, M., P. Boissy, H. Moffet, H. Corriveau, F. Cabana, F. Marquis and J. Simard Patients' satisfaction of healthcare services and perception with in-home telerehabilitation and physiotherapists' satisfaction toward technology for post-knee arthroplasty: an embedded study in a randomized trial. *Telemed J E Health, 17*(5): 376-382.

Tritilanunt, T. and W. Wajanavisit (2001). The efficacy of an aerobic exercise and health education program for treatment of chronic low back pain. *J Med Assoc Thai, 84 Suppl 2*: S528-533.

Tsao, H. and P. W. Hodges (2007). Immediate changes in feedforward postural adjustments following voluntary motor training. *Exp Brain Res, 181*(4): 537-546.

Ucok, K., A. Aycicek, M. Sezer, A. Genc, M. Akkaya, V. Caglar, F. Fidan and M. Unlu (2009). Aerobic and anaerobic exercise capacities in obstructive sleep apnea and associations with subcutaneous fat distributions. *Lung 187*(1): 29-36.

Uysal, N., K. Tugyan, B. M. Kayatekin, O. Acikgoz, H. A. Bagriyanik, S. Gonenc, D. Ozdemir, I. Aksu, A. Topcu and I. Semin (2005). The effects of regular aerobic exercise in adolescent period on hippocampal neuron density, apoptosis and spatial memory. *Neurosci Lett 383*(3): 241-245.

Valkeinen, H., K. Hakkinen, A. Pakarinen, P. Hannonen, A. Hakkinen, O. Airaksinen, L. Niemitukia, W. J. Kraemer and M. Alen (2005). Muscle hypertrophy, strength development, and serum hormones during strength training in elderly women with fibromyalgia. *Scand J Rheumatol, 34*(4): 309-314.

Van Houdenhove, B., F. Van Den Eede and P. Luyten (2009). Does hypothalamic-pituitary-adrenal axis hypofunction in chronic fatigue syndrome reflect a 'crash' in the stress system? *Med Hypotheses, 72*(6): 701-705.

van Uffelen, J. G., A. P. M. J. Chin, M. Hopman-Rock and W. van Mechelen (2008). The effects of exercise on cognition in older adults with and without cognitive decline: a systematic review. *Clin J Sport Med, 18*(6): 486-500.

Vera-Garcia, F. J., S. H. Brown, J. R. Gray and S. M. McGill (2006). Effects of different levels of torso coactivation on trunk muscular and kinematic responses to posteriorly applied sudden loads. *Clinical Biomechanics, 21*(5): 443-455.

Vlaeyen, J. W., A. M. Kole-Snijders, R. G. Boeren and H. van Eek (1995). Fear of movement/(re)injury in chronic low back pain and its relation to behavioral performance. *Pain, 62*(3): 363-372.

Vlaeyen, J. W. S. and S. J. Linton (2000). Fear-avoidance and its consequences in chronic musculoskeletal pain: a state of the art. *Pain, 85*: 317-322.

Voet, N. B., E. L. van der Kooi, Riphagen, II, E. Lindeman, B. G. van Engelen and A. Geurts (2010). Strength training and aerobic exercise training for muscle disease. *Cochrane Database Syst Rev*(1): CD003907.

Wakefield, E., A. Holtermann and P. J. Mork (2011). The effect of delayed onset of muscle soreness on habitual trapezius activity. *European Journal of Pain, 15*(6): 577-583.

Wall, P. D. (1996). Comments after 30 years of the gate control theory. *Pain Forum, 5*(1): 12-22.

Wall, P. D. and R. Melzack (2005). *Textbook of Pain*. London, Elsevier.

Wedekind, D., A. Sprute, A. Broocks, G. Huther, K. Engel, P. Falkai and B. Bandelow (2008). Nocturnal urinary cortisol excretion over a randomized controlled trial with paroxetine vs. placebo combined with relaxation training or aerobic exercise in panic disorder. *Curr Pharm Des, 14*(33): 3518-3524.

Weissbecker, I., A. Floyd, E. Dedert, P. Salmon and S. Sephton (2006). Childhood trauma and diurnal cortisol disruption in fibromyalgia syndrome. *Psychoneuroendocrinology, 31*(3): 312-324.

Wigers, S. H., T. C. Stiles and P. A. Vogel (1996). Effects of aerobic exercise versus stress management treatment in fibromyalgia. *Scandinavian Journal of Rheumatology, 25*: 77-86.

Wingenfeld, K., D. Wagner, I. Schmidt, G. Meinlschmidt, D. H. Hellhammer and C. Heim (2007). The low-dose dexamethasone suppression test in fibromyalgia. *J Psychosom Res, 62*(1): 85-91.

Wolfe, F. (2012). Sleep problems and risk of fibromyalgia — untenable conclusions: comment on the article by Mork et al. *Arthritis and Rheumatism, 64*(5): 1692-1693; author reply 1693-1694.

Wolff, M. S., T. H. Michel, D. E. Krebs and N. T. Watts (1991). Chronic pain — assessment of orthopedic physical therapists' knowledge and attitudes. *Phys Ther, 71*(3): 207-214.

Woods, J. A., M. A. Ceddia, B. W. Wolters, J. K. Evans, Q. Lu and E. McAuley (1999). Effects of 6 months of moderate aerobic exercise training on immune function in the elderly. *Mech Ageing Dev, 109*(1): 1-19.

Wu, G., L. Keyes, P. Callas, X. Ren and B. Bookchin (2010). Comparison of telecommunication, community, and home-based Tai Chi exercise programs on compliance and effectiveness in elders at risk for falls. *Arch Phys Med Rehabil, 91*(6): 849-856.

Yamamoto, U., M. Mohri, K. Shimada, H. Origuchi, K. Miyata, K. Ito, K. Abe and H. Yamamoto (2007). Six-month aerobic exercise training ameliorates central sleep apnea in patients with chronic heart failure. *J Card Fail, 13*(10): 825-829.

Yanagida, H. (1995). Sympathetic nervous system and pain: introduction. *The Pain Clinic, 8*(1): 1-3.

Zhang, K. R., H. T. Liu, H. F. Zhang, Q. J. Zhang, Q. X. Li, Q. J. Yu, W. Y. Guo, H. C. Wang and F. Gao (2007). Long-term aerobic exercise protects the heart against ischemia/reperfusion injury via PI3 kinase-dependent and Akt-mediated mechanism. *Apoptosis, 12*(9): 1579-1588.

Notes

Chapter 7

Putting It All Together

7.1: Introduction

In chapter 1, we introduced a chronic pain patient that we wrote up as a case study (Louw, Puentedura et al., 2012). In this chapter, we will use that case as a clinical example of how TNE can be applied to a complex patient, along with the clinical implementation.

7.2: History

The patient is a 64-year-old female who presented to physical therapy with a three-year history of chronic low back pain (CLBP). She had previously worked as a registered nurse but had not been working due to her persistent pain. She reported that the onset of her LBP had been insidious with no known injury or cause. The LBP, and resultant disability, progressively increased to the point where she stopped working approximately 18 months prior to the initial physical therapy examination.

She was never placed on disability nor received workman's compensation. Since the onset of her LBP, she had been treated by numerous healthcare providers, including physical therapists, chiropractors, massage therapists, acupuncturists, spine surgeons, her general practitioner, various pain management specialists, psychologists, a neurologist and a physiatrist. The most common treatments received included therapeutic exercise (various forms), massage, chiropractic adjustments, physical modalities, epidural steroid injections, education about her back pain, relaxation exercises, and various medications, including pain medications and muscle relaxants.

At the time of her initial physical therapy visit, she reported that she was taking Hydrocodone (7.5 mg Hydrocodone Bitartrate and 500 mg Acetaminophen every 4-5 hours), Oxycontin (10 mg every 4 hours), Skelaxin (800 mg 3-4 times per day) and Celebrex (100 mg 2 times per day). These medications offered only short term relief and did not result in any long term improvements in her symptoms.

Her most recent treatments included a series of three epidural steroid injections and a multi-level radiofrequency nerve ablation, which had not eased her pain. She was then referred to the physical therapy, specifically for TNE. Her most recent MRI revealed "multi-level disc degeneration," which she believed was the main cause of her pain.

During the subjective history, the patient reported that her general health was good and she had no other orthopedic injuries or concerns about other joints. Prior to the initial physical therapy evaluation, the patient completed a medical screening questionnaire (MSQ) to screen for potential red and yellow flags that may require further workup and/or referral. The MSQ includes a review of systems with special questions designed to screen for organ system involvement based on subjective symptoms perceived by the patient. The MSQ was reviewed by the primary therapist with the patient and did not reveal any red flags at the time of the initial evaluation.

Over the previous 18 months, she had steadily decreased her activities of daily living (ADL) due to pain and an increased fear of pain. Of particular concern to her was her inability to clean her house. She reported increased pain with vacuuming more than half a room at a time. If she vacuumed more than half a room, her back pain would increase considerably ("flare") to where she needed to take extra pain medication, lay down and usually was unable to do any further house work.

She reported that she enjoyed exercising ("working out") but had decreased her walking distance and frequency due to her CLBP. At the time of the initial examination, she reported that she was unable to stand at a stove and cook a meal, or sit at a desk for more than 30 minutes. The pattern of her pain was assessed by having her complete a body chart (Figure 7.1), which was then discussed.

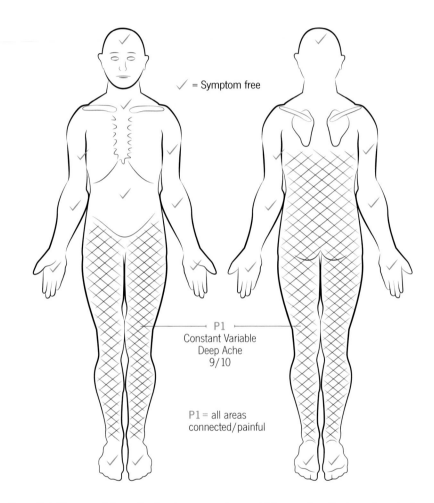

Figure 7.1: The area of the patient's primary symptoms, which were described as a "constant variable deep ache" and rated 9 out of 10 on the pain rating scale.

The examining therapist did not find any red flags when she was questioned about her pain pattern, and it appeared to be consistent with that of a patient with central sensitization in that pain was widespread (diffuse area). She rated her current pain as 9 out of 10 on the Numeric Pain Rating Scale (NPRS) (Moseley, 2002; Cleland, Childs et al., 2008). The patient reported that her easing factors included lying down on either side (left or right), frequent periods of sitting down or taking her medication. Her most recent MRI (2005) revealed multi-level "bulging" discs (most notably at L2/3, L4/5 and L5/S1) and multi-level degenerative disc disease – findings that, based on the interview, created a lot of anxiety for the patient. The patient's goals for attending physical therapy were to return to part-time work (2-3 half-days per week in her husband's office), be able to stand in the kitchen and cook a whole meal, clean her house and return to her regular exercise program, which included aerobics, walking, and yoga.

7.3: Questionnaires

Prior to the patient being further evaluated for physical therapy services, she was asked to complete questionnaires pertaining to pain, disability, fear-avoidance beliefs, and depression. These questionnaires were chosen based on her early communication with the primary therapist, prior to setting up the appointment, and her CLBP history. These same questionnaires were completed by the patient immediately following the TNE session (75 minutes later) and at seven-month follow-up. The four self-report questionnaires used for this case report included the Numeric Pain Rating Scale (NPRS), Oswestry Disability Index (ODI), Fear-Avoidance Beliefs Questionnaire (FABQ) and Zung Depression Scale.

The NPRS, ODI and FABQ are described in detail in Chapters 1 and 2. The Zung Self-Rating Depression Scale is a short self-administered 20-item survey to quantify the depressed status of a patient and has been used in measuring depression related to spinal disorders (Zung, 1965; Ronnberg, Lind et al., 2007). Zung Depression Scale scores range from 20 to 80, with a score of 55 or higher suggesting possible depression (Zung, 1965).

7.4: Physical Examination

A lower-quarter screening examination was performed, aimed at identifying any potential red flags and nervous system involvement. The lower-quarter screen included a neuromuscular examination of the lower extremities, consisting of myotome strength, sensation along dermatomes and peripheral nerves, and deep tendon reflexes of the lower extremities (Butler, 1991; Butler, 2000). The screening examination did not identify any abnormal findings. Adjacent peripheral joints (hip and knee) and spinal regions (cervical and thoracic) were subjected to active range of motion (ROM) assessments in all planes. The adjacent joints and spinal regions, although "sensitive" to movement, did not reveal significant ROM deficits or exacerbation of her primary complaint of widespread LBP.

The rest of the physical examination was focused, as the therapist felt that including too many tests and measures would likely yield little useful data and may exacerbate the patient's pain state. This type of examination is consistent with what has been proposed in the physical examination of patients with chronic pain (Butler, 2000). Nattrass and others stated that there was no evidence for a relationship between impairments and disability in CLBP, and it is "illogical" to evaluate impairment in CLBP patients using a spinal range of motion model when aiming to measure disability (Nattrass, Nitschke et al., 1999).

The patient presented with signs and symptoms associated with central sensitivity. The presentation of central sensitivity with a generalized upregulation of the central nervous system (CNS) (secondary hyperalgesia) influences the results of physical examinations and limits the validity of tests and measures aimed at finding specific physical dysfunction (Smart, Blake et al.; Butler, 2000). Identifying specific physical impairments may have limited value when examining patients with widespread and prolonged pain (Butler, 2000; Moseley, 2003; Fernandez-de-las-Penas, de la Llave-Rincon et al., 2009).

The tests and measures section of the physical examination began with active movement testing. The therapist deemed this important because it was important to assess the quantity and quality of functional movement present, as well as any aberrant movements, as this finding has been purported to predict success with lumbar stabilization exercises (Hicks, Fritz et al., 2005). The patient was instructed to "bend forward while keeping your knees straight and to stop whenever you feel like you need to stop" (Figure 7.2). It is important to point out here that the patient was not asked to bend forward until pain onset, pain increase or pain limit. In fact, the word 'pain' was not used during testing instructions. The patient was only able to achieve 10 degrees of flexion, as measured by a single inclinometer.

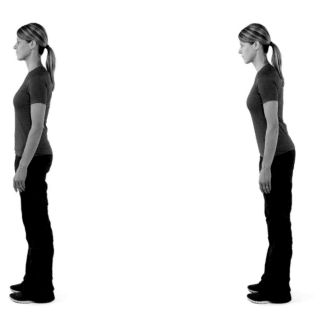

Figure 7.2: Active lumbar range of motion was examined by asking the patient to bend forward while keeping the knees straight and to stop whenever she felt like she needed to stop. She was able to achieve 10 degrees of flexion, as measured by a single inclinometer (clinical images recreated).

Fritz and others reported that single inclinometer measurements of lumbar flexion and extension had intraclass correlation coefficients (ICC) of 0.60 and 0.61 for inter-rater reliability, respectively (Cleland, Whitman et al., 2005).

During the forward bend, the patient reported that she was afraid to move beyond the 10 degrees for fear her pain would get worse. When questioned about "her pain," the therapist asked the patient to relate the pain she was fearful of reproducing to her body chart. She related that she was afraid that further forward flexion would bring on the "entire" pain area depicted on the body chart. Because of the expressed anxiety about active movement, no further active lumbar ROM movements were performed, in order to avoid exacerbating the patient's condition.

Neurodynamic testing followed, which included the straight leg raise (SLR) test (Butler, 1991; Butler, 2000) on the left and the right, to the first point of resistance. Her SLR averaged 70 degrees on both legs (goniometer measurement – average for three measurements) with reported symptoms of "pulling" in both her legs, left equal to right. The "pulling" in her legs was not her primary complaint and did not correlate with the pain pattern outlined on the body chart. Slump testing (Butler, 1991; Butler, 2000) was limited due to her inability to "slouch" without pain and anxiety. A modified slump was performed in a slightly slumped position but revealed decreased knee extension of -30° from full extension bilaterally, with a sensation of "pulling" in the leg and low back. The modified slump test elicited her primary pain complaint of back and leg pain, and this did correlate with the pain pattern outlined on the body chart.

7.5: Diagnosis

Although the patient presented with a complex pain diagram, the primary therapist concluded that the patient's signs and symptoms were consistent with a chronic pain state with central sensitization. "Central sensitization" is defined as a condition in which peripheral noxious inputs to the central nervous system (CNS) lead to an increased excitability where the response to normal inputs is greatly enhanced (Smart, Blake et al.; Merskey and Bogduk, 1994). This is not to imply that the symptoms were non-organic, but rather a complex neurophysiological process was in play whereby the CNS had become "hyper-excitable" to input received from the periphery (Butler, 2000; Woolf, 2007).

Although no standardized or validated screening tools exist to identify patients with central sensitivity, a number of theoretical clinical decision-making strategies exist, based on the recognition of characteristic signs and symptoms (Butler, 2000; Lidbeck, 2002). The patient in this case report demonstrated several of the signs and symptoms that are typically associated with central sensitivity, including a high FABQ score, diffuse area of pain as seen in her body diagram, spontaneous pain ("it comes on when it wants to"), pain associated with emotional disturbances and maladaptive cognitions, history of failed treatments, and diffuse/non-anatomic areas of pain and tenderness on palpation (George and Zeppieri, 2009).

Table 7.1 provides a list of signs and symptoms typically observed with central sensitization and found to be present in this patient.

It is important to note that at the initial evaluation, the patient presented with a score of 58 on the Zung Depression Scale. Most people with depression are reported to score between 50 and 69 (Romera, Delgado-Cohen et al., 2008). As this score was elevated and would have suggested the potential need for a referral to a psychological health care provider, the primary therapist discussed this with the patient. The patient related a history of treatment for depression by a psychologist. It was suggested to the patient that she may benefit from further examination by a psychological health care provider, but she declined and reported that her previous treatment (three months prior) had not helped. The patient felt that her "depression" was caused by her pain and limited function, and she was hoping that physical therapy might be able to improve her CLBP. The therapist and the patient agreed to monitor these symptoms and proceed with physical therapy. If her depressive symptoms worsened, she would be referred to a psychological health care provider.

Table 7.1: The list of signs and symptoms typically observed with central sensitization and notation about their presence in this patient

Signs and symptoms	Reference	Present in this patient
"Hyper-excitable" to input from the periphery	(Butler, 2000; Woolf, 2007)	✔
High FABQ score	(Cleland, Fritz et al., 2008; Nijs, Van Houdenhove et al., 2010)	✔
Diffuse area of pain	(Butler, 2000; George and Zeppieri, 2009)	✔
Spontaneous pain	(Fernandez-de-las-Penas, de la Llave-Rincon et al., 2009; Nijs, Van Houdenhove et al., 2010)	✔
Pain associated with emotional disturbances and maladaptive cognitions	(Nijs, Van Houdenhove et al., 2010)	✔
History of failed treatments	(Butler, 2000; Meeus and Nijs, 2007)	✔
Visiting many healthcare providers	(Butler, 2000; Meeus and Nijs, 2007)	✔
Diffuse/non-anatomic areas of pain and tenderness on palpation	(Fernandez-de-las-Penas, de la Llave-Rincon et al., 2009; Nijs, Van Houdenhove et al., 2010)	✔
Depression	(Romera, Delgado-Cohen et al., 2008)	✔
Latency	(Butler, 2000; Fernandez-de-las-Penas, de la Llave-Rincon et al., 2009; Nijs, Van Houdenhove et al., 2010)	✔

7.6: Intervention

Upon completion of the examination, the treating therapist decided that the patient would benefit from a TNE session, as the patient's clinical presentation fit the clinical presentation of central sensitization (Butler, 2000; Butler and Moseley, 2003; Wall and Melzack, 2005; Woolf, 2007) for which TNE has been shown to be a useful intervention (Moseley, 2003; Moseley, 2004; Moseley, Nicholas et al., 2004; Moseley, 2005). Based on the patient's high level of fear, especially related to spinal movements, it was decided that physical therapy interventions would focus more on a CBT approach to address her underlying fear of movement, as manual therapy treatments aimed at improving physical impairments were not likely to succeed. Previous sessions in physical therapy had utilized various forms of exercise, suggesting a graded exercise or graded exposure program may have limitations since the patient had already "failed" with these approaches. By utilizing TNE and having her gain a better understanding of her pain, especially the increased sensitivity of her nervous system, it was argued the patient would not only be able to move better but be more inclined to participate and follow through with other active movement components of the intervention. Additionally, TNE education was chosen as opposed to other educational models like Back School, as it spends some time and detail on describing anatomical and/or biomechanical models of pain, which is contrary to the TNE approach of de-emphasizing anatomical and/or biomechanical findings.

The material that was presented was based on current knowledge of the neurophysiology of pain, according to Wall and Melzack (McMahon and Koltzenburg, 2006) and the 'Explain Pain' book, written by Butler and Moseley (Butler and Moseley, 2003). The TNE lasted 45 minutes in a private room and was administered by a physical therapist familiar with TNE. The TNE was accompanied by the use of pictures, examples, and metaphors (Butler and Moseley, 2003; Moseley, 2007). Given the significant pain presentation, it was decided to limit the first session to a comprehensive TNE-only session. Subsequent sessions would then allow for revisiting of the TNE while performing movement-based strategies, such as exercise, in her plan of care (chapters 5 and 6).

What follows is a series of drawings used to educate the patient about the neurophysiology and biology of her pain experience. For additional insight and more specific clinic and patient language, therapists are referred to chapter 4.

7.6a: Tissues and Areas That Hurt in the Patient

The therapist started drawing a body, emphasizing the main areas the patient was experiencing pain (Figure 7.3). By doing so, the therapist not only showed the patient that he had listened to her but started the preparation of explaining the widespread sensitivity of her nervous system. Additionally, the goal was not to focus on one particular area, or more importantly, one single tissue, i.e., a disc.

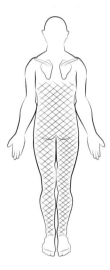

Figure 7.3: The pain drawing provided by the patient was the starting point for development of the individualized TNE session.

7.6b: Nerves in These Areas

The next addition to the drawing was a discussion on the nervous system, specifically its role as an alarm system. The patient was educated on the fact that each area she was experiencing pain in had nerves. "The body contains 45 miles of nerves and they travel all over the body like a road system." There are nerves in her back, hips, legs, upper back, neck and arms. The patient was also introduced to the fact that nerves work like an alarm system and "tell" her when there is something happening in the area. An example was given that if the therapist were to hit her in the arm, something would need to alert her there was someone unfriendly in her area and she needed to take action. The nerves in and around the arm would thus send the message to her brain to make her aware of it, so she could take appropriate action.

Furthermore, with the addition of arrows to the drawing, the patient was told that nerves constantly send messages. Some we react to and some we don't (Figure 7.4). For example, sitting on the chair and listening to the therapist, the nerves in her back would be sending messages that there's a hard back to the chair she's sitting in. If needed, action may be taken to move or reposition. Nerves constantly send impulses or information to the brain for interpretation. "This is normal and happens in everyone."

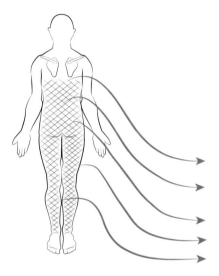

Figure 7.4: Arrows were drawn from the pain drawing to signify nerves sending 'messages.'

7.6c: How Do Nerves Work?

Once the patient understood that each area she experienced pain in had nerve endings, the patient was educated more on how we view the nervous system. In this case, the nervous system was compared to an alarm system. First, the patient was shown a drawing of normal electrical activity of the nervous system (Figure 7.5). "All nerves have electricity in them." However, the electrical activity is way below the firing level, which if reached, would result in a message being sent to the brain.

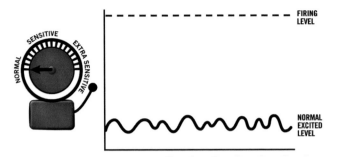

Figure 7.5: The drawing shown to the patient to explain normal electrical activity of the nervous system.

Once the patient understood that all nerves (including the ones in the areas she experienced pain) had electrical activity in them, she was introduced to action potentials (Figure 7.6). As described in chapter 4, she was asked if she stepped on a rusted nail, would she want to know about it; her answer was a resounding "yes." The patient was shown that stimulation of the nerves results in an action potential and a message, in this case to remove the nail, get medical attention and wear shoes to prevent repeated injury from rusted nails.

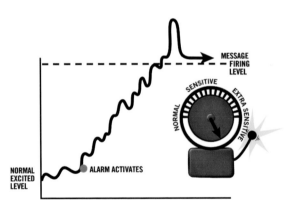

Figure 7.6: The drawing to explain action potentials.

The next part was deemed very important in her understanding of central sensitization. She was told that nerves, after activating the alarm system and sending messages, would normally come down to their pre-firing resting level, ready for action. Unfortunately, it is believed that in one in four people (current chronic pain epidemic) the alarm system stays elevated at an extra-sensitive level. We believe this is a large part of why she was experiencing so much pain, had not been able to do as much as before, and developed some sensitivity to movement, stress and temperature changes. More importantly, the patient was told this sensitization is quite normal in people experiencing long-lasting pain.

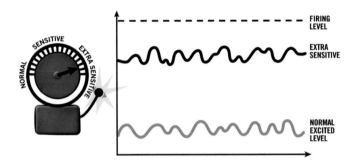

Figure 7.7: The drawing to explain increased sensitivity of the nervous system.

At this point, patients receiving TNE usually have some questions regarding sensitization. Especially since it pertained to her diagnosis of central sensitization, more education was provided in this regard. The patient was asked if she had any questions or comments at this point, and she replied with one encouraging comment: "So you think my nerves are extra sensitive?" The patient was told 'yes.' Three years ago, possibly due to an injury or overload, perhaps during a stressful time in her life, the alarm in her low back went off. We know this because she subsequently took action, i.e., seeing her doctor, getting treatments and tests, and ultimately bringing herself to this session. The alarm system had therefore done its job. The patient was told that three common questions come up during this discussion with patients and need to be addressed:

1. How do we know this?

2. Why did the nerves stay extra sensitive?

3. What can be done about it?

The standard answers to the three questions (chapter 4) were provided, helping the patient understand more about her nerve sensitivity. A summary is provided here:

1. How do we know this?
- The patient has, in essence, told us via the story of sensitization
- Physical examination supports this
- Medical treatments such as pharmacological approaches support this

2. Why did the nerves stay extra sensitive?
- Failed treatments
- Different explanations of her pain
- Fear
- Living daily in pain
- Poor outlook on life, specifically goals

3. What can be done about it?
The answers to the treatment were not provided at this point. The patient was advised that this will be discussed, and although we were excited to share this with her, there was more information about her pain she needed to know prior to discussing her treatment plan.

7.6d: Information to the Spinal Cord and Brain

Next the patient was introduced to central processing. She clearly understood that the nerves in her back had increased their activity, ultimately sending danger messages to get help and have since remained sensitive. The next step was to educate her on where the messages end up. All of the nerve messages are sent to the spinal cord and, ultimately, to the brain for interpretation (Figure 7.8). Before the patient could scoff at the notion, "oh, you think it's in my head," the therapist explained to her that the pain was real, but all information has to be processed in the brain. This point was elaborated on with a discussion of nociception, such as a scrape on the leg that's bleeding but you wonder where the blood came from because there is no pain.

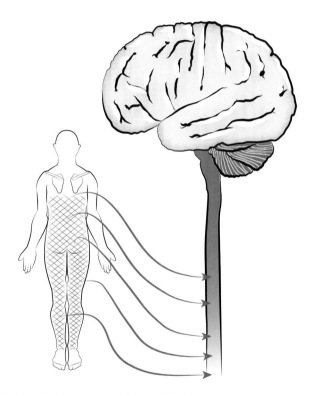

Figure 7.8: The drawing to introduce central sensitization.

7.6e: Central Sensitization

In chapters 3 and 4, action potential windup was discussed. A critical part of the TNE was to help the patient understand a great deal of her pain was due to an amplification of her 'danger messages.' She was told that the information from her back, hips and legs was being sent to her spinal cord and, ultimately, to the brain. Due to her long-lasting pain, however, the brain was acting like a 'worried CEO:' it wanted to know more and closely analyzed the reports it was getting, especially from the troubled low back, hips and legs. Two examples were provided: a magnifying glass enlarging everything reported to the brain or the notion of pressing one "X" on a keyboard, but having "XXXX" show up on the screen (Figure 7.9). She responded to the therapist with a poignant statement: "So, the pain I feel is not necessarily the pain I got." In many clinical cases, this could be seen as the "ah-ha" moment. She understood sensitivity. Sure, she had pain, but it wasn't a true reflection of her tissues' state of health. Tissues heal.

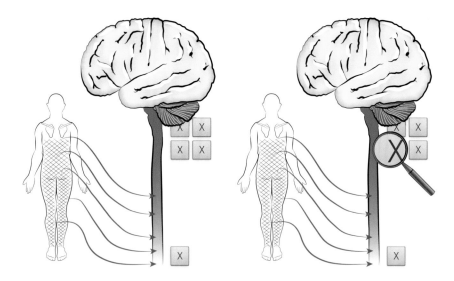

Figure 7.9: The drawing to explain action potential windup.

7.6f: Neuromatrix

The next step in the discussion centered on the brain's processing of nociception. This patient specifically had trouble understanding why she, since developing pain, struggled with focus and concentration. From a therapeutic perspective, she had already received a significant amount of spinal stabilization exercises, and it was sensed that she felt embarrassed she could not do her core exercises despite a long history of exercise, which included Pilates™.

Once the patient understood the information was sent to the brain for processing and her pain was real, biological and not "made up," she was introduced to the neuromatrix. As with the examples in chapters 3 and 4, she was asked to close her eyes and remember her grandmother, which resulted in the discussion of various parts of her brain being used to process her grandmother experience. The same thing occurred with her experiences of pain. She was shown pictures of the neuromatrix, with a focus on what typical tasks these regions fulfill when not used by pain (Figure 7.10). Special reference was made to the anterior cingulate, regarding focus and concentration, and the motor cortex with spinal stabilization. This explanation seemed to make a lot of sense to her. She was reminded to see the various areas as a 'board meeting,' which might explain why some activities were slightly more difficult for her since her pain started three years ago.

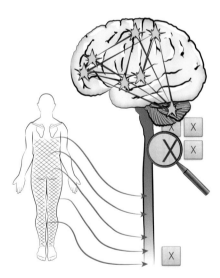

Figure 7.10: The drawing to explain the pain neuromatrix.

7.6g: Output Effect on the Brain

The next step of the TNE was aimed at further clarifying her signs and symptoms from a neuroscience perspective, specifically in regards to the various output systems such as endocrine, immune, motor and more. The patient was presented with the metaphorical example of a lion entering the room and the subsequent immediate responses. For this patient, discussion was specifically targeted towards the endocrine system and catecholamines because the therapist believed these were a big part of her memory changes, fatigue, mood swings and general fatigue. The picture was progressed with an arrow showing stress chemicals as a response to the threat (Figure 7.11). In this scenario, the arrow was extended to a cloud poised over the patient to depict how the altered cortisol, over time, would impact the patient and, more specifically, the brain. The altered cortisol was linked to mood swings, depression and problems with focus and concentration. This bigger, wider model of pain, showing a significant system involved in protecting was seen as a means to help the patient develop a greater understanding of her pain, but also pull her further away from a single faulty tissue model of pain, such as the bulging discs in her back she had been so focused on.

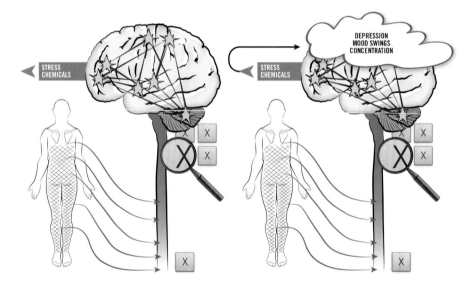

Figure 7.11: The drawing to explain output mechanism effects on the brain in response to continued pain.

7.6h: Output Related to Tissue Effects

The next step of the TNE was to complete the circle. An additional arrow was added to the "stress chemicals," tying it back to the original areas in which the patient experienced pain (Figure 7.12). The goal was to show her that the stress chemicals also had an effect on the tissues in the areas in which she experienced her pain and left the tissues sore, tired, sensitive, fatigued and deconditioned. In her case, leading up to explaining the treatment options, a big emphasis was placed on the need to improve blood and oxygen to these areas because they were sore and sensitive.

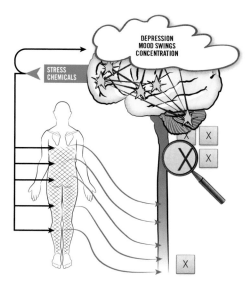

Figure 7.12: The drawing to explain output related tissue effects of persistent pain.

The final part of the TNE was aimed at returning to the question in section 7.5.3 regarding how we calm the nervous system down. Per chapters 3 through 6, the patient was instructed on how education (knowledge), aerobic exercise and medication are the mainstay in calming the nervous system and would form the mainstay of the therapy plan. The patient was asked, as an example, to think how she would react to a lion cub entering the room, followed by a discussion of how a decreased threat produces less of a widespread protective response. She was told this was the essence of the TNE program.

In the published case study, we provided a detailed description of the TNE, which is reprinted here as a means of showing the therapist the language and goals used in TNE in "real-life" clinical practice (Louw, Puentedura et al., 2012).

THE PERIPHERAL NERVOUS SYSTEM

- Your nervous system is a continuous system. This explains how low back pain can spread and become leg, upper back and neck pain over time.

- The nervous system is an alarm system – designed to warn you of danger, for example, a sprained ankle or thumbtack. Warning you about danger is normal and a part of survival.

- Nerves have electrical current inside them and "buzz" all the time. This is normal. (Drawing of electrical activity in a nerve)

- When nerves become excited they have more activity (electricity).

- There is a threshold – when the electricity reaches this, your nerves "fire" and send a message, probably a danger message.

- With persistent pain and issues such as failed treatment, different (or no) explanations of your pain, fear, stress, job and family issues, the nerves "wake up" and "buzz" at a higher level – closer to the threshold of firing. Now, just a little stress, fear, movement or thought can raise the activity to the level needed to make your nerves "fire."

- Although unpleasant, this "waking up" is a normal part of the nervous system's alarm function.

- Inside nerves there are sensors. These sensors are there to tell you about your environment. Unfortunately, we now know that when pain persists and your nerves become "sensitive," they can become sensitive to odd things like temperature, stress, anxiety, movement or pressure to name a few. This is normal. As you will see later, we can calm nerves down so they don't become so sensitive.

Take home message (for the patient)

- Let's summarize: In your case, you developed back pain and, based on many issues (pain, treatment, explanations, job and family), the nerves in your back have become very sensitive, but because your nervous system is one large, attached system that connects your low back to your hip, legs, neck and shoulders, the "system" wakes up. The good news is that we can explain this, and the more you understand about this, the more your nerves will calm down.

Practical (for the therapist)

- Show the patient a picture of a body nervous system.

- Draw a graph with nerve activity, time and action potential.

- Palpate the ulnar nerve at the cubital tunnel and tibial nerve at the posterior tarsal tunnel. Increased sensitivity to palpation should be tied back to the discussion of nerve sensitization.

THE CENTRAL NERVOUS SYSTEM AND NEUROMATRIX

- With the sensitized (and easily firing) nerves in your body, the central nervous system and your brain cannot help but get interested (excited). Again – this is normal.

- To understand pain you need to understand the brain.

- There are no pain areas in the brain.

- When you experience pain, pain uses multiple areas in the brain.

- These areas start communicating with each other.

- You develop a 'pain map.' When all of these areas "fire" and you 'run the map,' you experience pain.

- Over years of having pain, these maps become more entrenched and, therefore, difficult to get rid of.

- The good news is these maps can be changed. The more you understand about your pain and the less fear you have, the more these maps lose their power. Where a map would get ignited and result in pain, a map can actually be engaged and NOT have you experience pain – since the meaning of the experience is different. You understand it more.

- Let's apply this to your back. Let's examine you before and after this educational session:

- **Before education**—Pain is a response to a threat. During your evaluation you were asked to bend over. You bent down a little and said "it hurts." Because you are afraid of bending over, the nerves in your back fire a lot quicker. Remember – they are more sensitive than normal. These danger messages are sent straight to the brain and the brain processes the danger messages. You run your pain map and, because forward bending is a threat (of giving out, hurting, the unknown, etc.), your brain's summary of the threat is pain. Needless to say – you stop and say "it hurts." This is normal.

- **Understanding pain better**—You now realize that the danger messages you got during the forward bending are not a signal of tissue injury or damage. Your back may be sore, sensitive or even deconditioned, but not broken. Tissues heal. Now we ask you to bend forward – you get danger messages. The danger messages run up to the brain and it runs the map, but you are not threatened by this. You now understand that hurt does not equal harm. The map still runs. The map still gives you a sum result, but it may not be pain or if it is, the pain is better understood and, thus, less threatening. You can therefore go ahead and bend further.

Take home message (for the patient)
- Pain is a response by the brain based on the perceived threat. Your pain is real. The pain you experience, though, may not be a true reflection of your tissues.

- Your whole brain is involved in processing the pain.

Practical (for the therapist)
- Show the patient a functional MRI (fMRI) scan. A good example is the fMRI case study by Moseley, which shows both a pre-neuroscience fMRI (lit up/lots of activity) and then post-neuroscience fMRI showing the brain "calmed down."

OUTPUT SYSTEMS

- With all this "input" there has to be consequences. The brain will call upon systems to defend you – again quite normal.

- The lion metaphor – if a lion jumps into this room right now, what would you do? You will call upon systems to defend you, such as your heart (beating faster), breathing (faster and shallower), muscles (use big muscles to run/hit), shift blood (to areas you need and away from other areas you don't need right now, for example, muscles dealing with posture and stability), immune system (you can worry about the scratchy throat tomorrow, when the lion is gone), systems healing tissues (do that tomorrow), sleep (not while there's a lion in the room), language and more.

- These systems are very well designed to work for short times while there's a threat, and once the threat (the lion) goes away, everything returns back to normal.

- Here's the big issue: with persistent pain, issues at home, no/little explanation of your pain, failed treatment, stress, etc., you basically have a huge lion in your life – day in and day out.

- These systems have been turned on for years. So what happens? Muscles dealing with posture get sore, tired, fatigued and sensitive. Your breathing is shallow, allowing for less blood and oxygen, again making tissues sore, tired and sensitive. You're in a constant stress mode. You have problems with sleep, are getting aches/flu easier and so forth.

- Stress chemicals – for your body to protect you, it uses stress chemicals. Two main stress chemicals are adrenaline and cortisol. They shunt blood, get you breathing faster, increase vigilance and more. The problem is that over time they cause your tissues to become sore, sensitive and fatigued. Prolonged high levels of these have also been linked to issues such as memory changes, mood swings, appetite changes, weight gain, sleep disturbances and depression

Take home message (for the patient)

- These systems are there to protect you. It is normal. However, these systems need to be restored to normal resting levels.

- Why are they active? Threat. Every time you experience pain and do not understand it (which we already discussed), your systems will activate. Can you now see why understanding your pain better can help? Basically, the large lion (big threat) becomes a small lion cub, which is less threatening; therefore, you need not call on these systems to protect you as much.

Practical (for the therapist)

- Have ready a single piece of paper with a lion picture in the center. Present it to the patient and ask what they would do if a lion came into the room. Write down all the systems you identify in this patient as having been activated to protect her.

- Tie it back to the introduction: with tissues now more sore, fatigued and sensitive, the nerves will become even more sensitive, thus a vicious cycle develops

TREATMENT OPTIONS

- Hopefully, by now, you have a better (different) understanding of why you still hurt. But how do we treat it?

- **Education**–The studies show that the more you understand about your pain, the better you will do. Hopefully, with the discussion we've had thus far, you will realize why this will help. Understanding causes your nerves to "buzz down." Calming them down.

- **Aerobic exercise**–Aerobic exercise helps pump blood and oxygen through your body. This will allow your fatigued tissues to become less fatigued. Also, studies have shown that exercise also calm nerves down, which is a big focus of our treatment. Aerobic exercise also helps with depression, mood, sleep, memory and appetite. Aerobic exercise "burns" the stress chemicals out of your system. Imagine running a marathon – in the first few miles, adrenaline is flowing and you probably think you could "win it all." As the race progresses, adrenaline levels decrease and you know the rest.

- **Medication**–This is the realm of your physician, but realize medications are also used in calming nerves down – such as anti-seizure medication and anti-depressants.

Take home message (for the patient)

- There are many ways we can make your tissues healthier, better conditioned and less sensitive. Since they're not injured, they don't need to be "fixed."

- What if you experience pain during exercise/therapy? By now you should realize that the pain you feel is not necessarily a true reflection of your tissues' health. As you participate in therapy (hands-on and various forms of exercise), you will most likely experience pain. Your tissues have become so sensitive over the years, it will take a while to calm them down. They are basically "telling you" what the exercise is doing. As you stretch or work on some tissue, the nerves are still so sensitive that they will keep sending danger messages, but hopefully by now you understand this and the brain will produce chemicals to dampen those danger messages down. The good news is that you can (and will), over time, increase activity and function as the pain steadily decreases.

Practical (for the therapist)

- It is imperative that the patient develops a greater understanding and appreciation of how therapy may benefit him/her.

- There is no magic exercise or technique; rather, by understanding better how pain works and how therapy can help, the pain process can be reversed and the patient will increase his/her function.

Subsequent therapy visits (for the therapist)

In the first session, the patient underwent a subjective examination, objective examination and an introductory neuroscience educational session.

In the therapy sessions to follow, the therapist should do the following:

- Use any available time (during exercise, manual therapy, etc.) to reinforce the neuroscience message.

- Have the patient explain back to you their understanding of the sections above.

- Focus on cardiovascular exercise.

- Develop a home exercise program.

- Work on setting goals for their job, ADL's, exercise, recreation and social interaction.

- Set goals for therapy – especially prognosis.

7.7: Subsequent Therapy

The initial session (examination and TNE) was subsequently followed by a series of seven physical therapy visits, which included additional TNE and other treatment strategies that have been reported to improve outcomes in patients with chronic pain, such as aquatic therapy (Assis, Silva et al., 2006), cardiovascular exercise (Gowans, deHueck et al., 2001; Sim and Adams, 2002; Goldenberg, Burckhardt et al., 2004; Bonifazi, Suman et al., 2006; Busch, Barber et al., 2007; Rooks, Gautam et al., 2007; Brosseau, Wells et al., 2008; Carville, Arendt-Nielsen et al., 2008), and strengthening (Valkeinen, Hakkinen et al., 2005; Brosseau, Wells et al., 2008).

The therapeutic activities are listed below:

DESCRIPTION OF SUBSEQUENT THERAPY SESSIONS (2 TIMES PER WEEK, 4 WEEKS)

Subsequent therapy visits (for the therapist)

In the first session, the patient underwent a subjective examination, objective examination and an introductory neuroscience educational session (described above).

In the therapy sessions that followed, the therapy sessions consisted of the following:

- **Continued neuroscience education**—Before starting the exercise sessions, the patient received five minutes of formal education, which was used to answer questions, address goals and concerns, or to ask the patient to explain her understanding of certain aspects of her pain, e.g., nerve sensitivity. The neuroscience education was also reinforced during exercises, manual therapy, and/or modalities.

- **Cardiovascular exercise**—The patient started with treadmill walking and later progressed to the elliptical trainer. For both treadmill and elliptical, the speed was steadily increased to help increase heart rate.

- **Neural mobilization exercises**—Since the neuroscience education discussed issues related to the nervous system, a series of neural mobilization exercises were used for the upper extremities, lower extremities and trunk, e.g., slump sliders.

- **Basic trunk mobility exercises and stretches**—The patient performed exercises like single-knee to chest, trunk rotations, prayer stretch and piriformis stretch.

- **Strengthening exercises**—The exercises focused on higher repetitions using lighter weight (dumbbells, Theraband™), timed repetitions (clocks) and, over time, increasing the time of the sessions (endurance).

- **Aquatic therapy**—The patient also attended a 30-minute aquatic therapy session in which she performed exercises focusing on trunk mobility, "unloading," and strengthening.

- **A modality**—The final part usually consisted of a modality (usually heat) for 10 minutes, in which time the patient was asked to focus on relaxation, breathing, and reflection on her treatment plan and goals. This was also used as a time for the therapist to provide a summary of goals, progress, and plans associated with the next therapy session and home exercise program.

- **A home exercise program (HEP)**—The HEP was a continuation of the therapy session with focus on the exercises performed in the therapy sessions (neural glides, trunk exercises, light weights, and walking program).

After the initial TNE educational session, the following seven sessions comprised a CBT graded exercise/exposure approach. The patient completed a total of eight sessions of physical therapy over the course of four weeks. The dosage and frequency was chosen based on a previous study utilizing TNE (Moseley, 2002), as well as clinical experience. During the four weeks of physical therapy, the patient was advised to continue with the use of her medication as prescribed by her physician. Any questions regarding her taking, not taking or changing medication was deferred to her physician. The patient was asked to inform her therapist of any changes (increase or decrease) in the use of medication.

Although previous studies utilizing TNE included manual therapy, it was decided not to include manual therapy as a primary treatment approach in this case, based on several factors. First, with a primary clinical presentation of central sensitivity, it was decided that a manual therapy approach focusing on passive joint movements would not be effective in helping this patient with widespread pain. Second, a biomechanical approach contradicts the neuroscience model, which de-emphasizes a specific tissue or joint and focuses on the central sensitization. Third, the patient had seen several other manual therapy providers, including chiropractors, and improvements were transient and may have actually contributed to the fear avoidance beliefs by focusing the patient on joint and tissue "faults." Finally, the therapist's goal was to help the patient become less dependent on healthcare professionals and focus more on independent management and active approaches, such as exercise.

Upon completion of the initial TNE session (75 minutes, which included the examination), the patient related that she felt she had a much better understanding of her current condition. At this time, she was asked to complete the same questionnaires and once again perform active forward flexion. The patient was discharged from PT after eight sessions with a complete home exercise program (HEP). The HEP consisted of basic stretches, neural tissue mobilization and a walking program. The primary therapist kept in contact with the patient by monthly phone calls to monitor progress and answer questions. After seven months, the patient returned to PT for a follow-up assessment.

7.8: Outcomes

7.8a: Immediate Effects

Active forward flexion (with the same verbal instructions given as before) improved dramatically from 10 degrees to 72 degrees immediately following TNE (Figure 7.13). The patient was not asked to rate her pain during the active forward flexion, as the TNE session was designed to "de-focus" pain, i.e., knowing there would be pain, but the meaning of the pain (not signaling damage) had been changed (Moseley, 2003; Moseley, 2007).

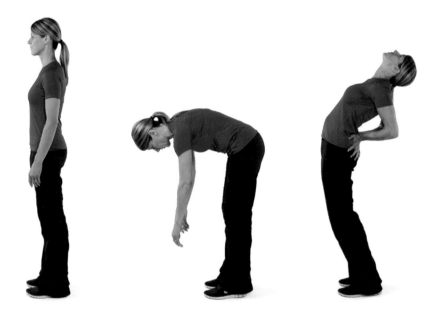

Figure 7.13: Active forward flexion and extension immediately after the initial TNE session (75 minutes, which included the examination) (clinical images recreated).

Two of the outcome measures did not show any apparent change. These were the NPRS and the ODI. The FABQ, however, dropped substantially. The FABQ-PA dropped from a 20/24 to 1/24, and the FABQ-W score dropped from 25/42 to 2/42 after the TNE session. The standard errors of measurement (SEM) for the FABQ-PA and FABQ-W have been reported as 2.0 and 2.4, respectively (George, Valencia et al., 2010). Furthermore, the minimal detectable change (MDC) for the FABQ-PA and FABQ-W was reported as 5.4 and 6.8, respectively (George, Valencia et al., 2010). The Zung depression scale dropped from a score of 58 to 48 after the TNE.

7.8b: Long Term Effects

The initial plan was to have the patient complete the questionnaires after four weeks of physical therapy. Unfortunately, after four weeks, the patient called and cancelled her appointment due to a death in the family. At that stage, the patient reported that she felt that her HEP, progressive increase in function and increased "understanding" of her LBP was beneficial and she planned to continue with her home program. After three months, the therapist called the patient to assess her progress, at which time she continued to express satisfaction with her progress. At seven months post initial visit, the patient called, was still reporting progress, and was willing to return for a formal re-evaluation.

At the seven-month follow-up, the patient subjectively reported substantial progress in regards to her ability to perform house work (now able to vacuum two rooms comfortably without a "flare" and able to stand 60 minutes to cook a meal), exercise (walking 4-5 times a week for 30 minutes at a time and returned to a step-aerobics class), office work (able to return to three half-days as a receptionist and sit at a desk 30 minutes at a time without having a "flare") and general feeling of well-being. Her general sense of well-being seemed to correlate well with her outcomes measures: her FABQ-PA was 6/24 (initial 20/24; immediate post-treatment 1/24), and her FABQ-W had risen to 12/42 (initial 25/42; immediate post-treatment 2/42), both of which were still reduced compared to her initial scores during the initial session seven months before. Her ODI improved from an initial score of 54% to 40%, while her Zung depression scale had decreased from a 58 at the initial examination to a 38 at the seven-month follow-up. Her NPRS was still a 7/10, but was reduced from a 9/10 at the initial examination. The patient's forward flexion was still markedly improved from the initial measurement (10 degrees) to 70 degrees, which was only slightly less than her measurement following the pain science education. The results of her questionnaires and active forward flexion are illustrated in Figure 7.14. Her new body chart image revealed a "fist sized" area of "discomfort" over the L4/5 spinal region only.

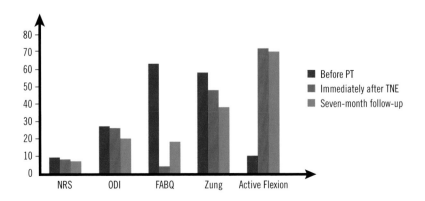

Figure 7.14: Results of the questionnaires over time.

7.9: Discussion

The TNE session resulted in an immediate change in the patient's scores and self-report questionnaires, most noticeably the FABQ. Her active forward flexion also showed notable improvement. The physical therapy program combining the TNE session with various forms of exercise and therapeutic activities resulted in clinically meaningful changes in pain, function, depression and active movement.

While one cannot presume cause and effect from a single case report, the findings of this case report suggest that TNE may have contributed to an immediate and long term reduction in disability, fear avoidance beliefs and depressive feelings as well as an increase in function and physical movement in a patient with CLBP. Although care should be taken when interpreting data from a single case report, the results from this clinical episode suggest that the current findings are important. Our goals for this case report were to present TNE in a more clinically manageable timeframe (45-minute session versus three hours), demonstrate a clinical reasoning process in which the clinician can make an informed decision for when to apply TNE in patient management, and describe in detail the exact content of an abbreviated TNE session aimed at explaining the chronic pain state in a non-threatening way to a patient with central sensitivity. This case report may provide clinicians with insights into the clinical application of the latest neuroscience research, and our findings suggest that altering a patient's thoughts and beliefs regarding CLBP may lead to immediate improvements in function and mobility.

The findings of this case report are consistent with previous research, which has demonstrated that TNE results in altered pain cognitions along with an increased ability to perform physical tasks (Moseley, Nicholas et al., 2004; Moseley, 2005). In contrast to our patient's outcomes, subjects in the Moseley et al., study did not report improvements in perceived disability, while our patient reported improvements in her ODI at seven months (Moseley, Hodges et al., 2004). It should be noted that although the patient's ODI decreased from 54% to 40% and the NRS decreased from 9/10 to 7/10 at the seven-month follow-up, these scores still indicate moderate levels of pain and disability. This may be due to the fact that other interventions were used and may suggest that a multimodal approach involving pain science education and formal physical therapy may maximize outcomes. Although it is not clear why NE may lead to the changes described above, it is hypothesized that this form of education "de-threatens" the situation for the patient (Moseley, 2005). TNE should be seen as a form of CBT, as it addresses issues related to the nervous system and "how pain works." It may be that when a patient has a more realistic understanding of his/her pain, he/she becomes less "afraid' of their pain, which leads to a more normalized perception of pain and improved physical performance.

Several functional MRI (fMRI) studies have shown that areas such as the motor and premotor areas are involved in processing pain (Flor, 2000; Moseley, 2005; Tsao and Hodges, 2007). It could be argued that the "de-threatening" of pain may lead the motor area (and other areas) to become less involved in processing pain, and once freed from contributing to a chronic pain response, may be able to once again focus on their primary functions. In the present case, the most pronounced immediate change occurred with the FABQ. The patient's initial FABQ-PA and FABQ-W were very high, and these scores dropped sharply following her NE session. It is hypothesized that the educational session may have reduced her fear associated with movement, which allowed her to function at a higher level. This finding is consistent with previous research (Moseley and Hodges, 2002; Moseley, 2002; George, Fritz et al., 2003; Hodges and Moseley, 2003; Moseley, Hodges et al., 2004; Moseley, 2005).

Although the focus of this case was to report on the immediate and long-term outcomes for a patient with CLBP following TNE, it is important to acknowledge that this patient also received aquatic therapy (Assis, Silva et al., 2006), cardiovascular exercise (Gowans, deHueck et al., 2001; Sim and Adams, 2002; Goldenberg, Burckhardt et al., 2004; Bonifazi, Suman et al., 2006; Busch, Barber et al., 2007; Rooks, Gautam et al., 2007; Brosseau, Wells et al., 2008; Carville, Arendt-Nielsen et al., 2008) and strengthening exercises (Valkeinen, Hakkinen et al., 2005; Brosseau, Wells et al., 2008), which have been shown to be effective interventions for patients with centralized pain states. We contend that the interaction of exercise and TNE is very important. The educational sessions aimed at reinforcing the idea that her tissues healed, but had become "sensitive" and "deconditioned" secondary to the central sensitization. Exercises were described and prescribed using the same TNE wording. For example, as she performed exercises she was constantly reminded that any pain and/ or discomfort were more associated with the fact that her nerves had become "sensitive." Aerobic exercise education was focused on teaching her that aerobic exercises increase blood flow and oxygen to tissues, thus making them healthier. Additionally, aerobic exercises would "flush out" chemicals such as adrenaline and cortisol, which are thought to make nerves more sensitive (Geiss, Rohleder et al., 2005). The patient was also educated on how gradual exposure to discomfort would allow her to not only increase her activities, but improve her "pain tolerance" level (graded exposure). During all of the exercises, the patient was presented with a central and recurring theme: the pain she was experiencing was not indication of tissue injury, but rather sensitivity.

Chronic pain rates are increasing, with data now showing that almost one in every four Americans are experiencing a chronic pain state (Magni, Marchetti et al., 1993; Butler and Moseley, 2003; Wall and Melzack, 2005) and physical therapists, with their extensive knowledge of anatomy, physiology, neuroscience, and exercise, are ideally equipped to manage patients in chronic pain. This case report adds to the current literature suggesting that TNE should be considered in the treatment of patients with CLBP (Moseley, 2002; Moseley, 2003; Moseley, 2003; Moseley, 2004; Moseley, Nicholas et al., 2004; Moseley, 2005). Finally, this case report illustrates that an abbreviated session of TNE can be an effective adjunct to more traditional treatments, as the 2-3 hour sessions utilized in research studies (Moseley, 2005) are not "practical" in clinical practice.

7.10: Conclusion

This case report describes the immediate and long-term results of TNE on a patient with a three-year history of CLBP. The results suggest that TNE may help to reduce disability, fear of movement, and depression while increasing active spinal ROM. These outcomes were evident immediately after the first session and were maintained at a seven-month follow-up. The immediate and long-term changes concur with similar studies using TNE for patients with CLBP.

Chapter 7 References

Assis, M. R., L. E. Silva, et al. (2006). A randomized controlled trial of deep water running: clinical effectiveness of aquatic exercise to treat fibromyalgia. *Arthritis Rheum, 55*(1): 57-65.

Bonifazi, M., A. L. Suman, et al. (2006). Changes in salivary cortisol and corticosteroid receptor-alpha mRNA expression following a 3-week multidisciplinary treatment program in patients with fibromyalgia. *Psychoneuroendocrinology, 31*(9): 1076-1086.

Brosseau, L., G. A. Wells, et al. (2008). Ottawa Panel evidence-based clinical practice guidelines for aerobic fitness exercises in the management of fibromyalgia: part 1. *Phys Ther, 88*(7): 857-871.

Brosseau, L., G. A. Wells, et al. (2008). Ottawa Panel evidence-based clinical practice guidelines for strengthening exercises in the management of fibromyalgia: part 2. *Phys Ther, 88*(7): 873-886.

Busch, A. J., K. A. Barber, et al. (2007). Exercise for treating fibromyalgia syndrome. *Cochrane Database Syst Rev*(4): CD003786.

Butler, D. and L. Moseley (2003). *Explain Pain*. Adelaide, Noigroup Publications.

Butler, D. S. (1991). *Mobilisation of the Nervous System*. Melbourne, Churchill Livingstone.

Butler, D. S. (2000). *The Sensitive Nervous System*. Adelaide, Noigroup.

Carville, S. F., S. Arendt-Nielsen, et al. (2008). EULAR evidence-based recommendations for the management of fibromyalgia syndrome. *Ann Rheum Dis, 67*(4): 536-541.

Cleland, J. A., J. D. Childs, et al. (2008). Psychometric properties of the Neck Disability Index and Numeric Pain Rating Scale in patients with mechanical neck pain. *Arch Phys Med Rehabil, 89*(1): 69-74.

Cleland, J. A., J. M. Fritz, et al. (2008). Psychometric properties of the Fear-Avoidance Beliefs Questionnaire and Tampa Scale of Kinesiophobia in patients with neck pain. *Am J Phys Med Rehabil, 87*(2): 109-117.

Cleland, J. A., J. M. Whitman, et al. (2005). Manual physical therapy, cervical traction, and strengthening exercises in patients with cervical radiculopathy: a case series. *J Orthop Sports Phys Ther, 35*(12): 802-811.

Deyo, R. A., M. Battie, et al. (1998). Outcome measures for low back pain research. A proposal for standardized use. *Spine (Phila Pa 1976), 23*(18): 2003-2013.

Fernandez-de-las-Penas, C., A. I. de la Llave-Rincon, et al. (2009). Bilateral widespread mechanical pain sensitivity in carpal tunnel syndrome: evidence of central processing in unilateral neuropathy. *Brain, 132(Pt 6)*: 1472-1479.

Flor, H. (2000). The functional organization of the brain in chronic pain. *Prog Brain Res, 129*: 313-322.

Fritz, J. M. and J. J. Irrgang (2001). A comparison of a modified Oswestry Low Back Pain Disability Questionnaire and the Quebec Back Pain Disability Scale. *Phys Ther, 81*(2): 776-788.

Geiss, A., N. Rohleder, et al. (2005). Predicting the failure of disc surgery by a hypofunctional HPA axis: evidence from a prospective study on patients undergoing disc surgery. *Pain, 114*(1-2): 104-117.

George, S. Z., J. M. Fritz, et al. (2003). The effect of a fear-avoidance-based physical therapy intervention for patients with acute low back pain: results of a randomized clinical trial. *Spine (Phila Pa 1976), 28*(23): 2551-2560.

George, S. Z., C. Valencia, et al. (2010). A psychometric investigation of fear-avoidance model measures in patients with chronic low back pain. *J Orthop Sports Phys Ther, 40*(4): 197-205.

George, S. Z. and G. Zeppieri (2009). Physical therapy utilization of graded exposure for patients with low back pain. *J Orthop Sports Phys Ther, 39*(7): 496-505.

Goldenberg, D. L., C. Burckhardt, et al. (2004). Management of fibromyalgia syndrome. *JAMA: The Journal of the American Medical Association, 292*(19): 2388-2395.

Gowans, S. E., A. deHueck, et al. (2001). Effect of a randomized, controlled trial of exercise on mood and physical function in individuals with fibromyalgia. *Arthritis Rheum, 45*(6): 519-529.

Grotle, M., N. K. Vollestad, et al. (2006). Clinical course and impact of fear-avoidance beliefs in low back pain: prospective cohort study of acute and chronic low back pain: II. *Spine, 31*(9): 1038-1046.

Hakkinen, A., H. Kautiainen, et al. (2007). Changes in the total Oswestry Index and its ten items in females and males pre- and post-surgery for lumbar disc herniation: a 1-year follow-up. *Eur Spine J, 16*(3): 347-352.

Hicks, G. E., J. M. Fritz, et al. (2005). Preliminary development of a clinical prediction rule for determining which patients with low back pain will respond to a stabilization exercise program. *Arch Phys Med Rehabil, 86*(9): 1753-1762.

Hodges, P. W. and G. L. Moseley (2003). Pain and motor control of the lumbopelvic region: effect and possible mechanisms. *J Electromyogr Kinesiol, 13*(4): 361-370.

Lidbeck, J. (2002). Central hyperexcitability in chronic musculoskeletal pain: a conceptual breakthrough with multiple clinical implications. *Pain Res Manag, 7*(2): 81-92.

Louw, A., E. L. Puentedura, et al. (2012). Use of an abbreviated neuroscience education approach in the treatment of chronic low back pain: a case report. *Physiotherapy Theory and Practice, 28*(1): 50-62.

Magni, G., M. Marchetti, et al. (1993). Chronic musculoskeletal pain and depressive symptoms in the National Health and Nutrition Examination. I. Epidemiologic follow-up study. *Pain, 53*(2): 163-168.

McMahon, S. B. and M. Koltzenburg, Eds. (2006). *Wall and Melzack's Textbook of Pain*. Philadelphia, PA, Elsevier Churchill Livingstone.

Meeus, M. and J. Nijs (2007). Central sensitization: a biopsychosocial explanation for chronic widespread pain in patients with fibromyalgia and chronic fatigue syndrome. *Clinical rheumatology, 26*(4): 465-473.

Merskey, H. and N. Bogduk (1994). *Classification of Chronic Pain*. Seattle, IASP Press.

Moseley, G. L. (2002). Combined physiotherapy and education is efficacious for chronic low back pain. *Aus J Physioth, 48*(4): 297-302.

Moseley, G. L. (2003). Joining forces - combining cognition-targeted motor control training with group or individual pain physiology education: a successful treatment for chronic low back pain. *J Man Manip Therap, 11*(2): 88-94.

Moseley, G. L. (2003). A pain neuromatrix approach to patients with chronic pain. *Man Ther, 8*(3): 130-140.

Moseley, G. L. (2004). Evidence for a direct relationship between cognitive and physical change during an education intervention in people with chronic low back pain. *Eur J Pain, 8*(1): 39-45.

Moseley, G. L. (2005). Widespread brain activity during an abdominal task markedly reduced after pain physiology education: fMRI evaluation of a single patient with chronic low back pain. *Aust J Physiother, 51*(1): 49-52.

Moseley, G. L. (2007). Reconceptualising pain according to modern pain science. *Physical Therapy Reviews, 12*(3): 169-178.

Moseley, G. L. and P. W. Hodges (2002). Chronic pain and motor control. *Grieves Modern Manual Therapy of the Vertebral column*. G. Jull and J. Boyling. Edinburgh, Churchill-Livingstone.

Moseley, G. L., P. W. Hodges, et al. (2004). A randomized controlled trial of intensive neurophysiology education in chronic low back pain. *Clinical Journal of Pain, 20*: 324-330.

Moseley, G. L., M. K. Nicholas, et al. (2004). A randomized controlled trial of intensive neurophysiology education in chronic low back pain. *Clin J Pain, 20*(5): 324-330.

Moseley, L. (2002). Combined physiotherapy and education is efficacious for chronic low back pain. *Aust J Physiother, 48*(4): 297-302.

Moseley, L. (2003). Unraveling the barriers to reconceptualization of the problem in chronic pain: the actual and perceived ability of patients and health professionals to understand the neurophysiology. *The Journal of Pain: Official Journal of the American Pain Society, 4*(4): 184-189.

Moseley, L. (2007). *Painful Yarns*. Minneapolis, OPTP.

Nattrass, C. L., J. E. Nitschke, et al. (1999). Lumbar spine range of motion as a measure of physical and functional impairment: an investigation of validity. *Clin Rehabil, 13*(3): 211-218.

Nijs, J., B. Van Houdenhove, et al. (2010). Recognition of central sensitization in patients with musculoskeletal pain: Application of pain neurophysiology in manual therapy practice. *Man Ther, 15*(2): 135-141.

Poiraudeau, S., F. Rannou, et al. (2006). Fear-avoidance beliefs about back pain in patients with subacute low back pain. *Pain, 124*(3): 305-311.

Romera, I., H. Delgado-Cohen, et al. (2008). Factor analysis of the Zung self-rating depression scale in a large sample of patients with major depressive disorder in primary care. *BMC Psychiatry, 8*: 4.

Ronnberg, K., B. Lind, et al. (2007). Patients' satisfaction with provided care/information and expectations on clinical outcome after lumbar disc herniation surgery. *Spine, 32*(2): 256-261.

Rooks, D. S., S. Gautam, et al. (2007). Group exercise, education, and combination self-management in women with fibromyalgia: a randomized trial. *Arch Intern Med 167*(20): 2192-2200.

Sim, J. and N. Adams (2002). Systematic review of randomized controlled trials of nonpharmacological interventions for fibromyalgia. *Clin J Pain, 18*(5): 324-336.

Smart, K. M., C. Blake, et al. Clinical indicators of 'nociceptive', 'peripheral neuropathic' and 'central' mechanisms of musculoskeletal pain. A Delphi survey of expert clinicians. *Man Ther, 15*(1): 80-87.

Tsao, H. and P. W. Hodges (2007). Immediate changes in feedforward postural adjustments following voluntary motor training. *Exp Brain Res, 181*(4): 537-546.

Valkeinen, H., K. Hakkinen, et al. (2005). Muscle hypertrophy, strength development, and serum hormones during strength training in elderly women with fibromyalgia. *Scand J Rheumatol, 34*(4): 309-314.

Waddell, G., M. Newton, et al. (1993). A Fear-Avoidance Beliefs Questionnaire (FABQ) and the role of fear-avoidance beliefs in chronic low back pain and disability. *Pain, 52*(2): 157-168.

Wall, P. D. and R. Melzack (2005). *Textbook of Pain*. London, Elsevier.

Woolf, C. J. (2007). Central sensitization: uncovering the relation between pain and plasticity. *Anesthesiology, 106*(4): 864-867.

Zung, W. W. (1965). A Self-Rating Depression Scale. *Arch Gen Psychiatry, 12*: 63-70.

Notes

Chapter 8

Conclusion, Summary and The Future of Therapeutic Neuroscience Education

8.1: Conclusions

We may have written this book for therapists but, ultimately, we believe it is also very much for, and about, the patient. The patient comes first. We truly believe that a patient-centered approach is what therapeutic neuroscience education (TNE) is all about (Maitland, 1986). Pain is personal, and a personalized biological explanation of the pain experience, applied to the individual situations and needs, is vital. The evidence for TNE is compelling and should provide hope for even the most impacted patients, those patients with chronic pain. TNE helps patients reconceptualize their pain, take charge of their life and steadily progress back to reclaiming their lives. TNE is not merely about helping patients to 'manage' their pain. TNE is an effective 'treatment' for pain.

As we stated earlier, we wrote this book for therapists, especially the therapists we encounter week after week at seminars and conferences. Those therapists who say they are tired, frustrated and worn out. Chronic pain takes a toll on therapists and they continue to struggle with the treatment of patients with chronic pain conditions. Dr. Patrick Wall believed that physiotherapy/physical therapy was the ideal profession to treat pain. TNE is at the core of this belief and a consequence of Wall's belief in the profession. Therapists should be energized and see the numerous opportunities to help the patient with chronic pain, including changes in beliefs and cognitions, as well as a more movement-based approach that includes exercise, manual therapy and more. The reality is that therapy has much to offer the patient with chronic pain. Therapists should be energized and empowered by the neuroscience of pain, which in turn changes their beliefs and attitudes about chronic pain.

TNE comes with some challenges and opposition. Current orthopedic therapy is still deeply rooted in the biomedical approach, and we have a long way to go in embracing a true biopsychosocial model of pain. The majority of therapists are still stuck in the Cartesian model of pain, targeting 'pain fibers' and figuratively stopping at the C0-C1 joint because the territory above 'belongs to another profession.' Sure, there are some therapists out there who embrace the biopsychosocial model, but perhaps they do so only when everything else has failed. There is a mindset that the biopsychosocial model is only really needed for those truly chronic type patients. We believe this is a real tragedy because the neuroscience view of pain is powerful and liberating for therapists. Only through fear or stubbornly held beliefs do we hold ourselves back.

Consider the example of a therapist facing a patient with paraplegia who's complaining of severe leg pain. The patient sees themself as disabled and their legs as not being part of them. The therapist that still clings to the Cartesian model of pain might see this situation as a potentially long, drawn-out slog through therapy for months, even years, and 'hopefully the patient's pain can be managed.' Contrast this with a neuroscience view: a therapist ready to engage the brain, change how the brain "sees" the legs and change painful, unwanted and disabled legs into functional legs via mirror therapy. And what if that pain is abolished in only 15 days (Moseley, 2007)? We can cite many other amazing examples of the way TNE induces change for the better, including changing the size of a body part instantly changes pain (Moseley, Parsons et al., 2008), crossing hands impacts pain, temperature and swelling (Gallace, Torta et al., 2011), thoughts determine straight leg raise (Moseley, 2004; Louw, Puentedura et al., 2012), physical movements improving with education alone (Moseley, 2004; Louw, Puentedura et al., 2012), sham surgery in orthopedics producing similar outcomes as real orthopedic surgery in conditions such as compression fractures and more (Louw et al. – submitted for publication). It is amazing to watch how a therapist who embraces the neuroscience and biopsychosocial approach interacts with their patients. It's about time that all therapists became more enthusiastic about seeing these patients.

TNE is a relatively effective and low-tech, low-cost approach; this alone should capture the attention of therapists, patients, third-party payers and healthcare policy makers. Globally, healthcare costs are increasing and solutions that do not require elaborate and expensive testing and interventions will likely become increasingly appealing. TNE is significantly less expensive than drugs, injections or surgery and this aspect will need to be explored in future research. We are just completing a multi-center randomized controlled trial (Louw et al. – submitted for publication) and can report that patients who received a TNE approach prior to lumbar surgery for radiculopathy, had 38% less costs in the six-month postoperative period, in terms of further medical tests, doctors' visits and rehabilitation compared to a control group who did not receive the new designed preoperative TNE program (Louw, Butler et al., 2013). The fact that TNE may be a more cost-effective alternative to expensive drugs and surgery is likely to bring challenges. Surgeons, interventional pain physicians, drug companies and surgery companies are likely to scoff at the notion that such a "simple" cognitive therapeutic approach might significantly impact pain and disability.

The material covered in this book's chapters, as well as the aforementioned discussion of TNE, also provides direction for potential future paths for TNE. Three are featured here.

8.2: Group TNE

In chapter 5, we discussed the evidence suggesting one-on-one being superior in outcomes to group therapy, but group therapy sessions do result in a more cost-effective strategy (Moseley, 2003; Louw, Diener et al., 2011). The superiority of one-on-one sessions is easily understood, considering that pain is based on an individual's specific pain neuromatrix and each person's pain experience is individualized. A one-on-one TNE program would allow for individualizing that education.

It could also be argued that group sessions may have a limiting effect on patients' willingness to express very personal issues and, thus, limit a deep learning process. In contrast to this potential limitation of sharing personal information, it is important to realize that group sessions may indeed create an opportunity for sharing experiences that have shown benefit in spine surgery patients after lumbar fusion (Christensen, Laurberg et al., 2003). In the TNE study utilizing group therapy, groups of 7-10 patients were instructed using a single four-hour session (Moseley, 2003). It is highly recommended that clinicians and researchers explore other group designs to optimize outcomes and provide a cost effective approach. It is recommended that group sizes be limited to 4-10 patients.

An additional strategy to consider, in regards to cost-effectiveness, is homework. Provide written material and self-study to enhance the learning experience (Moseley, 2002; Louw, 2013). Future research should explore the optimal size of a group receiving TNE and even potential variables that may make a group more compatible, able and willing to share their experiences, and open up and gain access to a deeper learning process, which is essential in TNE.

8.3: TNE for the General Population

Current epidemiological data shows that at least 1 in 4 people experience persistent pain in their daily lives. In the US alone, this constitutes more than 75 million people. TNE, as an individualized approach, is likely to only have minimal impact on the sheer numbers of people with chronic persistent pain. The problem here is that for each patient with chronic pain who is successfully treated with TNE and reconceptualizes their pain, more than one extra patient with pain will be added.

In section 8.2, group sessions are discussed as a means to impact a greater number of patients and also provide a more cost-effective approach. The ultimate goal should be educating large numbers of patients and even the general population as a whole. Large scale educational programs have achieved some level of success with epidemics such as polio, AIDS and more recently, the West Nile virus. When a government or global organization such as the World Health Organization (WHO) mobilizes a large scale educational campaign, the effects are easily seen, for example, polio vaccines or using necessary precautions to prevent the spread of AIDS. Given the global epidemic of pain, it could be argued that regional, national and, ultimately, global educational campaigns should be considered.

A great example of such a campaign is the multimedia campaign that was launched during 1997 in Victoria, Australia, positively advising patients with LBP to stay active and exercise, not to rest for prolonged periods, and to remain at work (Buchbinder, Jolley et al., 2001; Buchbinder, Jolley et al., 2001). The campaign's impact on the population's beliefs about back pain and fear-avoidance beliefs was measured by telephone surveys. The effect of the campaign on the potential management of low back pain by general practitioners was assessed by eliciting their likely approach to two hypothetical scenarios in mailed surveys. Demographically identical population groups in Victoria and the control state, New South Wales, were surveyed at three times: before, during, and after the educational ad campaign in Victoria. There were large, statistically significant improvements in back pain beliefs over time in Victoria (mean scores on the Back Beliefs Questionnaire, 26.5, 28.4, and 29.7), but not in New South Wales (26.3, 26.2, and 26.3, respectively). Among those who reported back pain during the previous year, fear-avoidance beliefs about physical activity improved significantly in Victoria (mean scores on the Fear-Avoidance Beliefs Questionnaire for physical activity, 14, 12.5, and 11.6), but not in New South Wales (13.3, 13.6, and 12.7, respectively). General practitioners in Victoria reported significant improvements over time in beliefs about back pain management, as compared with their interstate colleagues. There were statistically significant interactions between state and time for 7 of 10 responses on management of acute low back pain and for 6 of 10 responses on management of sub-acute low back pain.

Another consideration in educating the general population about TNE is the importance of making it readily available to all people, including those in more remote regions. An easy starting point for patients and therapists could be a recent randomized controlled trial, based on TNE, that utilized a patient book on metaphors for pain (Gallagher, McAuley et al., 2013). In this randomized, single-blind, partial cross-over controlled trial, 79 people with chronic pain received either a booklet of metaphors and stories conveying key pain biology concepts or a booklet containing advice on how to manage chronic pain according to established cognitive-behavioral principles. The primary outcome variables, pain biology knowledge (NPQ) and catastrophizing, were measured before randomization, at three weeks and at three months, at which time the control group was crossed over to receive the metaphors and stories booklet. Pain and disability were secondary outcome variables. The Metaphors group showed larger changes in both catastrophizing and pain biology knowledge. Gains were maintained for at least three months. Changes were replicated in the Advice group when they crossed over. There was, however, no change in pain or self-reported disability in either group. The research group concluded that providing educational material through metaphors and stories in a book can assist patients to reconceptualize pain and reduce catastrophizing.

Additionally, there is an increase in patients accessing the Internet for healthcare information, including information about pain (Hering, Harvan et al., 2005; Garcia, Messerschmitt et al., 2009; Morr, Shanti et al., 2010). With the increased utilization of electronic media, clinicians and researchers should examine potential avenues to educate patients via distance (Hurling, Catt et al., 2007). In a recent case study (Louw et al., 2013 – submitted for publication), a patient with chronic pain due to thoracic outlet surgery received a single one-on-one clinic session with a therapist who examined the patient and delivered a TNE session. After the initial and only 'in-person' consultation, the patient was monitored, educated, advised and progressed in regards to exercise, movement and goals via email (Figure 8.1).

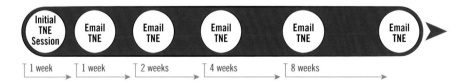

Figure 8.1: Timeline for a patient who received a single 'in-person' TNE consultation and was then followed and progressed in treatment via email communication.

In this case, the patient not only had a significant recovery, but also had the financial benefit of limiting the expenses involved with travel and time (Figure 8.2).

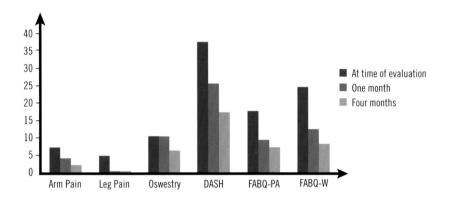

Figure 8.2: Outcome measures for the patient treated with a single 'in person' TNE consultation and then followed remotely via email communication.

It is proposed that approaches such as this may be of significant benefit for patients in remote areas, and future research should aim to investigate such avenues. With the rapid growth of technology, tele-health and the provision of remotely monitored health care services should be further studied. This includes the delivery of TNE (Tousignant, Boissy et al.; Thomas, Burton et al., 2004).

8.4: Preventive TNE

All healthcare professionals will acknowledge that prevention is better than cure and will remember Benjamin Franklin's famous quote, "An ounce of prevention is better than a pound of cure." If we consider the devastating effects of persistent nociception, it could be argued that the best way to treat chronic pain is to prevent it (Woolf, 2007). Therapists will often consider TNE as a last resort or 'special tool' for treating patients with chronic pain. We would like to encourage therapists to change their thinking and consider the potential benefits of preemptive TNE on pain. Martin H. Fischer, a German-born American physician and author (1879-1962) is famous for many medical quotes, and one that we think applies handsomely is, "In the sick room, ten cents' worth of human understanding equals ten dollars' worth of medical science." For therapists treating patients with chronic pain, we would suggest that ten cents' worth of TNE equals ten dollars' worth of physical modalities.

To date, most of the preemptive education in orthopedic therapy has centered on anatomy, biomechanics, pathoanatomy and procedural information. This approach has been shown to have little to no effect on pain and disability (Louw, Diener et al., 2013). Preemptive education can, however, be quite helpful if certain questions are adequately answered for the patient. What is wrong with me? How long will it take? What can I do for this? What will treatment entail? (Chapter 1 and Forward by Louis Gifford).

A great example of this was provided by a whiplash study examining the role of early education in patients with whiplash injuries (Oliveira, Gevirtz et al., 2006). That study was a randomized controlled trial which sought to determine the effects of a short psycho-educational video on pain and medical utilization. One hundred and twenty six patients who attended the Emergency Department or Urgent Care within 48 hours post-motor vehicle accident were randomized to receive usual care or usual care plus an 11-minute video addressing the important issues patients with whiplash need to know. The results showed that patients viewing the video had dramatically lower pain ratings at a one-month follow-up (6.09 [10.6] vs. 21.23 [17.4], $P < 0.001$) and remained lower for the three- and six-month follow-up period. Similarly, for 17 of 21 items asked at follow-up, the video group showed superior outcomes (Chi-square ranged from 5 to 35, $P < 0.05$, all). For example, 4% of patients in the video group were using narcotics at six-month post ED visit, compared with 36% of the control group. The brief psycho-educational video had a profound effect on subsequent pain and medical utilization.

In contrast, it is now well established that 1 in 3 patients will develop chronic pain from whiplash (Spitzer, Skovron et al., 1995; Bogduk, 2000). Current research indicates that a significant source of persistent pain in patients with WAD can be attributed to the immediate up-regulation of the nervous system after injury (Scott, Jull et al., 2005; Jull, Sterling et al., 2007; Sterling and Kenardy, 2008). An argument could be made that appropriate early education may, in part, help to desensitize (calm down) the nervous system. This could account for the findings of decreased pain and disability in the video group in the Oliveira et al. study. WAD is a classic example of an environment where early TNE may be effective. It could be argued that patients 'injured' in environments such as motor vehicle accidents, surgery, work and war may be helped by preemptive TNE.

Another example where TNE may be beneficial as a preemptive approach may be in surgery, such as lumbar surgery. The primary surgical intervention for lumbar radiculopathy is lumbar laminectomy or lumbar laminotomy, with or without discectomy (Ostelo, de Vet et al., 2002; Ostelo, de Vet et al., 2003). Studies on lumbar disc surgery for radiculopathy have shown that this surgical intervention has between a 60-90% success rate (Lurie, Birkmeyer et al., 2003; Ostelo, de Vet et al., 2003; Weinstein, Lurie et al., 2006), leaving 10-40% of patients with residual pain, loss of movement and disability (Ostelo, de Vet et al., 2003). With persistent pain and disability after surgery, rehabilitation is often prescribed and is proposed to decrease disability, increase movement and facilitate return to regular activities (Danielsen, Johnsen et al., 2000; Dolan, Greenfield et al., 2000; Ostelo, de Vet et al., 2003; McGregor, Dicken et al., 2006; Ostelo, Costa et al., 2008). However, postoperative rehabilitation has shown little effect on reducing postoperative disability and pain (Ostelo, de Vet et al., 2003; Ostelo, Costa et al., 2008), and surgeons do not readily send patients to rehabilitation following spinal surgery (McGregor, Dicken et al., 2006; Louw, Butler et al., 2011). This may indicate that many patients suffer long-term disability following lumbar disc surgery.

To date, only a handful of studies have been conducted on the outcome of preoperative education for lumbar surgery. Unfortunately, that preoperative education focused on procedural information (about the surgery to come) and informed consent, and those studies showed that it added little to no benefit for post-surgical outcomes (Douglas, Mann et al., 1998; Krupp, Spanehl et al., 2000; LaMontagne, Hepworth et al., 2003; Johansson, Nuutila et al., 2005; Walters and Coad, 2006). Three studies surveyed patients who had undergone spinal surgery to determine their preferences regarding preoperative education for spinal surgery (McGregor, Burton et al., 2007; Ronnberg, Lind et al., 2007; Louw, Louw et al., 2008; Louw, Louw et al., 2009). A study by Louw, Louw et al. (2009) showed that patients wanted more preoperative information regarding the surgical procedure, the potential risks, and the limitations and benefits of surgery, but also more information on their pain and how surgery would impact it. McGregor, Burton et al. (2007) also showed that patients wanted preoperative information, but provided little information on the exact content of this information. Finally, Ronnberg, Lind et al. (2007) showed that patients undergoing disc surgery were, in general, satisfied with the care given to them preoperatively, but not with the content of the information regarding their impending spinal surgery.

Most education programs for the orthopedic patient population utilize anatomical and biomechanical models for addressing pain (Maier-Riehle and Harter, 2001; Butler and Moseley, 2003; Moseley, 2004; Brox, Storheim et al., 2008), which not only have shown limited efficacy (Koes, van Tulder et al., 1994; Maier-Riehle and Harter, 2001; Butler and Moseley, 2003; Waddell, 2004; Brox, Storheim et al., 2008) but may even increase patient fears, anxiety and stress, thus negatively impacting their outcomes (Nachemson, 1992; Hirsch and Liebert, 1998; Maier-Riehle and Harter, 2001; Poiraudeau, Rannou et al., 2006). Several educational strategies are advocated for patients with LBP, including biomechanical/back school type of education, evidence-based guideline education such as the Back Book (Burton, Waddell et al., 1999), cognitive behavioral therapy (Johnson, Jones et al., 2007; Rundell and Davenport, 2010), and more recently, neuroscience education (Moseley, 2002; Moseley, 2004; Moseley, Nicholas et al., 2004). In response to the emerging evidence for TNE, a preoperative TNE program was recently developed to determine if it would reduce pain and disability after lumbar surgery for radiculopathy (Louw, Butler et al., 2013).

The preoperative TNE program was based on the results of the systematic review by the same research team (Louw, Diener et al., 2011), and the program was designed to de-emphasize anatomical and pathoanatomical reasons for pain from lumbar radiculopathy. Although the preoperative TNE program described the anatomy of the nervous system, it was primarily done as a means to describe pathways for the communication of nerve sensitivity. A neuroscience message focusing on peripheral neuropathic pain mechanism was developed based on the understanding of the current mechanisms associated with lumbar radiculopathy.

This message was used to develop a program that could be administered in a clinically meaningful time period. The preoperative neuroscience education program was designed to include prepared pictures (Moseley, 2004; Moseley, Nicholas et al., 2004; Meeus, Nijs et al., 2010; Ryan, Gray et al., 2010; Van Oosterwijck, Nijs et al., 2011), examples (Moseley, Nicholas et al., 2004; Meeus, Nijs et al., 2010; Van Oosterwijck, Nijs et al., 2011), and metaphors (Van Oosterwijck, Nijs et al., 2011). The sensitivity of the nervous system metaphorically described as an alarm system (Van Oosterwijck, Nijs et al., 2011) accompanied by drawings of action potentials (Moseley, 2004; Van Oosterwijck, Nijs et al., 2011) was used to describe peripheral sensitization (Moseley, 2004; Moseley, Nicholas et al., 2004; Van Oosterwijck, Nijs et al., 2011), central sensitization (Moseley, 2004; Moseley, Nicholas et al., 2004; Van Oosterwijck, Nijs et al., 2011), and plasticity of the nervous system (Moseley, Nicholas et al., 2004; Van Oosterwijck, Nijs et al., 2011). The sensitization of the nervous system was further described in relation to various stressors associated with lumbar surgery, including diagnosis, hospital procedures, surgery, anesthesia and recovery (Louw, 2012).

The preoperative TNE booklet received favorable responses from patients, surgeons, pain scientists and clinicians in its development (Louw, Butler et al., 2013) and at the time of the writing of this textbook was being trialed in a case series examining the immediate post-education effect, fMRI measurement of brain activation, and a multi-center RCT. This approach underscores the need for therapists and researchers to work together to explore the potential impact of early pain neuroscience education on long-term outcomes.

8.5: Conclusion

TNE is here to stay. We encourage clinicians to take on the pain message. Take it to your patients. Patients are interested in pain and the evidence indicates they are much better for it on so many levels. Education is therapy. Know pain; know gain.

Chapter 8 References

Bogduk, N. (2000). Epidemiology of whiplash. *Ann Rheum Dis, 59*(5): 394-395; author reply 395-396.

Brox, J. I., K. Storheim, M. Grotle, T. H. Tveito, A. Indahl and H. R. Eriksen (2008). Systematic review of back schools, brief education, and fear-avoidance training for chronic low back pain. *Spine J, 8*(6): 948-958.

Buchbinder, R., D. Jolley and M. Wyatt (2001). 2001 Volvo Award Winner in Clinical Studies: Effects of a media campaign on back pain beliefs and its potential influence on management of low back pain in general practice. *Spine (Phila Pa 1976), 26*(23): 2535-2542.

Buchbinder, R., D. Jolley and M. Wyatt (2001). Population based intervention to change back pain beliefs and disability: three part evaluation. *BMJ 322(7301)*: 1516-1520.

Burton, A. K., G. Waddell, K. M. Tillotson and N. Summerton (1999). Information and advice to patients with back pain can have a positive effect. A randomized controlled trial of a novel educational booklet in primary care. *Spine, 24*(23): 2484-2491.

Butler, D. and L. Moseley (2003). *Explain Pain.* Adelaide, Noigroup Publications.

Christensen, F. B., I. Laurberg and C. E. Bunger (2003). Importance of the back-cafe concept to rehabilitation after lumbar spinal fusion: a randomized clinical study with a 2-year follow-up. *Spine, 28*(23): 2561-2569.

Danielsen, J. M., R. Johnsen, S. K. Kibsgaard and E. Hellevik (2000). Early aggressive exercise for postoperative rehabilitation after discectomy. *Spine, 25*(8): 1015-1020.

Dolan, P., K. Greenfield, R. J. Nelson and I. W. Nelson (2000). Can exercise therapy improve the outcome of microdiscectomy? *Spine, 25*(12): 1523-1532.

Douglas, T. S., N. H. Mann and A. L. Hodge (1998). Evaluation of preoperative patient education and computer-assisted patient instruction. *Journal of Spinal Disorders, 11*(1): 29-35.

Gallace, A., D. M. Torta, G. L. Moseley and G. D. Iannetti (2011). The analgesic effect of crossing the arms. *Pain, 152*(6): 1418-1423.

Gallagher, L., J. McAuley and G. L. Moseley (2013). A randomized-controlled trial of using a book of metaphors to reconceptualize pain and decrease catastrophizing in people with chronic pain. *The Clinical Journal of Pain, 29*(1): 20-25.

Garcia, R. M., P. J. Messerschmitt and N. U. Ahn (2009). An evaluation of information on the Internet of a new device: the lumbar artificial disc replacement. *J Spinal Disord Tech, 22*(1): 52-57.

Hering, K., J. Harvan, M. Dangelo and D. Jasinski (2005). The use of a computer website prior to scheduled surgery (a pilot study): impact on patient information, acquisition, anxiety level, and overall satisfaction with anesthesia care. *AANA J, 73*(1): 29-33.

Hirsch, M. S. and R. M. Liebert (1998). The physical and psychological experience of pain: the effects of labeling and cold pressor temperature on three pain measures in college women. *Pain, 77*(1): 41-48.

Hurling, R., M. Catt, M. D. Boni, B. W. Fairley, T. Hurst, P. Murray, A. Richardson and J. S. Sodhi (2007). Using internet and mobile phone technology to deliver an automated physical activity program: randomized controlled trial. *J Med Internet Res, 9*(2): e7.

Johansson, K., L. Nuutila, H. Virtanen, J. Katajisto and S. Salantera (2005). Preoperative education for orthopaedic patients: systematic review. *J Adv Nurs, 50*(2): 212-223.

Johnson, R. E., G. T. Jones, N. J. Wiles, C. Chaddock, R. G. Potter, C. Roberts, D. P. Symmons, P. J. Watson, D. J. Torgerson and G. J. Macfarlane (2007). Active exercise, education, and cognitive behavioral therapy for persistent disabling low back pain: a randomized controlled trial. *Spine, 32*(15): 1578-1585.

Jull, G., M. Sterling, J. Kenardy and E. Beller (2007). Does the presence of sensory hypersensitivity influence outcomes of physical rehabilitation for chronic whiplash?--A preliminary RCT. *Pain, 129*(1-2): 28-34.

Koes, B. W., M. W. van Tulder, W. M. van der Windt and L. M. Bouter (1994). The efficacy of back schools: a review of randomized clinical trials. *J Clin Epidemiol, 47*(8): 851-862.

Krupp, W., O. Spanehl, W. Laubach and V. Seifert (2000). Informed consent in neurosurgery: patients' recall of preoperative discussion. *Acta Neurochir (Wien), 142*(3): 233-238; discussion 238-239.

LaMontagne, L., J. T. Hepworth, M. H. Salisbury and F. Cohen (2003). Effects of coping instruction in reducing young adolescents' pain after major spinal surgery. *Orthop Nurs, 22*(6): 398-403.

Louw, A. (2012). *Your Nerves Are Having Back Surgery.* Minneapolis, OPTP.

Louw, A. (2013). *Your Fibromyalgia Workbook: A Neuroscience Approach.* Minneapolis, OPTP.

Louw, A., D. S. Butler, I. Diener and E. J. Puentedura (2011). Preoperative education for lumbar radiculopathy: a survey of US spine surgeons. Submitted for publication.

Louw, A., D. S. Butler, I. Diener and E. J. Puentedura (2013). Development of a Preoperative Neuroscience Educational Program for Patients with Lumbar Radiculopathy. *American Journal of Physical Medicine & Rehabilitation/ Association of Academic Physiatrists.*

Louw, A., I. Diener, D. S. Butler and E. J. Puentedura (2011). The effect of neuroscience education on pain, disability, anxiety, and stress in chronic musculoskeletal pain. *Archives of Physical Medicine and Rehabilitation, 92*(12): 2041-2056.

Louw, A., I. Diener, D. S. Butler and E. J. Puentedura (2013). Preoperative education addressing postoperative pain in total joint arthroplasty: Review of content and educational delivery methods. *Physiotherapy Theory and Practice, 29*(3): 175-194.

Louw, A., Q. Louw and L. C. C. Crous (2009). Preoperative Education for Lumbar Surgery for Radiculopathy. *South African Journal of Physiotherapy, 65*(2): 3-8.

Louw, A., Q. A. Louw and L. C. Crous (2008). *Preoperative education for lumbar surgery for radiculopathy.* Masters Article - submitted for publication, University of Stellenbosch.

Louw, A., E. L. Puentedura and P. Mintken (2012). Use of an abbreviated neuroscience education approach in the treatment of chronic low back pain: a case report. *Physiotherapy Theory and Practice, 28*(1): 50-62.

Lurie, J. D., N. J. Birkmeyer and J. N. Weinstein (2003). Rates of advanced spinal imaging and spine surgery. *Spine, 28*(6): 616-620.

Maier-Riehle, B. and M. Harter (2001). The effects of back schools--a meta-analysis. *Int J Rehabil Res, 24*(3): 199-206.

Maitland, G. D. (1986). *Vertebral Manipulation.* London, Butterworths.

McGregor, A. H., A. K. Burton, P. Sell and G. Waddell (2007). The development of an evidence-based patient booklet for patients undergoing lumbar discectomy and un-instrumented decompression. *Eur Spine J, 16*(3): 339-346.

McGregor, A. H., B. Dicken and K. Jamrozik (2006). National audit of post-operative management in spinal surgery. *BMC Musculoskelet Disord, 7*: 47.

Meeus, M., J. Nijs, J. Van Oosterwijck, V. Van Alsenoy and S. Truijen (2010). Pain Physiology Education Improves Pain Beliefs in Patients With Chronic Fatigue Syndrome Compared With Pacing and Self-Management Education: A Double-Blind Randomized Controlled Trial. *Arch Phys Med Rehabil, 91*(8): 1153-1159.

Morr, S., N. Shanti, A. Carrer, J. Kubeck and M. C. Gerling (2010). Quality of information concerning cervical disc herniation on the Internet. *Spine J, 10*(4): 350-354.

Moseley, G. L. (2002). Physiotherapy is effective for chronic low back pain. A randomised controlled trial. *Aus J Physioth, 48*: 297-302.

Moseley, G. L. (2003). Joining forces - combining cognition-targeted motor control training with group or individual pain physiology education: a successful treatment for chronic low back pain. *J Man Manip Therap, 11*(2): 88-94.

Moseley, G. L. (2004). Evidence for a direct relationship between cognitive and physical change during an education intervention in people with chronic low back pain. *Eur J Pain, 8*(1): 39-45.

Moseley, G. L. (2007). Using visual illusion to reduce at-level neuropathic pain in paraplegia. *Pain, 130*(3): 294-298.

Moseley, G. L., M. K. Nicholas and P. W. Hodges (2004). A randomized controlled trial of intensive neurophysiology education in chronic low back pain. *Clin J Pain, 20*(5): 324-330.

Moseley, G. L., T. J. Parsons and C. Spence (2008). Visual distortion of a limb modulates the pain and swelling evoked by movement. *Current Biology: CB, 18*(22): R1047-1048.

Moseley, L. (2002). Combined physiotherapy and education is efficacious for chronic low back pain. *Aust J Physiother, 48*(4): 297-302.

Nachemson, A. L. (1992). Newest knowledge of low back pain. A critical look. *Clinical Orthopaedics and Related Research*(279): 8-20.

Oliveira, A., R. Gevirtz and D. Hubbard (2006). A psycho-educational video used in the emergency department provides effective treatment for whiplash injuries. *Spine, 31*(15): 1652-1657.

Ostelo, R. W., L. O. Costa, C. G. Maher, H. C. de Vet and M. W. van Tulder (2008). Rehabilitation after lumbar disc surgery. *Cochrane Database Syst Rev*(4): CD003007.

Ostelo, R. W., H. C. de Vet, J. W. Vlaeyen, M. R. Kerckhoffs, W. M. Berfelo, P. M. Wolters and P. A. van den Brandt (2003). Behavioral graded activity following first-time lumbar disc surgery: 1-year results of a randomized clinical trial. *Spine, 28*(16): 1757-1765.

Ostelo, R. W., H. C. de Vet, G. Waddell, M. R. Kerckhoffs, P. Leffers and M. van Tulder (2003). Rehabilitation following first-time lumbar disc surgery: a systematic review within the framework of the cochrane collaboration. *Spine, 28*(3): 209-218.

Ostelo, R. W., H. C. de Vet, G. Waddell, M. R. Kerckhoffs, P. Leffers and M. W. van Tulder (2002). Rehabilitation after lumbar disc surgery. *Cochrane Database Syst Rev*(2): CD003007.

Poiraudeau, S., F. Rannou, G. Baron, A. Le Henanff, E. Coudeyre, S. Rozenberg, D. Huas, C. Martineau, I. Jolivet-Landreau, J. Garcia-Mace, M. Revel and P. Ravaud (2006). Fear-avoidance beliefs about back pain in patients with subacute low back pain. *Pain, 124*(3): 305-311.

Ronnberg, K., B. Lind, B. Zoega, K. Halldin, M. Gellerstedt and H. Brisby (2007). Patients' satisfaction with provided care/information and expectations on clinical outcome after lumbar disc herniation surgery. *Spine, 32*(2): 256-261.

Rundell, S. D. and T. E. Davenport (2010). Patient education based on principles of cognitive behavioral therapy for a patient with persistent low back pain: a case report. *The Journal of Orthopaedic and Sports Physical Therapy, 40*(8): 494-501.

Ryan, C. G., H. G. Gray, M. Newton and M. H. Granat (2010). Pain biology education and exercise classes compared to pain biology education alone for individuals with chronic low back pain: a pilot randomised controlled trial. *Man Ther, 15*(4): 382-387.

Scott, D., G. Jull and M. Sterling (2005). Widespread sensory hypersensitivity is a feature of chronic whiplash-associated disorder but not chronic idiopathic neck pain. *Clin J Pain, 21*(2): 175-181.

Spitzer, W. O., M. L. Skovron, L. R. Salmi, J. D. Cassidy, J. Duranceau, S. Suissa and E. Zeiss (1995). Scientific monograph of the Quebec Task Force on Whiplash-Associated Disorders: redefining "whiplash" and its management. *Spine (Phila Pa 1976), 20*(8 Suppl): 1S-73S.

Sterling, M. and J. Kenardy (2008). Physical and psychological aspects of whiplash. Important considerations for primary care assessment. *Man Ther, 13*: 93-102.

Thomas, K., D. Burton, L. Withrow and B. Adkisson (2004). Impact of a preoperative education program via interactive telehealth network for rural patients having total joint replacement. *Orthop Nurs, 23*(1): 39-44.

Tousignant, M., P. Boissy, H. Moffet, H. Corriveau, F. Cabana, F. Marquis and J. Simard Patients' satisfaction of healthcare services and perception with in-home telerehabilitation and physiotherapists' satisfaction toward technology for post-knee arthroplasty: an embedded study in a randomized trial. *Telemed J E Health, 17*(5): 376-382.

Van Oosterwijck, J., J. Nijs, M. Meeus, S. Truijen, J. Craps, N. Van den Keybus and L. Paul (2011). Pain neurophysiology education improves cognitions, pain thresholds, and movement performance in people with chronic whiplash: A pilot study. *J Rehabil Res Dev, 48*(1): EPub ahead of print

Waddell, G. (2004). *The Back Pain Revolution*. Edinburgh, Elsevier.

Walters, M. and J. Coad (2006). Preparation of children for spinal surgery: an exploratory study. *Paediatric Nursing, 18*(10): 27-29.

Weinstein, J. N., J. D. Lurie, T. D. Tosteson, J. S. Skinner, B. Hanscom, A. N. Tosteson, H. Herkowitz, J. Fischgrund, F. P. Cammisa, T. Albert and R. A. Deyo (2006). Surgical vs nonoperative treatment for lumbar disk herniation: the Spine Patient Outcomes Research Trial (SPORT) observational cohort. *JAMA, 296*(20): 2451-2459.

Woolf, C. J. (2007). Central sensitization: uncovering the relation between pain and plasticity. *Anesthesiology, 106*(4): 864-867.